ORGAN SHORTAGE: THE SOLUTIONS

Transplantation and Clinical Immunology

Symposia Fondation Marcel Mérieux

VOLUME 26

Organ Shortage: The Solutions

Proceedings of the 26th Conference on Transplantation and Clinical Immunology, 13–15 June 1994

organized by
Fondation Marcel Mérieux and Université Claude Bernard-Lyon I

Edited by

J.L. Touraine
J. Traeger
H. Bétuel
J.M. Dubernard
J.P. Revillard
C. Dupuy

SPRINGER-SCIENCE+BUSINESS MEDIA, B.V.

Library of Congress Cataloging-in-Publication Data

Conference on Transplantation and Clinical Immunology (26th : 1994)
    Organ shortage : the solutions : proceedings of the 26th
  Conference on Transplantation and Clinical Immunology, 13-15 June
  1994 / edited by J.L. Touraine ... [et al.].
        p.   cm. -- (Transplantation and clinical immunology ; v. 26)
    Includes bibliographical references and index.
    ISBN 978-94-010-4091-4   ISBN 978-94-011-0201-8 (eBook)
    DOI 10.1007/978-94-011-0201-8
    1. Donation of organs, tissues, etc.--Congresses.
  2. Transplantation of organs, tissues, etc.--Congresses.
  3. Donation of organs, tissues, etc.--Social aspects--Congresses.
  4. Transplantation of organs, tissues, etc.--Congresses.
  I. Touraine, J. L. (Jean Louis) II. Title. III. Series.
  RD120.7.I56a vol 26
  [RD129.5]
  617.9'5 s--dc20
  [362.1'783]   94-37471

ISBN 978-94-010-4091-4

Printed on acid-free paper

Table of Contents

List of Contributors   XV

Part 1: Organ shortage in various countries   1

1. How severe is organ shortage in Eurotransplant?   3
   G.G. Persijn, J. de Meester, B. Cohen

2. Organ shortage in France: present status, causes and the future   11
   J.P. Romano

3. Is there a shortage of organs in Argentina?   19
   P.M. Raffaele

4. How to increase the search for organs in Argentina within the respect of ethics   27
   A. Fagalde

5. Effect of transplantation laws on organ procurement   33
   P. Michielsen

6. Causes and socio-psychological dimensions in donation refusal   41
   J. Traeger, J.J. Colpart

7. Disappointing rate of altruism in the population   49
   G. Schütt, G. Duncker

Part 2: Expanding the donor pool   53

8. Organ procurement from non-heart-beating donors   55
   J.W. Daemen, Y. Ming, G. Kootstra

9. Heart transplant from non-beating heart donor: past experience and report of one clinical case   61
   G. Dureau

10. Total body cooling for organ procurement   67
    R. Valero, M. Manyalich, C. Cabrer, L. Salvador, L.C. Garcia-Fages

11. The living donor program in Scandinavia   73
    U. Backman, D. Albrechtsen, H. Løkkegaard, K. Saalmela

12. Pancreas transplants from living related donors   77
    R.W.G. Gruessner, J.S. Najarian, A.C. Gruessner, D.E.R. Sutherland

13. Expanding the donor supply by using high risk donors: the use of pulsatile kidney perfusion for evaluation of high risk kidney donors   85
    R.J. Tesi, E.A. Elkhammas, E.A. Davies, M.L. Henry, R.M. Ferguson

14. Relative effect of HLA matching and cold ischemia time   93
    J.Yuge, P.I. Terasaki

15. Are kidneys of very young donors suitable for transplantation?   99
    P. Cochat, L. Dubourg, A. Hadj-Aïssa, M. Dawahra, M.H. Saïd, L. David

16. Organ procurement from cadaveric children   103
    H. Nivet, C. Cheliakine, S. Benoit, G. Deschênes, Y. Lebranchu

17. Influence of donor age on the result of heart transplantation   111
    G. Dureau, J.P. Gare, M. Chuzel, O. Jegaden, J.F. Obadia, J.F. Chassignolle, P. Mikaeloff

18. Results of kidney transplantation using high risk donors   121
    D. Cantarovich, M. Giral, M. Hourmant, J. Dantal, G. Blancho, G. Karam, J.N. Le Sant, P. Daguin, J.P. Soulillou

19. Anesthesia and resuscitation of the genetically related living donor in liver transplantation   127
    D. Gille, O. Boillot, M.C. Graber, P. Sagnard, C. Beaude, B. Chabrol, C. Kopp, D. Long, B. Delafosse, G. Bagou

Part 3: Optimization of organ procurement   133

20. Potential donors and brain death epidemiology in the region of
    Madrid   135
    A. Navarro

21. Logistics and management for improvement of multiorgan
    procurement from potential brain dead donors   143
    J.J. Colpart, B. Guillot, G. Saury, B. Maillefaud, B. Bouttin,
    A. Marion, D. Minarro, C. Micaud, J.F. Moskovtchenko

22. Optimal use of cadaver kidneys for transplantation   161
    G. Opelz, Th. Wujciak

23. Organ procurement in Spain: the national organization of
    transplantation   167
    R. Matesanz, B. Miranda, C. Felipe, M.T. Naya

24. Integrated ways to improve cadaveric organ donation   179
    B. Miranda, R. Matesanz, C. Filipe, M.T. Naya

25. Training the Transplant Procurement Management (TPM)
    coordinator   191
    M. Manyalich, C.A. Cabrer, L.C. Garcia-Fages, R. Valero,
    L. Salvador, J. Sanchez

26. Surgical optimization of multi-organ procurement   197
    M. Dawahra, X. Martin, P. Cloix, L. Tajra, J.M. Dubernard

27. The place of anatomy in liver transplantation: multiplicity of
    possibilities and optimization of the utilization of cadaveric and
    living donor's organs   207
    T. Van Minh

28. Detection of anti-HLA class 1 IgG antibodies by ELISA   213
    I. Mercier, L. Glanville, L. Ellingson, L. Igoudin,
    N. Vanpouille, A. Segers, P. Pouletty, R. Buelow

Part 4: Ethics and recipient selection   221

29. The foundations of the right to be grafted   223
    A.M. Moulin

30. The graft survival curve: Ideology & rhetoric – Part II   235
    R.D. Guttmann

31. The nature of the selection of candidates for cardiac transplant   243
    S. Wait, R.D. Guttmann, J.J. Caro

32. Should we review the indications for transplants because of the
    shortage of organs?   253
    P. Deteix

33. Can we select candidates for combined kidney and heart or liver
    transplantation?   261
    J.L. Garnier, A.C. Marrast, C. Pouteil-Noble, X. Martin,
    G. Dureau, G. Champsaur, J. Ninet, P. Boissonnat, J.P. Gare,
    P. Chossegros, J.M. Dubernard, J.L. Touraine

34. When to refer a patient for lung transplantation   267
    I. Paradis, J.D. Manzetti, D.E. Foust, G.S. Bauldoff,
    B.P. Griffith

35. Must the choice of surgical procedure for lung transplantation
    be guided by organ shortage?   277
    J.F. Mornex, M. Bertocchi, T. Wiesandanger, F. Thévenet

36. Is cardiac transplantation justified in patients over 60 years of
    age?   281
    J. Robin, J. Ninet, E. Bonnefoy, J. Neidecker, P. Boissonnat,
    G. Champsaur

37. The media and organ shortage   287
    B. Cuzin, J.M. Dubernard

Part 5: Alternatives to human organ transplant   295

38. Gene therapy as an alternative to organ transplantation?   297
    H. Gilgenkrantz

39. Xenochimerism and tolerance   301
    M. Sykes

40. Transgenic pigs and xenotransplantation   309
    C.A. Carrington, E.C. Cozzi, G.A. Langford, A.C. Richards,
    A. Rosengard, N. Yannoutsos, D.G. White

41. The endothelial cell as a target of xenogeneic hyperacute
   rejection   317
   Y. Calmus, J. Cardoso, L. Gamblez, Ch. Chéreau, D. Houssin,
   B. Weill

Part VI: Posters

ORGAN DONATION

The follow up of the French grafts   327
Ph. Romano, M. Busson, J. Hors

Outcome of 490 kidneys procured from brain dead donors in one
center   328
G. Benoit, P. Blanchet, D. Devictor, H. Bensadoun, C. Richard,
J. Depret, A. Decaux, J. Decaris, B. Charpentier

Organ shortage and a local waiting list allow a local kidney
allocation policy to ensure both short ischemia time and good
HLA-1, B, DR matching   329
E. Bertoni, P.L. Tosi, S. Bandini, A. Rosati, F. Pradella,
P. Mattiuz, G. Taddei, G. Nicita, M. Salvadori, P. Rindi,
G. Rizzo, M. Carmellini, F. Mosca

France transplant regional transplant coordination unit °3   330
J.J. Colpart, B. Guillot, G. Saury, B. Maillefaud, B. Bouttin,
A. Marion, D. Minarro, C. Micaud, J.F. Moskovtchenko

The organizative transplant model in Catalonia: The O.CAT.T   331
E. Fernandez, M.T. Aguayo, M.A. Viedma, J.M. Via

P.H.S.P.O.   332
C. Boisriveaud, Ph. Romano

Healthcare on the worksite: A strong means of communication to
promote organ donation   333
J.C. Drouet and coll., J. Borsarelli and coll., M. Blangero, G. Botti

Aspects of the legal regulation of living donor transplantion within
Europe   334
A. Garwood-Gowers, D. Price, A. Lea, P. Donnolly

A European Multicenter study of transplantation from living donors   335
A. Lea, D. Price, A. Garwood-Gowers, P. Donnolly

Kidney transplantation from living related donors   336
C. Mouquet, H. Benalia, B. Barrou, J. Luciani, M.O. Bitker,
P. Viars

Role of the donor in the post transplant renal function   337
L. Dubourg, P. Cochat, A. Hadj-Aïssa, B. Parchoux, X. Martin,
L. David

Older living related and cadaveric donors in renal transplantation 338
D. Gakis, V. Papanikolaou, A. Papagiannis, G. Imvrios,
D. Takoudas, A. Antoniadis

The high risk donor in kidney transplantation. Effect of sex and age
on the long term graft outcome   339
P. van Steenberge, P.P. Mulder, J.N. Ijzermans, W. Weimar

The lack of donor or lack of understanding and cooperation results
of the attitude survey among public medical and nursing profession 340
J. Walaszewski, W. Rowinski, M. Lao, G. Michalak, B.
Barcikowska

ORGAN PRESERVATION, SURGICAL TECHNIQUES AND IMMUNOLOGICAL PROTOCOLS

Jugular oxymetry and brain death during intensive care of comatose
patients   343
B. Page

Modifications of UW solution can improve metabolic and cellular
protection of hearts during long term hypothermic storage:
Evaluation by P-31 magnetic resonance spectroscopy and
biochemical analyses   344
M. Bernard, T. Caus, M. Sciaky, J.R. Monties, P.J. Cozzone

Hypophysis thyroid axis distrubances in human brain dead donors   345
J.J. Colpart, S. Ramella, M. Bret, B. Coronel, D. Dorez,
A. Mercatello, A. Hadj-Aïssa, J.F. Moskovtchenko

Normothermic preservation of "multiple organ blocks" with a new
perfluorooctyl bromide emulsion   346
E.J. Voiglio, L. Zarif, F. Gorry, M.P. Krafft, J. Margonari,
S. Balter, X. Martin, J.G. Riess, J.M. Dubernard

Evaluation of a high sodium-low potassium cold-storage solution
using the isolated perfused rat kidney 347
S.G. Ramella, A. Hadj-A—ssa, A. Barbieux, J.P. Steghens,
J.J. Colpart, P. Zech, N. Pozet

Organ preservation by vitrification 348
J.L. Descotes, E. Payen, E. Chapelier, J.J. Rambeaud

Immunological factors together with ischaemia result in primary non-
function of cadaveric kidney grafts 349
B. Łągiewska, M. Pacholczyk, W. Rowiński, K. Ostrowski, S. Cajzner,
J. Wałaszewski

The new technique of rapid en bloc removal of both kidneys in non-
heart beating donors 350
Z.L. Min, L.M. Wang

The anatomic feasibility studies on the technique of splitting-liver
transplantation (SLT) 351
Z.X. Wen, S.S. Xia, D.G. Liu

Combined kidney transplantation (Tx) with heart, liver or pancreas 352
A.C. Marrast, J.L. Touraine, J.M. Dubernard, G. Dureau,
O. Boillot, J.L. Garnier, J. Finaz, C. Pouteil-Noble, P. Paillard,
N. Lefrançois

Combined hepatic and renal transplantation in primary
hyperoxaluria type I: Report of four cases 353
A. Déglise-Favre, G. Manganella, D. Samuel, H. Bismuth

RISKS, COMPLICATIONS AND TREATMENTS IN GRAFT RECIPIENTS

HCV RNA in patients undergoing kidney transplantation 357
G. Lunghi, A. Archenti, R. Cardone, A. Aroldi, A. Pagano

Indication for transplant and efficacy of itraconazole in aspergillus
fumigatus infection reconsidered 358
L. Van Elsland, E. Cassuto-Viguier, J.R. Mondain, J.C. Bendini,
J. Bracco, M. Gari-Toussaint, M. Franco, H. Gaid, D. Barrillon

Out-center dialysis and renal transplantation 359
E. Delawari, M. Laville, W. Arkouche, E. Abdullah, R. Sibai,
J. Traeger

Spontaneous regression of a metastatic adenocarcinoma transmitted
by a cadaver kidney graft: Support for "immunotherapy"?   360
F. Vincent, V. Levy, D. Glotz, A. Duboust, J. Bariety

Posttransplant malignant lymphomas (PTL) treated with
doxorubicin-based chemotherapy   361
M. Altieri, F. Maloisel, R. Herbrecht, C. Sosa, M.P. Chenard,
B. Lioure, M.L. Woehl-Jaegle, B. Ellero, K. Boudjema, D. Jaeck,
F. Oberling, Ph. Wolf

Malignancies in children with renal replacement therapy (RRT)   362
S. Carl, M. Wiesel, A.M. Wingen, O. Mehls, G. Staehler

Endothelial activation in xenografts' rejection: Evaluation of the
role of heparan-sulphate   363
R. Di Stefano, G. Bonanomi, M. Scavuzzo, A. Pinna, D. Donati,
F. Mosca

Systemic IL-10 release, after a single pre or per operative large dose
of ATG-fresenius in human kidney transplantation   364
Y. Saint Hillier, B. Hory, E. Racadot, C. Bresson, D. David,
F.A.L. Freijat, P. Vautrin, V. Fournier, E. Berger, M. Jamali

Prolongation of skin allograft survival in mice following
administration of new 20-epi vitamin D3 analogues   365
R. Pamphile, P. Veyron, L. Binderup, J.L. Touraine

A model for self tolerance induction based on intrathymic anergy,
reversible in the absence of the tolerogen   366
A. Aitouche, J.L. Touraine

SUPPLEMENTAL POSTERS

Breaking the donor age barrier to face the organ shortage in liver
transplantation
L. Aldrighetti, I.R. Marino, H.R. Doyle, C. Doria, C. Scotti-Foglieni,
J.A. Kovalak, A.G. Tzakis, J.J. Fung, T.E. Starzl   369

Successful transplantation of pediatric donor kidneys in adult recipients
G. Kirste, M. Blümke, P. Pisarski   371

Public campaign to increase donor availability in a regional transplant
center
G. Kirste, M. Blümke, F. Schaub, R. Dreier   372

Morphologic findings in baseline renal transplant biopsies
R. Cahen, F. Dijoud, C. Couchoud, M. Devonec, P. Trolliet,
P. Adeleine, J.P. Fendler, P. Joubert, P. Perrin, B. François   373

Systemic IL-10 release, after a single pre- or per-operative large dose
of ATG-fresenius in human kidney transplantation
Y. Saint Hillier, B. Hory, E. Racadot, C. Bresson, D. David,
F. Al Freijat, P. Vautrin, V. Fournier, E. Berger, M. Jamali, H. Bittard   374

The feasibility of organ preservation at warmer temperatures
L. Brasile, J. Clarke, E. Green, C. Haisch   375

In Situ preservation without traditional hypothermia
L. Brasile, J. Clarke, E. Green, C. Haisch   376

Name Index   377

List of contributors

U. BACKMAN
Department of Medicine
Renal Unit
University Hospital
S 751 85 Uppsala
Sweden

O. BOILLOT
Pavillon V
Hopital Edouard Herriot
Place d'Arsonval
69374 Lyon 3
France

Y. CALMUS
Groupe Hospitalier Cochin
Clinique Chirurgicale
27 Rue du Fbrg St Jacques
75679 Paris 14
France

D. CANTAROVICH
Service Transplantation et
Réanimation
Hopital Necker
161 Rue de Sèvres
75743 Paris
France

C.A. CARRINGTON
Department of Surgery
University of Cambridge Clinical
School
Douglas House
18 Trumpington Road
Cambridge CB2 2AH
UK

G. CHAMPSAUR
Chirurgie Vasculaire et Cardiaque
Hopital Cardio-Vasculaire et
Pneumologique Louis Pradel
28 Av. du Doyen Lépine
69500 Bron
France

P. COCHAT
Pavillon S-Néphrologie
Hopital Edouard Herriot
Place d'Arsonval
69437 Lyon 3
France

J.J. COLPART
Pavillon P
Hopital Edouard Herriot
Place d'Arsonval
69437 Lyon 3
France

B. CUZIN
Pavillon V
Hopital Edouard Herriot
Place d'Arsonval
69437 Lyon 3
France

M. DAWAHRA
Pavillon P
Hopital Edouard Herriot
5 Place d'Arsonval
69437 Lyon 3
France

P. DETEIX
Service de Néphrologie
CHRU de Clermont-Ferrand
Hopital Gabriel Montpied
Place Henri Dunant – BP. 69
63003 Clermont Ferrand
France

JM. DUBERNARD
Pavillon V
Hopital Edouard Herriot
Place d'Arsonval
69437 Lyon 3
France

G. DUREAU
Chirurgie Vasculaire et Cardiaque
Hopital Cardio-Vasculaire et
Pneumologique Louis Pradel
28 Av. du Doyen Lépine
69500 Bron
France

A. FAGALDE
La prida
54500 Cordoba
Argentina

J.L. GARNIER
Pavillon P
Hopital Edouard Herriot
Place d'Arsonval
69437 Lyon 3
France

H. GILGENKRANTZ
CHU Cochin
Inserm U 129
24 Rue du Fbg St Jacques
75014 Paris
France

R. GRUESSNER
Department of Surgery
Medical School
University of Minnesota
Philipps-Wagensteen Building
516 Delaware Street S.E.
Minneapolis MN 55455
USA

R.D. GUTTMANN
Centre d'Immunobiologie Clinique
et de Transplantation Université McGill
687 Avenue des Pins Ouest
Montréal Québec H3A 1A1
Canada

D. HOUSSIN
Clinique Chirurgicale
Groupe Hospitalier Cochin
27 Rue du Fg St-Jacques
75679 Paris CEDEX 14
France

G. KOOTSTRA
Academisch Ziekenhuis Maastricht
P. Debyelaan 25
Postbus 5800
6202 AZ Maastricht
The Netherlands

M. MANYALICH I VIDAL
Hospital Clinic i Provincial de
Barcelona
C/Vilarroel 170
08036 Barcelona
Spain

X. MARTIN
Pavillon P
Hopital Edouard Herriot
5 Place d'Arsonval
69437 Lyon 3
France

R. MATESANZ ACEDOS
National Transplant Coordinator
Ministerio de Sanidad Y Consumo
Organizacion Nacional de
Trasplantes
C/Sinesio Delgado 8
28029 Madrid
Spain

I. MERCIER
SangStat Medical Corporation
1505 Adams Drive
Menlo Park
California
USA

P. MICHIELSEN
Acacialaan 54
B3020 Herent
Belgium

B. MIRANDA
Ministerio de Sanidad Y Consumo
Organizacion Nacional de
Trasplantes
C/Sinezio Delgado 8
28029 Madrid
Spain

J.F. MORNEX
Hopital Cardio-Vasculaire et
Pneumologique Louis Pradel
BP. Lyon Montchat
69394 Lyon 3
France

A.M. MOULIN
Inserm U 158
Hopital des Enfants Malades
149 Rue de Sèvres
75743 Paris CEDEX 15
France

A. NAVARRO IZQUIERDO
Regional Coordinator
Organizacion Nacional de
Trasplantes
C/Sinesio Delgado 8
28029 Madrid
Spain

H. NIVET
Centre Hospitalier de Tours
Service Nephrologie
2 Bd Tonnelé
37044 Tours CEDEX
France

G. OPELZ
Institut für Immunologie
der Universität Heidelberg
Im Neuenheimer Feld 305
69120 Heidelberg
Germany

I. PARADIS
Medical Center
University of Pittsburgh
3458 Fifth Avenue
Pittsburgh PA 15213–3241
USA

G. PERSIJN
Eurotransplant Foundation
P.O. Box 2304
2301 CH Leiden
The Netherlands

P. RAFFAELE
Dardo Rocha 235
1842 Monte Grande
Buenos Aires
Argentina

P. ROMANO
France Transplant
1 Av. Claude Vellefaux
75475 Paris
France

R. SCHÜTT
Organisationszentrale des DSO
Chirurgische Universitätsklinik
Arnold Heller Strasse 7
24105 Kiel
Germany

M. SYKES
Transplantation Biology Research
Center
Massachusetts General Hospital
MGH-East Building 149–9019
13th Street
Boston MA 02129
USA

P. TERASAKI
Department of Surgery
University of California
1000 Veterans Avenue
Los Angeles CA 90024–1652
USA

R.J. TESI
Division of Transplantation
The Ohio State University
259 Means Hall
1654 Upham Drive
Columbus OH 43210–1228 USA

J.L. TOURAINE
Pavillon P
Hopital Edouard Herriot
Place d'Arsonval
69437 Lyon 3
France

J. TRAEGER
Aural
8–10 Impasse Lindberg
69003 Lyon
France

T. VAN MINH
Faculté de Medecine de Hanoi
Département d'Anatomie
Hanoi
Vietnam

R. VALERO
Hospital Clinic I Provincial
Calle Casanova 543
08036 Barcelona
Spain

S. WAIT
8 Rue Fondary
75015 Paris
France

PART ONE

Organ shortage in various countries

1. How severe is organ shortage in Eurotransplant?

G.G. PERSIJN, J. DE MEESTER & B. COHEN

1. Introduction

In 1967, a proposal was made to set up an international structure to be called Eurotransplant for the organization of organ exchange and transplantation (Van Rood 1967). The main reason for this proposal was the prediction that optimal tissue typing, i.e. typing for the antigens of the Major Histocompatibility Complex – the so-called HLA-antigens – and the matching of donor and recipient for these antigens, would improve the outcome of organ transplants. Data from experimental skin transplants as well as kidney transplants performed between family members formed the scientific basis for this proposal. The original goals of Eurotransplant were:

– to ensure optimal use of donor organs,
– to help to improve transplant results through HLA-typing and matching of donors and recipients, and
– to support these aims through careful follow-up analyses of the transplantation results.

Since its start, more than 43,000 cadaveric kidney transplants have been performed in 66 transplantation collaborating centers (current number) in Austria, Belgium, Germany, Luxembourg and the Netherlands, covering an area of approximately 113 million inhabitants. Due to optimal HLA-A, -B and -DR matching as well as the use of the immunosuppressive agent Cyclosporin, the 5-year kidney patient and graft survival rates have reached 87% and 75%, respectively.

In the early eighties there was renewed interest in performing heart and liver transplants. This was mainly because of better patient and graft survival due to the introduction of new immunosuppressive regimens as well as refined techniques to diagnose rejection episodes. In the mid-eighties, several centers started combined pancreas plus kidney transplants for treatment of diabetic patients with end stage renal failure. Due to better surgical techniques and better graft survival results, some centers began with single- and double-lung

J.L. Touraine et al. (eds.), *Organ Shortage: The Solutions*, 3–10.

transplants. Currently, 31 heart, 30 liver, 21 pancreas and 15 lung centers are actively performing these transplants in the Eurotransplant area.

All these developments have led to increasing lists of patients awaiting kidney, heart, lung, liver and pancreas transplants. Of course, this has resulted in the active involvement of Eurotransplant for organ procurement to meet the demands. As a result of these efforts, 61% of all kidney donors reported in 1993 were used as so-called "multi-organ" donors. Although the figures obtained for organ procurement and transplantation results look very impressive so far, problems still exist.

The improved graft survival results obtained during the last decade have led to the increased willingness of many patients to be registered on waiting lists for organ transplantation. Huge waiting lists have resulted and, thus, longer waiting times for kidney, heart, liver, lung and pancreas patients. Society is now confronted with the greatest problem in organ transplantation: the increasing gap between the supply and demand of organs and tissues for transplantation. (Matesanz et al. 1993).

2. Results

2.1. *Patients*

Figure 1 clearly demonstrates the demand and supply for kidney patients in the Eurotransplant area. The same phenomenon is observed by all other national or international transplant programs. The "gap" between numbers of transplants performed and patients registered on the waiting list has doubled over the last 10 years. As of December 31, 1993, 11,956 kidney patients were registered in the Eurotransplant central computer in Leiden, the Netherlands. It is also interesting to note that the percentage of patients awaiting a retransplant is now 15%. During the years 1992 and 1993, respectively, 4,114 and 4,388 new kidney patients were reported as potential transplant candidates while only 3,101 and 3,293 renal transplants were performed. The number of renal patients dying while awaiting a transplant was 404 and 412 kidney patients in 1992 and 1993, respectively.

Figure 2 shows the curves of patients awaiting a heart, heart plus lungs, lungs, liver, pancreas plus kidney or a pancreas alone. The number of patients as of December 31, 1993 were 1,076, 72, 222, 314, 143 and 57, respectively. These numbers, however, do not reflect new patients registered during the entire year 1993, amounting to 1,368, 78, 223, 1,067, 89 and 32, respectively. Here, also, the number of transplants performed does not keep up with the need. In 1993, 767 hearts, 28 heart plus lungs, 119 lungs, 878 livers, 92 kidney plus pancreas and only 2 pancreases alone were transplanted. Interesting to note is that 6 patients also received pancreatic islets as a transplant.

As patients awaiting a thoracic organ of a liver graft do not have the

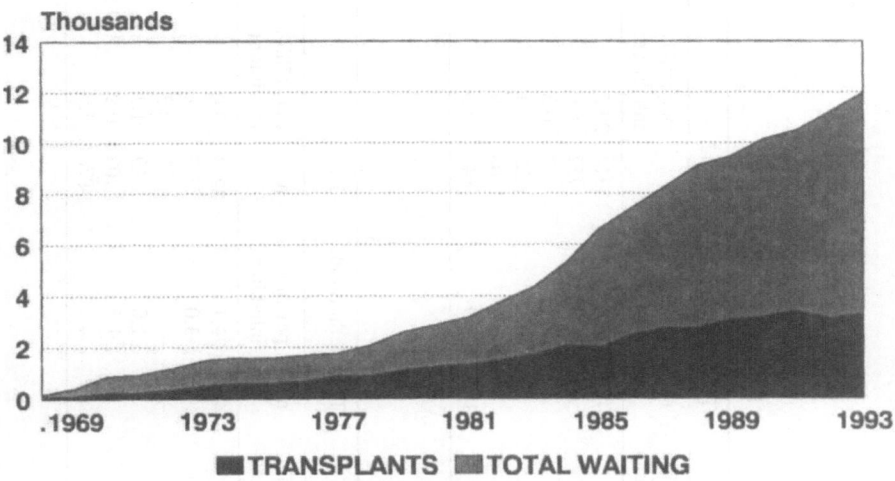

Figure 1. Renal patients in Eurotransplant.

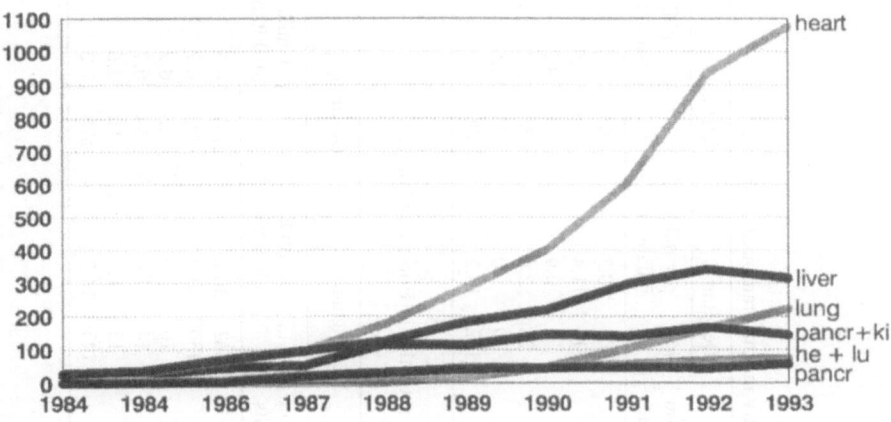

Figure 2. Patients on the waiting list of Eurotransplant.

alternative that renal patients have, i.e. (haemo)dialysis treatment, they die if a graft does not become available in time. The number of heart and liver patients that died while waiting for a transplant were 293 and 113, respectively. Also, 26 heart plus lung and 40 lung transplant candidates died in 1993.

Table 1. Overview of organ availability in Eurotransplant 1993

	Austria		Belgium		Germany		Luxembourg		The Netherlands		Total	
	n	per million inhabitants	n	per million inhabitants	n	per million inhabitants	n	per million inhabitants	n	per million inhabitants	n	per million inhabitants
Kidney	397	49.6	403	40.3	2070	25.8	18	45.0	426	28.4	3314	29.2
Heart	101	12.6	114	11.4	466	5.8	7	17.5	64	4.3	752	6.6
Heart + lungs	6	0.8	9	0.9	16	0.2	–	–	1	0.1	32	0.3
Lungs	27	3.4	26	2.6	59	0.7	1	2.5	12	0.8	125	1.1
Pancreas	19	2.4	20	2.0	41	0.5	1	2.5	19	1.3	100	0.9
Livers	119	14.9	132	13.2	490	6.1	4	10.0	103	6.9	848	7.5

Table 2. Overview of transplantation activities in Eurotransplant 1993

	Austria		Belgium		Germany		Luxembourg		The Netherlands		Total	
	n	per million inhabitants	n	per million inhabitants	n	per million inhabitants	n	per million inhabitants	n	per million inhabitants	n	per million inhabitants
Kidney	380	47.5	362	36.2	2107	26.3	8	20.0	436	29.1	3293	29.0
Heart	105	13.1	130	13.0	493	6.2	–	–	45	3.0	773	6.8
Heart + lungs	5	0.6	10	1.0	13	0.2	–	–	–	–	28	0.3
Lungs	33	4.1	14	1.4	58	0.7	–	–	14	1.0	119	1.1
Pancreas	16	2.0	15	1.5	50	0.6	–	–	19	1.3	100	0.9
Livers	91	11.4	143	14.3	578	7.2	–	–	66	4.4	878	7.7

2.2. *Donors and transplantations*

Table 1 gives an overview of the donor availability in 1993 for the different Eurotransplant countries. It should be noted that the number of post-mortem kidneys available per million inhabitants differs substantially between the collaborating countries. Austria, Belgium and Luxembourg are on top with, respectively, 49.6, 40.3 and 45 kidneys per million, while Germany and the Netherlands have only 25.8 and 28.4 kidneys per million. A similar phenomenon is seen for the procurement rates of hearts and livers. Austria and Belgium rank the highest with, respectively, 12.6 and 11.4 hearts per million inhabitants, and 14.9 and 13.2 livers per million inhabitants, respectively.

Table 2 shows the actual number of transplants performed in the various countries collaborating within Eurotransplant. The top two performing countries are Austria and Belgium, regardless of organ transplantation type. The discrepancy between the number of organs procured and the number of organs transplanted can be explained by the exchange between the different countries. Thus, Austria, Belgium and Luxembourg were exporting kidneys while Germany and the Netherlands were "importers" in 1993. However, concerning liver and heart transplantation, Belgium is an importer while the Netherlands exports these organs. The low heart and liver transplantation rate per million inhabitants in the Netherlands might also be the result of more stringent patient selection criteria and, thus, the relatively small number of patients on the heart and liver transplantation waiting list. Germany imported 27 hearts and 88 livers in 1993.

3. Discussion

For patients suffering from end-stage organ failure the optimal treatment is organ transplantation. Major progress in many fields related to transplant immunology and medicine has been realized during the last decade, resulting in higher survival rates of grafts and patients. The factors which have contributed most to these developments are the better management of the recipient pre- and post transplantation (surgical, nephrological, cardiological, haematological as well as immunological), standardized and reliable HLA-A, -B and -DR typing and matching, screening and cross-match procedures, preservation techniques and careful application and monitoring of immunosuppressive drugs. Immunological developments, such as the introduction of very potent new immunosuppressive drugs, e.g. FK506, Rapamycin, etc., as well as better insight into the mechanisms of graft rejection and, thus, treatment will certainly result in better patient and graft survival. However, the potential impact of all the above-mentioned factors may be seriously restricted by one persistent problem, namely the shortage of organ donors. The data of all organ exchange organizations in Europe and the United States show that a solution to this problem has not yet been found.

Publicity campaigns, distribution of donor cards, appointment of transplant coordinators, introduction of donor protocols in hospitals, reimbursement of donor hospital costs for procurement, educational programs for hospital personnel such as the European Donor Hospital Education Programme (EDHEP), and many other initiatives have been introduced (Wight 1992). Although these factors all help, they are so far insufficient to increase donor supply and thus prevent patients dying while awaiting transplantation.

The most well-known factor is the introduction of the so-called "Presumed Consent" law, which provides that every citizen is a donor after death unless he/she has objected during life, as used for example in Austria and Belgium. Analyzing the data regarding donor procurement and efficacy, indeed it seems that in these countries the number of available kidneys, hearts and livers significantly increased compared to countries such as the Netherlands and Germany where no legislative measurements have yet been taken. Comparing donation and transplant results in countries with apparently the same legislative system should be undertaken with caution, especially with regard to the "Presumed Consent" law. There are many differences in how these regulations are handled and practiced by the donor hospitals and the doctors in charge of potential donors. Even within one country governed by one law there are many different approaches, e.g. whether or not the family is approached, whether or not a central registration system exists and so on.

Informed consent means that the deceased has given permission during life by means of a donor card or registration in a central database to be an organ donor. If no permission has been given, the next of kin of the deceased are approached and asked for permission to remove organs and tissues for transplantation purposes. Standardization, uniformity and clarity would be very helpful not only for the doctors in charge but for the general public as well.

Care should also be paid to the interpretation of transplantation activities in the different countries. For example, the availability of potential candidates for an organ transplant might be a reflection of the selection procedure of potential transplant candidates. However, it might also be due to the fact that governmental and financial restrictions play an important role. This is especially noteworthy in the Netherlands.

Interesting in this respect is the number of non-residents registered and transplanted in Belgium and Austria. The low percentage of "own" dialysis patients registered on the waiting list for a renal graft might be caused by local, regional or national policies.

Political reasons and personal circumstances of transplant doctors might affect donation and transplant activities. The growth in the number of transplant centers might reflect this factor. This is especially so with new centers which have started their own heart and/or liver transplant programs and thus require donor organs to give themselves a reason for existence. In France, this has certainly led to a greater number of available donor kidneys because the thinking is, if a liver or a heart can be used, why not then use the kidneys?

Another oft-heard argument explaining the high availability of donor organs is related to the number of road traffic accidents: many victims of traffic accidents are potentially suitable donors. This might be partially true, especially for Austria and Belgium where the number of fatal traffic accidents per million inhabitants in 1989 was above 200. But here, also, caution must be used in interpreting and comparing these traffic accident data. Victims who died at the scene of the accident are nearly always lost as an organ donor. Therefore, a better way would be to compare the number of traffic victims who are severely wounded and transported to a hospital. Interesting to note is that in the Eurotransplant area there is a trend over the last 5 years to use more patients who died from intracerebral hemorrhages (>60% of total).

The relationship between the number of transplant coordinators and the availability of donor organs might be an obvious one. Yet, some caution is again necessary, as the definition and tasks of a transplant coordinator differ from country to country. Some are more involved in administrative work such as registration of transplant candidates, looking after the logistical aspects (transportation arrangements, financial aspects etc.) and follow-up activities, while others are really involved with organ donation, assisting and advising local doctors in charge of a potential donor. Additionally, the professional background of transplant coordinators varies from nurses to anaesthesiologists, from psychologists to surgeons in training.

Another important factor in determining potential donors is the diagnosis of brain death. All European countries participating in the Council of Europe have accepted the brain death criteria. Nevertheless, the definition of brain death remains a difficult concept to understand, and not only for the general public. It is of the utmost importance that the criteria used for determining brain death are crystal-clear. Thus, as much uniformity and standardization as possible is of enormous importance for the acceptance of brain death as the definitive and irreversible end of life. One of the most frequent questions from lay people is: Because I carry a donor card do doctors declare me dead earlier than non-donor card holders?

Confusion and carelessness over the diagnosis of brain death have damaged organ donation and transplantation programs in the past. The "Panorama-effect" caused by a program on BBC-TV in the early eighties is the best and thus worst example of this. Recently, new turmoil has started in Germany where high ranking officials from the Catholic and Protestant Church have openly disputed the definition of brain death on television and accuse, in fact, transplantation surgeons of using brain death as an alibi for their work. The mass media play a crucial role in influencing the public. They should accept their responsibility and use their power to turn the existing negative attitude against organ donation into a positive one.

In summary, the problem of the widening gap between demand and supply of donor organs must be solved. If not, commercial activities, as already practiced in some countries, will be the consequence. Alternatives such as xenografts might be considered but will certainly not be feasible on a large scale within the next 10 years. Therefore, all measures should be taken, maybe even on a compulsory basis, to solve this long-lasting problem in modern medicine.

Acknowledgements

The authors are indebted to the physicians and their administrative and nursing staffs for providing the Eurotransplant Foundation with the data. Ms. Astrid Wijbrandts is greatly acknowledged for her secretarial assistance.

References

1. Matesanz R, Hors J, Persijn GG, Thayer C, Dupuy JM. Transplant. vol 05. Fondation Merieux-Lyon: Council of Europe-Conseil de l'Europe, 1993.
2. Van Rood JJ. A proposal for international cooperation in organ transplantation: Eurotransplant. Histocompatibility Testing 1967; 451.
3. Wight C. The European Donor Hospital Education Programme (EDHEP) In: Cohen B, Persijn G, editors. Eurotransplant Annual Report 1992. 1993, 67.

2. Organ shortage in France: Present status causes and the future

PHILIPPE J-P. ROMANO

Transplantation activity in France

There is an important need for organs for transplantation. The shortage of organs affects everyone involved. Between 1985 and 1993, 104 authorised teams performed 19,910 transplantations Fig. 1. In 1992 there was a negative evolution in the number of grafts Fig. 2. Until 1987, the number of transplants steadily grew each year. Since then, the rate of increase has slowed down. 1992 was the first year when there was an actual decline in the number of transplants, by 9.25% from the previous year (Fig. 3).

The evolution of the waiting lists confirms that the decrease is caused by an organ shortage (Table 1).

Behind the numbers, the real tragedy is the increasing number of people waiting for transplantation. Last year, only 31% of the patients waiting for transplants received them (Table 2). The shortage represents the lack of what is necessary. An organ shortage exists because there are not enough organs available to graft new waiting patients.

Why is there this scarcity?

There are many explanations for this situation. The sum of all these facts generates the organ shortage. Some factors are major, some are minor.

The scarcity is often incorrectly attributed to two minor factors: a decrease in both the number of road traffic accident injuries and the number of non-resident patients.

Road traffic accident injuries

Happily, there has been a decline in the number of road traffic accidents, but the number is still high in France. Last year, there were 137,000 corporal injuries, of which 9,052 victims died in the first week (the potential donors), and 9,568 died before the end of the first month. Of the 1,652 brain deaths

J.L. Touraine et al. (eds.), Organ Shortage: The Solutions, 11–17.
© 1995 *Kluwer Academic Publishers.*

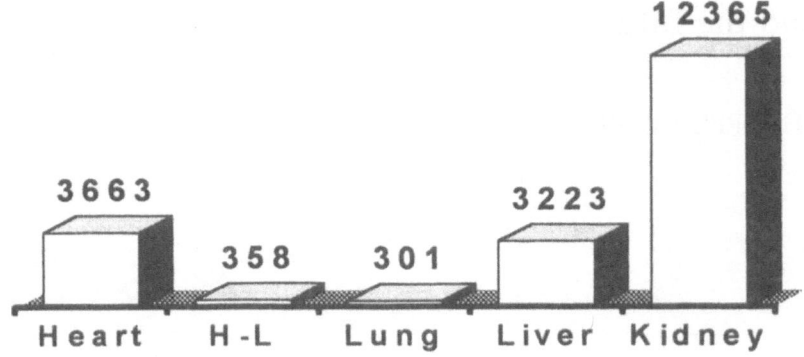

Fig. 1.

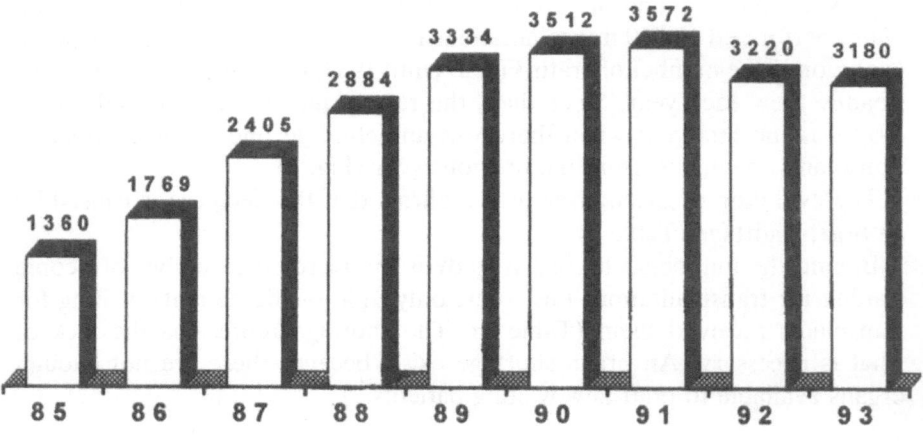

Fig. 2.

taken in charge, 25% are caused by road traffic accidents. Twenty-five percent of the 977 harvested organs also resulted from road traffic accidents
(Fig. 4).

Non-resident patients

It is often thought that the high number of non-resident patients is a significant factor but this is never officially announced. There are "too many
non-resident patients". Too many on the waiting lists and too many to be
transplanted!
But what is the real situation?
Physicians have always naturally refused to take care what the nationality

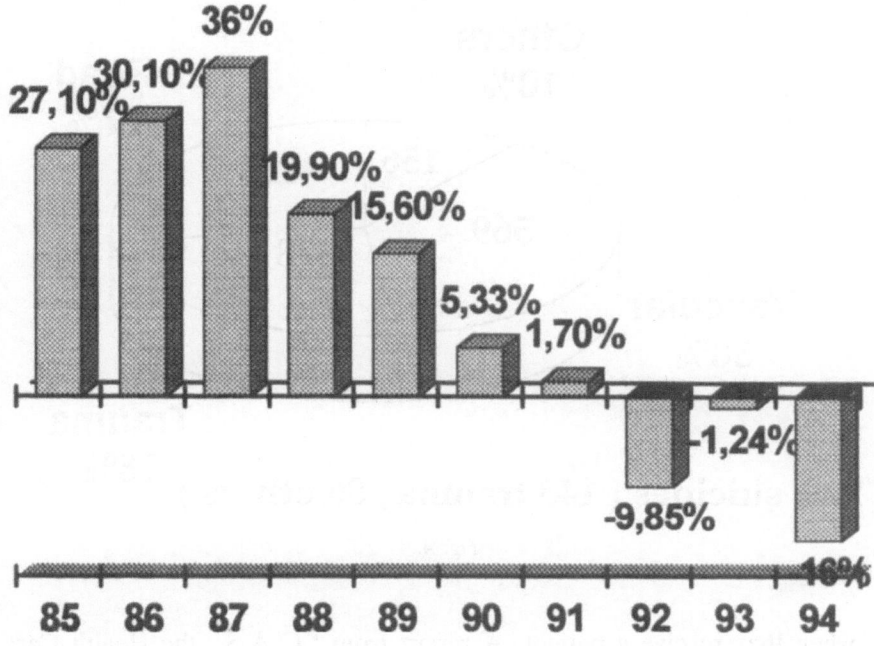

Fig. 3.

Table 1. Waiting list.

	1990	1991	1992	1993	1994
Heart	719	690	494	426	422
H-L	163	144	96	89	83
Lung	111	127	131	118	103
Liver	380	402	388	384	375
Kidney	4734	4886	4529	4565	4589
Total	6107	6249	5638	5582	5572

Table 2. Flow in 1993.

	01/01/93	1993	Sum	Grafted	%
Heart	494	711	1205	526	43
H-L	96	108	204	45	22
Lung	131	197	328	113	34
Liver	388	885	1273	662	52
Kidney	4529	2426	6955	1781	25
Total	5638	4327	9965	3127	31

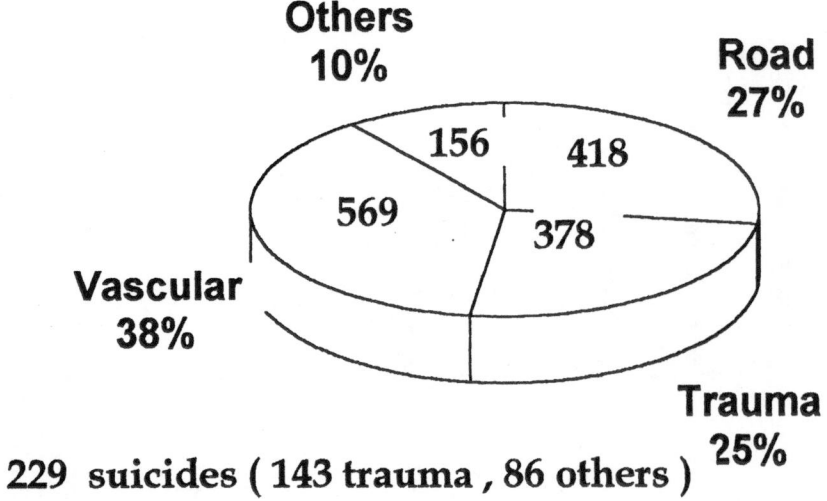

**Others
10%**

**Road
27%**

156   418

569   378

**Vascular
38%**

**Trauma
25%**

229 suicides (143 trauma , 86 others)

Fig. 4.

is, when they receive a patient. A report from I.G.A.S., the Health Care Ministry Inspectors, was carried out in June 1992, to analyse this situation and draw attention to the actions of a number of hospital teams. The findings were:

- 17.5% transplated are non-residents
- 10.3% for heart transplantations
- 34.6% for liver transplantations
- 13.6% for kidney transplantations
- 25% on waiting lists are non-residents
- 36% for liver list
- 28% for kidney list

In fact, we actually do not know what the real situation is.

Physicians and hospital administrators have not complied with new regulations that were passed on 24 September 1990, laying down new procedures for non-resident patients.

Arrêté du 24 septembre 1990, Articles 6 et 7:
. . . hospital administration put on waiting lists patients . . .
. . . non-residents are put on the waiting list only when they have received the agreement from the Regional Director of Sanitary Organisation . . .

Consequently, we do not know how many non-resident patients are on the national waiting lists. Nor do we know how many are grafted each year by each medical team and for each category of organs.

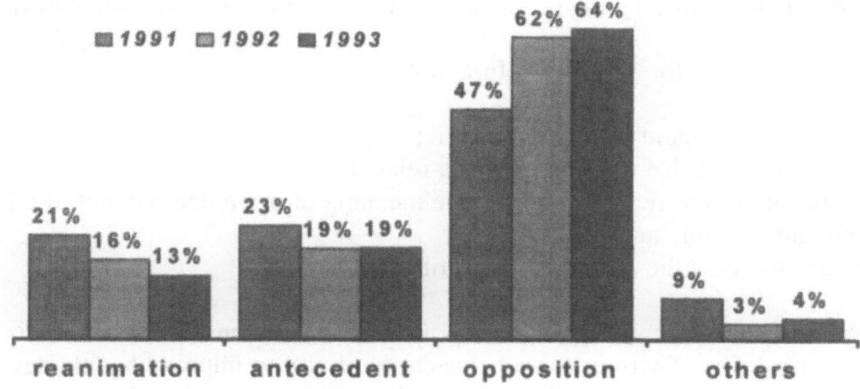

Fig. 5.

What are the more important real causes of the scarcity?

Two are found at the very beginning of the transplant procedure: namely, the donor and the medical team.

The donor

Typically, the wishes of the deceased are unknown. The medical team follows the relevant laws – "Decree no. 78–501 of 31st March 1978 and Circular of 3rd April 1978" – for such an eventuality, meeting with the family of the deceased and trying to learn from them his or her wishes.

> Décret no. 78–501 du 31 mars 1978 – Chapitre II, Article 9:
> . . . toutes les personnes pouvant témoigner qu'une personne hospitalisée a fait connaître qu'elle s'opposait à un prélèvement sur son cadavre, en particulier les membres de sa famille et ses proches . . .

> Circulaire du 3 avril 1978, Chapitre II – Information des personnes hospitalisées et de leur famille, aliné "B" Information des familles:
> . . . Il importe, en effet, d'éviter que les familles soient mises devant un fait accompli en leur donnant la possibilité effective d'apporter les preuves qu'elles détiennent de l'expression de la volonté du défunt, . . .

We are seeing an increase in "family" refusal.

This type of refusal typically reflects the opinion of the family and does not at all respect the wishes of the deceased, someone speaks of false witness. It is interesting to compare this fact with the results of opinion polls. For several years SOFRES, an opinion polling institute, has carried out surveys on the topic of organ sharing. The results, when the surveys are conducted amongst people who have no direct experience of a serious accident show significant variations. Young people are generally more in favour than elderly people.

The main reasons for "family" refusal are:

- religious, social and traditional factors;
- failure to recognize the wishes of the related;
- doubts about the reality of death; the meaning of brain death is not at all well understood; and
- refusal to allow the corpse to be mutilated.

There is also a degree of ignorance about and lack of consideration for this type of medicine. There is a gap between the desire to improve health care and the discrediting of medicine, particularly concerning hospital teams. Their reputation is further damaged by the media and newspapers in particular, which tend to give a great deal of attention to exceptions. This is compounded by a social retire within oneself.

Teams of the intensive care units

The other main cause of organ scarcity is the weakness of the second link in the chain of solidarity: the teams of the intensive care units. Potential donors are taken charge of within these structures. At present, emergency and intensive care departments are faced with many difficulties – a shortage of nurses, lack of physicians, lack of money. In addition, they suffer from a lack of consideration from other links in the transplantation procedure. These difficulties are symbolized by the number of unfilled posts: 405 at present, up from 280 last year. These teams are often demotivated because they feel appreciated by neither the transplant patients nor the surgeons. Generally they do not know the follow-up of the organs they have shared.

Yet, these men and women have surpassed themselves: after failing to save one life, they can try to save several more lives, thanks to an organ harvesting. It is they who must meet the relatives of the deceased and explain the procurement. And it falls upon them to convince these relatives of the importance of donating the organs. After several long hours, they organize the surgical operation in connection with their regional and national regulations.

The future

If these facts are, as we believe, the real causes of organ shortage, the situation will only get worse, unless something is done about it. There are two major points to be taken into consideration.

Informing the entire population about transplantation. Opinion polls show that 92% of the french population would like to benefit from the *equality* of transplants. namely, the opportunity to potentially lengthen their lives in return for accepting duties of *fellowship*. in other words, to agree to give their own organs from their corpse or those of their relatives. for this purpose, it is necessary to help everyone make their wishes known by way of a donor card: A "life card", which is supplemented by a computerised system.

These are decisions that each and every one of us should make for ourselves today. They are not decisions that should be left for our relatives in the event of an acute accident and a sudden death.

The second point is substantial help for the intensive care teams. This help should come from both hospital administrators and from the Ministry of Health Care. Further help could come from information and training courses on transplant coordination, such as those offered under the European Donor Hospital Educational Programme. The objectives should be:

- To help participants to acknowledge the importance of their own feelings and emotions when dealing with the family of the deceased
- To understand the dynamics of the reactions of distressed people and to positively help them
- To sensitize these personnel to the idea of organ donation and guide them in how they can assist the families in the decision-making process

In the future, the Etablissement Français des Greffes will take national responsibility for promoting the donation of organs.

We have to agree with the words of Jacques Prevert:

"The dead is in the life,
the life is in the dead."

3. Is there a shortage of organs in Argentina?

PABLO M. RAFFAELE

Introduction

I would like to give you a brief review of Argentina and its history before addressing our specific subject. In this way, it will be easier to understand its situation.

The causes of the Spanish occupation and colonization of the lands of the River Plate were mainly strategic. The foundation of the port of Buenos Aires by Don Pedro de Mendoza in 1536 evidenced of the need of the Spanish monarchy to limit the expansion of Portugal, its main rival.

The process of independence in Argentina began in the year 1810, determined by the events of the time, such as:

- the Independence of the United States of America
- the fall of the Hapsburgs from the throne of Spain for Napoleon invasion
- the surge of England as a naval and economic power

Our present society is the result of immigration policies. The impact of immigration, especially from Europe, is more important in the larger cities. The differences between the people that live in the interior of the country, the "Gaucho" population (a cross of breeds) and the ones that live in the cosmopolitan cities became stronger.

Therefore, we have to analyse the real situation of the procurement of organs in *two* Argentinas: that of the large cities, with heavy European influence, and that of the interior, the Argentina of Pampas, the Patagonia, the Tropics and the Andes, with a "mestizo" influence.

Organ procurement in Argentina

Early in the '60s, Professor A. Lanari carried out the first cadaveric kidney transplant in 1962, at the University of Buenos Aires. Unfortunately, in spite

J.L. Touraine et al. (eds.), *Organ Shortage: The Solutions*, 19–26.
© 1995 *Kluwer Academic Publishers.*

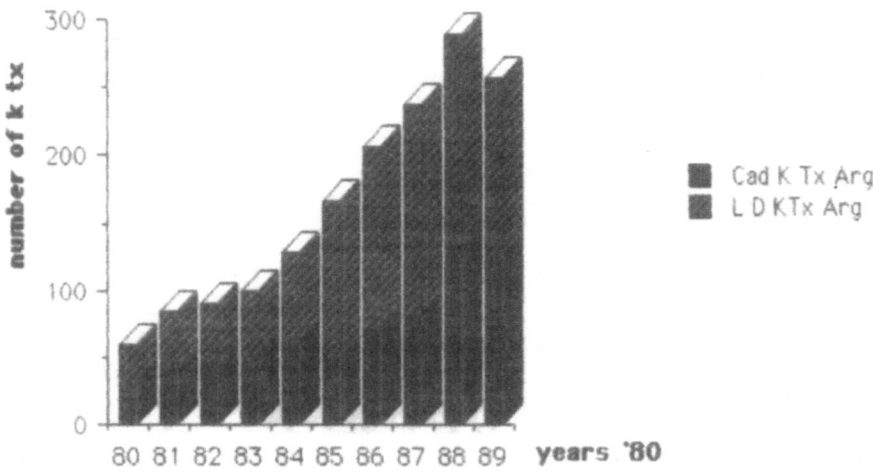

Fig. 1. Kidney transplantation in Argentina (cadaveric & living donor transplant).

of the first promising steps, after '80s Argentina didn't accompany the rest of the evolution of transplant activity.

I will analyse the data of Argentina and compare this information with that of France. I take France as an example because she is the host country and a good model for international transplant activity.

You see in Figure 1 kidney transplant activity in the '80s in Argentina. Only half of these kidney transplants were done with cadaveric donors. At the end of the '80s, 27 years after Professor Lanari performed the first cadaveric kidney transplant, Argentina presented an index of under 5 cadaveric kidney transplants per million inhabitants (pMInh). In France, in the same period, this index was over 35 (Figure 2).

In Figure 3 we can see the evolution of cardiac transplantation in Argentina.

Although we see an increase in cardiac transplantation since 1987, the panorama is discouraging. This is more evident if we express in terms of cardiac transplants p MInh and we then compare Argentina and France: in 1989, 13 cardiac transplants pMInh were carried out in France; by contrast, only 0.38 were carried out in Argentina (Figure 4).

We can make similar comparisons if we look at hepatic transplantation (Figures 5 and 6).

Situation in Argentina today

If we look at the evolution of national kidney procurement in the '90s, there is an improvement in 1993 – approximately 8 kidneys procured pMInh (Figure 7).

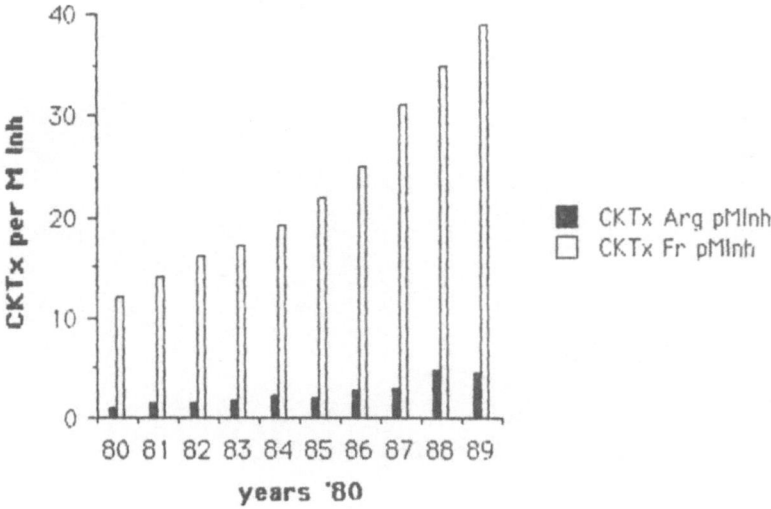

Fig. 2. Cadaveric kidney Tx France/Argentina.

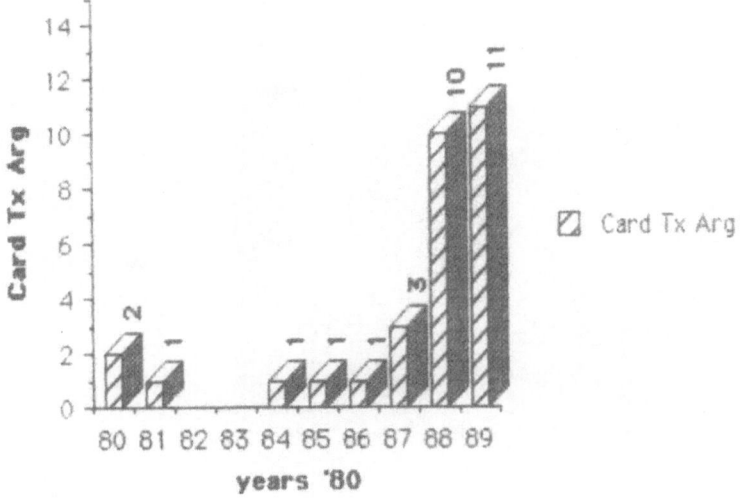

Fig. 3. Cardiac Tx in Argentina.

In our analysis, an important factor in improving organ procurement is the regionalization of our National Institute of Organs procurement, the INCUCAI, 2 years ago (Table 1).

In the northwest region, difficulty in communication, social and economic factors determine very poor kidney procurement results (0.8 kidney pMinh).

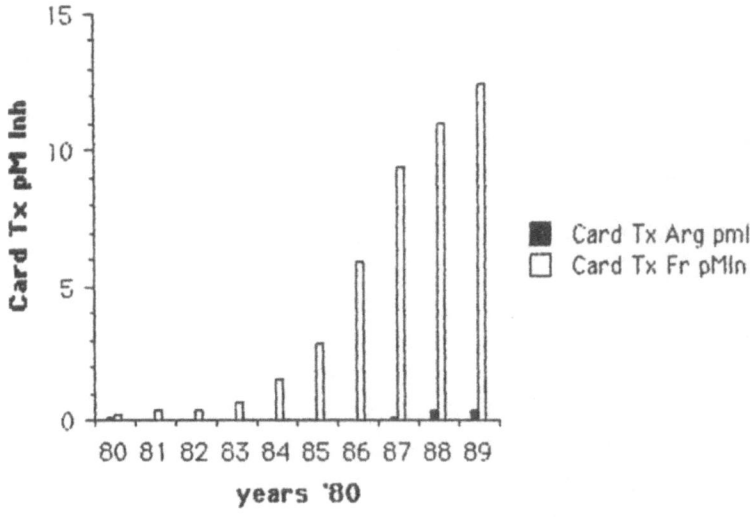

Fig. 4. Cardiac Tx pMInh France/Argentina.

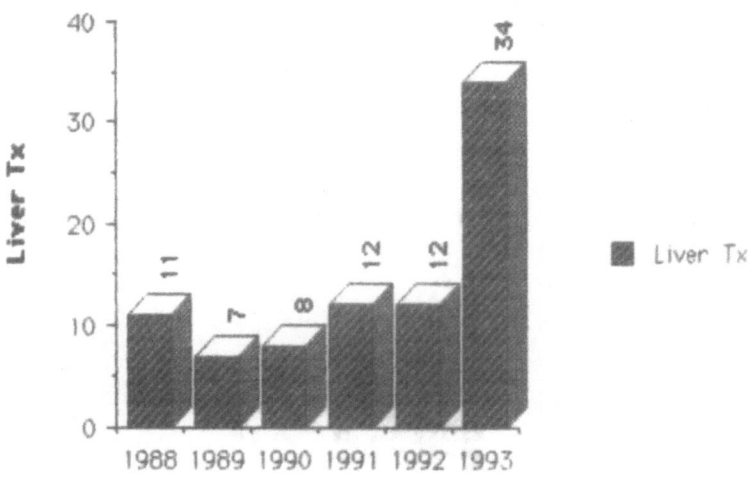

Fig. 5. Liver transplantation in Argentina.

This region has the widest differences in climate, landscape and culture (indigenous influence). The plateau in the north descends abruptly from 4,000 m.a.s.l. to 300 m.a.s.l. There are more peaks over 6,000 m.a.s.l. than in any other part of the world, with the exception of Asia.

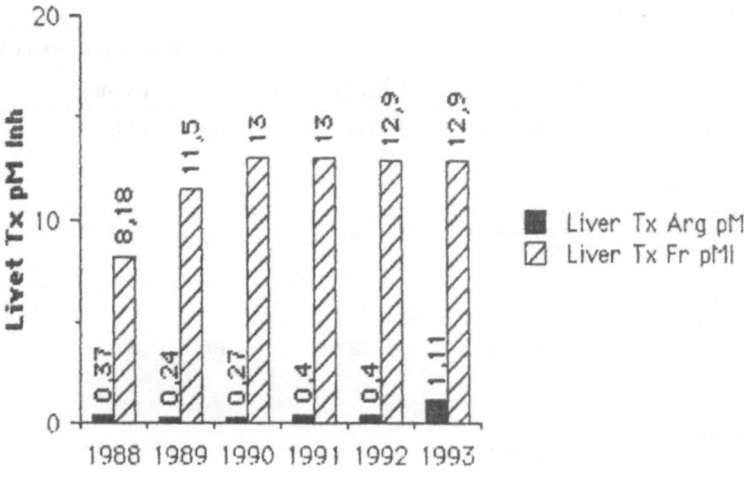

Fig. 6. Liver transplantation pMInh France/Argentina.

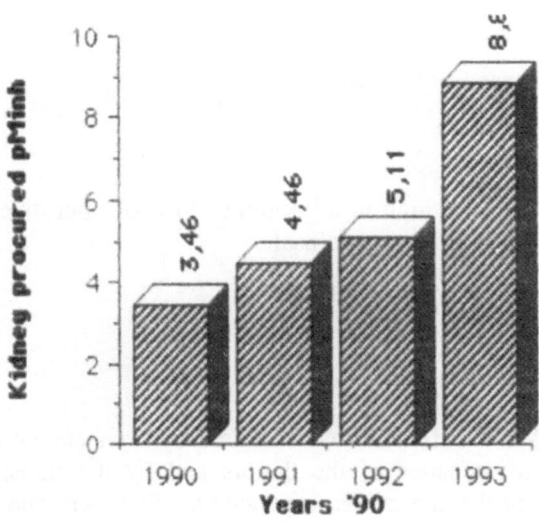

Fig. 7. Kidney procuration pMinh in Argentina '90's.

Table 1. The different INCUCAI regions

Region	No. inhabitants	Inhabitants/km^2	1993 kidney procurement	
			No.	pMinh
Federal Capital Region	3,000,000	15,000	68	22.6
Central Region (Germany + Switzerland + Belgium + Holland + Luxemburg)	3,922,777	8	46	11.7
Pampean Region Italy + Denmark + Belgium + Holland + Luxemburg)	12,842,355	28	108	8.4
Litoral Region (Germany + Switzerland + Belgium + Holland + Luxemburg)	6,647,526	13.3	24	3.6
North Western Region United Kingdom	2,523,010	11	2	0.8
Cuyo Region (Italy + Luxemburg)	2,230.312	7	12	6.2
North Patagonia Region (United Kingdom + Denmark + Luxemburg)	895,730	3	8	8
South Patagonia Region (without Antartica and the South Atlantic Islands)	586,000	1.12	10	6.74

Intervening factors in organ procurement

Donation refusal

The donation refusal index is high in all regions. 40% of operatives discontinued in 1993 were due to donation refusal.

Deficient operative structure

Organ procurement is also affected by a deficiency in state procurement organisation, by the maintenance of the donors and by the transplantation teams. More than 20% of the operatives suspended in 1993 were due to donors causes.

Otherwise, in the North Patagonia region, 55% of the operatives failed were due to deficient procurement structure.

Notification of brain death

Another factor which play a negative role in organ procurement is the lack of notification of brain death to the INCUCAI. A study performed in a provincial hospital of the Pampean region found that of the 40 brain deaths that occured not one was reported to INCUCAI.

The high number of deaths caused by traffic accidents in Argentina (7,000 per year) is not proportional to organ procurement activity.

Other Causes

In the Pampean region with a high density population, 249 organs were procured in the period 1992–1993. 46 of them were refused by the transplantation team. The causes were:

– shortage of recipients 36%
– donor related 36%
– deficient operational structure of the transplantation team 23%
– without data 5%

In regions where population density and the procurement operative capacity are higher, we see another cause of organ loss: organs refused by the transplant team. These rejected organs include heart, liver and lungs. Analysis of the waiting lists for these organs, expressed in patient pMinh, shows a low rate of inscription, as compared to France (Table 2).

An economic factor underlies this situation. There is a deficiency in the registration for some organ waiting lists because the national health system does not ensure prompt payment of institute fees in the more expensive transplant activities (heart, liver, lungs). The very large kidney waiting list reflects poor transplant activity. Furthermore, transplant activities in Argentina are mostly carried out in private medical centers.

Table 2. Waiting lists

Organ	Argentina		France	
	No. patients	pMinh	No. patients	pMinh
Heart	150	4.5	490	9.24
Liver	60	1.8	400	7.50
Lungs	12	0.36	95	1.8
Kidney	5,500	166	4,500	85

Summary

– Donation refusal is high in all the regions of Argentina.
– The deficient operative structure is a negative reality that allows inadequate donor maintenance and organ procurement.
– In more developed regions, there are a high number of organs which are not utilized. This is true for heart, liver and lungs. Small waiting lists for these organs probably reflect an inadequate economic coverage for these organ transplant activities.
– There is a long waiting list for cadaveric kidney transplants, which reflect poor procurement and transplant activity.
– Lack of awareness by many physicians leads to the denouncing of brain deaths.

In spite of these factors, we can say that there has been a significant growth in organ procuration and transplantation in 1993, after the regionalization of the INCUCAI.

Conclusions

Is there a shortage of organs in Argentina? There may be.

But the situation in Argentina differs from that in Europe, as we have a pool of organs which are not utilized (donation refusal, operational deficits, lack of denouncing of brain deaths). Perhaps, in the future, when we are able to make good use of all the organs submitted for transplantation, we will be able to say objectively whether the number of organs is sufficient or not.

Acknowledgements

I would like to thank the University of Lyon and the Merieux Foundation, especially Professors Traeger, Touraine and Dr. Dupuy for the honour of being invited to talk about the issue of organ procurement.

Professors Traeger, Touraine and Dubernard have greatly contributed to the improvement of medical formation and training in transplant activity in Argentina.

I would like to thank, too, Lic Pedro Bilik, Dr. José Duhalde, Dr. Graciela Filanino, Dr. Daniel Neustadt, Dr. Ingrid Smulevici and Dr. Roberto Suarez Samper, from the INCUCAI regions, who answered by requests about organ procurement information.

4. How to increase the search for organs in Argentina within the respect of ethics

ALCIDES FAGALDE

Introduction

Argentina is a country with a large territorial extension of 2,500,000 km^2 on its continental side. The great majority of the population of 35 million people are of European descent. Buenos Aires is home to 40% of the population; most other Argentinians live in five other urban conglomerates: Cordoba, Rosario, Tucuman, Mendoza, Resistencia and Corrientes. There are large differences in the country from a regional point of view.

The area of Buenos Aires City has a population density of 2,300 inhabitants per km^2, while there are Patagonian provinces that have just 1.2 inhabitants per km^2.

The population has access to health through three systems: public, for those who completely lack social coverage and/or resources, representing approximately 30–35% of the population; varied social security funds, which cover 60% of the population; or the private sector, used only by a minimum of the population. High medical development is concentrated in the above-mentioned urban centers and, principally, in the private clinics which serve patients from social security funds and private patients.

Medicine in Argentina has always shown a particular interest in transplantation; in 1938 the first cornea transplant was done in the Rawson Hospital of Buenos Aires. Since 1948, Professor Ottolenghi has performed several cadeveric bone transplants, Professor Alfredo Lanari performed the first cadaveric renal transplant in 1962 and, a few months after the first cardiac transplant by Dr. Barnard, Dr. Bellizi accomplished a similar operation. In 1977, at the request of the nephrologist organization, the first Argentine transplant law was passed and the CUCAI (National Transplant Organization), dependent on the nation's Health Ministry, was established.

What then followed was the first organized effort to constitute the basis of such an organization. Although supported by an official structure, the organ procurement activities of the organization were not as successful as expected. This was due to the excessive centralization mentioned before the lack of political support from both national and provincial authorities (very

J.L. Touraine et al. (eds.), Organ Shortage: The Solutions, 27–31.
© 1995 *Kluwer Academic Publishers*.

Table 1. Cadaveric transplants evolution in Argentina

Cadaveric transplants	Years								
	1986	1987	1988	1989	1990	1991	1992	1993	1994*
Kidneys	70	82	134	126	104	118	156	270	96*
Hepatic			11	7	8	12	12	34	16*
Cardiac	1	3	10	11	19	35	17	33	19*

* Until 30/04/94.

Table 2. Theoretical annual necessities and patients on waiting list

Cadaveric organ	Waiting list	Theoretical necessities by years
Kidneys	4800	1500
Hepatic	100	600
Cardiac	90	600

important since Argentina is a federal country) and, also, development was restrained by a deep, decades-long economic crisis in Argentina that lasted until three years ago. Paradoxically, dialysis development continued with virtually no restrictions nor planning. However, it is regulated by a specific law and waiting lists of patients for transplants have been growing considerally.

How many transplants have been done under these conditions in Argentina?

The number of annual transplants can be seen in Table 1. In Table 2 the theoretical necessities and current patients' waiting lists are shown.

In view of this situation and because of action by the Argentine Transplant Society, legislators voted in a new law where CUCAI was transformed into the National Institute for Transplants. In this way the organization is much more independent and autonomous relating to the legal, administrative and eocnomic aspects, and it is provided with a strong budget. The institute became effective in April 1992, with the naming of the Actual Board of Directors.

How do we satisfy the transplant needs in Argentina within legal and ethical boundaries?

I will make an analysis not only from the procurement point of view but, also, by taking the patients' needs into consideration.

In the first place, we have to carry out a diagnosis of the situation within the characteristics of the health system and the different regional realities.

Second, we must apply the law of transplants, which provides a strong regulatory frame for all procurement and implantive activities. This law contemplates the diagnosis of brain death, the obligatory registry of all activity, records of which must be kept for 10 years, the dispositions relating to the donation of organs between living or deceased persons, and the necessary conditions for institutional professionals and equipment. Express consent is now in force, but it is foreseen that, before 1996, a survey will be conducted soliciting the opinions of persons over the age of 18 (70% of the population) regarding organ donation and presumed consent will then be established (although families will still be able to refuse donation). Donation among non-relative living persons will only be carried out in exceptional cases and with previous judicial intervention. The law also obliges the denunciation of presumptive brain-dead patients. Penalties for such violations are severe to the point that they have been criticized because they are harsher than those for equivalent infractions in the Penal Code. Previous and present laws expressly prohibit the tracing of organs, as well as donation by minors or the mentally disabled; the present law adds the impossibility of removing organs from deceased patients in psychiatric institutions.

Third, we have to achieve institutional consolidation of INCUCAI, our goal being that the institute become the transplant's policy rector and supportive to the provinces. We believe that the population feels safer it transplant activity is controlled by the government, even more so if the country is democratic. Medical training in the specific task of procurement will also create more security throughout the system. We have begun with a plan for placing medical coordinators in all provinces with the coperation of the Spanish ONT and Lyon's organization. A public institute casrries a heavy duty since there is a series of publics norms that cannot be forgotten. In the fourth place, we must support existing provincial organizations and the development of those in the process of formation. Decentralized operations and distribution will begin to define the regionalization which we consider to be the logical policy in a country like Argentina.

Fifth, meetings are held with each of the system's parts. I would like to mention that within INCUCAI there is a patients committee that can supervise activity in various ways; this, we believe, is of great importance because it ensures transparency in the appliance of pre-established norms of distribution, the approach used by those who defend the system when it is questioned. This is very well received by the public and restrain the tabloid press.

Sixth, we need to correct or attenuate inequalities of regional development. For example, there are regions that are able to obtain organs but do not have transplant capacities. The objective of the different provinces development plan is for each region's organs to be distributed among local patients, except when there are national priorities.

The majority of donors come from public sector hospitals and most transplants are carried out in the private sector. Therefore, we must make the following analysis: clinics and private hospitals have had to face the costs of organ removal which are constantly increasing by day, with the consequent economic loss when dispositions are not forseen to oblige health organizations that protect a receiving patient with an economic refund. Having undertaken cost studies, norms have been dictated so that both public and private hospitals, as well as regional procurement organizations, are able to finance part of their operations. Therefore, no excuses exist for not integrating the system.

Although it is not the specific issue of this presentation, I cannot fail to mention the ethical problems that we face at present. They are primarily related to the inequality of transplant opportunities regarding regional health and reality mentioned in the first part of the presentation.

The situation depends on the organ being considered. For kidney and cornea cases, there are private services in almost every region, but public services are only found in the Buenos Aires area, Cordoba and Mendoza. Treatment is covered by social security funds in the public sector or by government money marked for transplants. If the receiver's province does not have a public center for transplants, he can only be operated on in one of the above three cities. The patient then suffers not only from the inconvenience of a change of place, but also from the more serious inconvenience of not having easy access to posterior control and immunosuppressors.

For organs such as the heart, liver, lung or double transplants, almost all activity at the moment is concentrated in the country's capital, using private equipment, so patients must obtain money from social security and/or loans which the government grants with many requirements and a great deal of anxiety. In response to this situation we have encouraged the availability of public services. This has been achieved for pediatric transplants at the National Pediatric Hospital and for adult lung and heart transplants at Buenos Aires Public Center.

We are expecting a fund that will allow us to develop a public transplant center in every region, as foreseen by the law. The province of Buenos Aires already has the resources to cover the costs needed for transplant patients. Although this means hard administrative work for the regional organization, it replaces the deficit in social security.

We hope that the deep economic transformation, followed by an important health system change, allows us to develop a procurement plan to satisfy the necessity of transplants. And, further, that the transplantations are carried out *only* in accordance with medical and not economic requirements, so that we are able to fulfil the ethical principles of equal opportunity.

Summary

Argentina is a nation with an immense territory, an economy which, until recently, suffered severely, and a population grouped in urban centers with strong regional contrasts. This heterogeneous and complex organization is now trying to develop the procurement and transplantation of organs, based on a strong regulatory law framework, governing the entire activity. The government, in compliance with the law, created the National Institute of Procuration and Transplant two years ago, which carries out policy based on the support of provinces and regions, having the Hospital Medical Coordinator as a base for procurement. The ethical problems mostly relate to obtaining equal opportunity for all patients needing a transplant. To this end, regional public services are being developed through national and provincial economic funds.

Acknowledgements

I would like to acknowledge Pedro Bilik for his help.

5. Effect of transplantation laws on organ procurement

P. MICHIELSEN

"Opting-in" versus "opting-out" laws: an oversimplification

The laws on organ procurement are usually classified as two different types: "opting-in" or informed consent, where the explicit consent of the family of the deceased is needed for organ procurement and "opting-out" or presumed consent, where organs can be removed post-mortem without the consent of the family if the deceased did not object during his life. The United Kingdom, Sweden and Denmark have an "opting-in" law; Germany and the Netherlands have no specific transplant law, but follow "opting-in" rules; Austria, Belgium, Finland, France, Norway and Spain have adopted a presumed consent law [1].

In fact, this division into two types is an oversimplification. "Opting-in" legislations can differ on several points: on the possibility for the family to overrule an expressed will of the deceased, on the definition of the family members concerned by the consent procedure, on required request, etc. This diversity of rules and practices is still greater is presumed consent systems. Informed and presumed consent laws have in common the priority given to the decision made by the deceased during his life. This decision on post-mortem donation can be positive or negative. The laws differ, however, in the way in which citizens can register their decision. Only the Belgian transplant law has established a central computerised registry in which citizens can enter their decision to donate or oppose donation. This registry must be consulted by the transplant centres before the removal of any organs. In some presumed consent laws, as in Belgium, in the absence of a registered will of the donor, the family is granted the possibility to object against organ removal. In the Finnish and Norwegian laws (1), informing the family of the planned organ removal is a legal obligation. In the other presumed consent laws there are three legal possibilities: removal of organs without the knowledge of the family, removal of organs after informing the family and removal of organs after informed consent of the family. Only an exhaustive enquiry can indicate how the donor centres make use of these different possibilities in a given country. Any comparison of the efficiency of transplant laws in

J.L. Touraine et al. (eds.), Organ Shortage: The Solutions, 33–39.

various countries should take into account these differences, which can influence the way in which the law is applied. The impact of the introduction of a transplant law will therefore be easier to evaluate in a single country.

In addition, the final organ procurement score cannot be used indiscriminately for this evaluation. The transplant law can only determine the legal and psychological environment within which organ procurement can be organised. The final result will depend on several factors unrelated to the law [2]. The most obvious is the number of potential donors, which varies from country to country with the density and age stratification of the population, the number of intensive care beds, the number of traffic accidents etc. How many of these potential donors will become effective donors is dependent on the more or less efficient organisation of the retrieval of organs, the motivation and collaboration of the medical profession etc. Organ procurement is the final result of a chain of events and the final result will be determined by the weakest link. It is therefore incorrect to evaluate the merits of the different legal provisions on the basis of the score of organ procurement alone. Comparison between countries should be restricted to countries with a similar background.

Is organ procurement more efficient in countries with a presumed consent legislation?

In their recent review of the transplant laws in Europe, Land and Cohen [1] were unable to find an obvious correlation between high post-mortem organ removal rates and the existence of presumed consent laws. This was obviously due to the inclusion in the study of countries with less developed transplantation programs and different levels of medical care. Table 1 shows some relevant data for countries in which an effort to maximise organ retrieval has been accomplished. At first sight it is obvious that higher kidney procurement rates were obtained in the countries with an "opting-out" legislation.

The number of road deaths, however, is lower in countries with an "opting-in" legislation, and this cannot be excluded from possible factors contributing to the lower organ procurement, as traumatic head injury ($\frac{3}{4}$ of the cases due to road accidents) is one of the most commonly found causes of death in organ donors. Still, the influence of the number of traffic deaths on the pool of potential donors is not as overwhelming as could be inferred from the global traffic death numbers given in Table 1.

"Traffic deaths" include all deaths occurring within 30 days of a road accident. People who died "on the spot" in traffic accidents are, as a rule, not available as organ donors. The potential donors are persons wounded in a traffic accident and dying within the first few days after admission to an intensive care unit. In Belgium, as in most European countries, the incidence of traffic deaths has declined progressively over the years. Interestingly, when deaths on the spot and deadly wounded are considered separately

Table 1. Relevant data for countries with an active organ retrieval organisation

	Kidney procurement[a]		Road deaths[b]		
	1992	1993	1991	1992	Intensive care beds[c]
Opting-out					
Austria	40.8	52.4	197	187	92
Belgium	35.1	40.1	187	171	190
Spain	43.3	38.4	225	199	107
France	32.7	33	186	159	248
Opting-in					
Netherlands	29.7	28.8	86	91	104
UK	28.7	28.8	81	74	70
Germany	25.2	25.8	123	91	179

Data per million inhabitants. Source: [a]European Transplant Coordinators Organisation, [b]Belgian Institute for Traffic Safety, [c]European Society of Intensive Care Medicine.

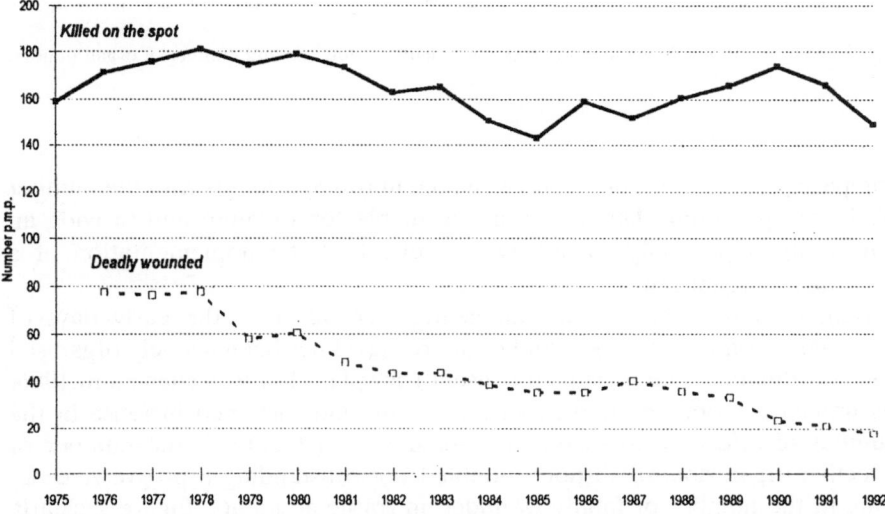

Fig. 1. Traffic deaths per million population in Belgium, subdivided in "killed on the spot" and "deadly wounded". Data from the Belgium Institute for Traffic Safety.

(Figure 1), only the latter decreased. The number of deadly wounded decreased from 80 pmp in 1976 to less than 20 in 1992. Consequently, for Belgium the number of road deaths that could provide donors was only 10% of the figure indicated in Table 1. Comparable data are not available for other countries and global traffic deaths cannot be used as a substitute to evaluate the pool of potential organ donors. Taking into account this difficulty in estimating the pool of potential donors, comparisons between countries are not a reliable measure of the efficiency of the organisation of organ retrieval. However, efficiency can be fairly accurately estimated by

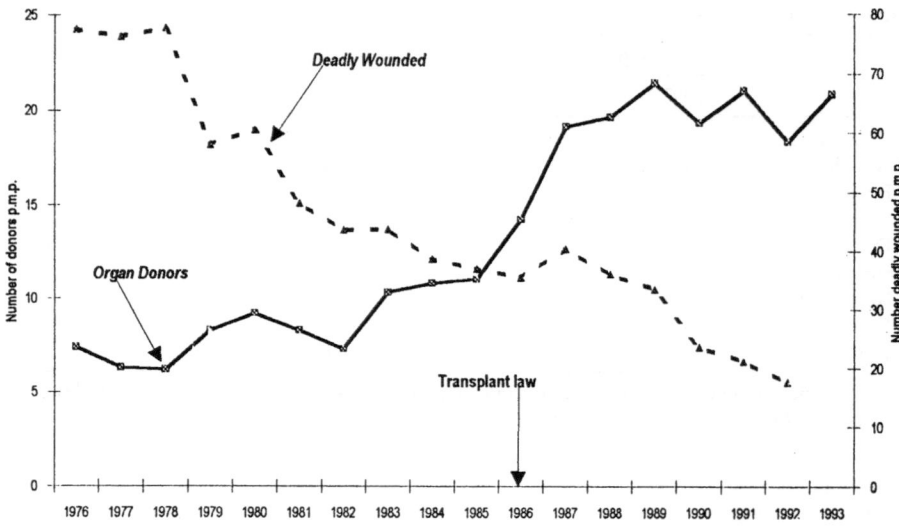

Fig. 2. Number of deadly wounded in traffic accidents in Belgium and number of organ donors.

comparing the number of deadly wounded in traffic acidents with the number of donors procured. These data are available for Belgium and provide an interesting opportunity to analyse the effect of the implementation of a presumed consent law.

Belgium has several transplant centres, active since the early days of transplantation in the sixties, and organ retrieval has been actively organised and coordinated. The presumed consent transplant law was enacted in 1986. Its implementation resulted in an immediate and sustained increase in the number of effective organ donors. As shown in Figure 2, the number of effective organ donors abruptly doubled notwithstanding a progressive decline in the number of fatally wounded in traffic accidents. Figure 2 clearly indicates that despite optimal conditions and the existence of a large potential donor pool, we were unable to increase significantly organ retrieval, until the law was implemented. Even with an extreme reduction of deadly wounded to 17.6 pmp per year in 1993, there was no decreasing trend in organ procurement.

The most convincing evidence of the role played by the transplant law in Belgium is given in Figure 3. As could be expected, there was no unanimity among the Belgian transplant centres. The presumed consent principle was heavily debated. The transplant centre of Antwerp was strongly opposed to and campaigned vigorously against the law. After its enactment, a strict "opting-in" policy was continued in Antwerp, together with a maximal effort for efficient transplant coordination and public information. In contrast, the

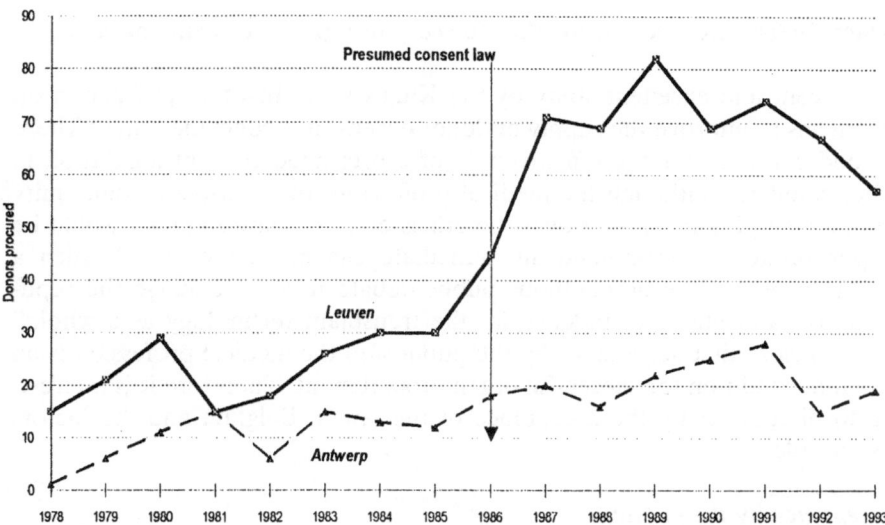

Fig. 3. Donor procurement in Antwerp, with a strict "opting-in" policy and in Leuven, with a flexible "presumed consent" policy.

transplant centre of Leuven was very active in promoting presumed consent and made full use of the possibilities offered by the law.

Although there was no uniform attitude among the hospitals collaborating with Leuven nor among the doctors in the same hospital, in general, removal without informing the family remained exceptional. It occurred when it was impossible to contact the family, or in circumstances where the attitude of the relatives suggested disinterest. The usual practice has been to inform the family to give them the opportunity to object to donation, but without asking explicitly for permission. Every effort is made to relieve the family of the burden of responsibility of allowing what is usually perceived as mutilation of the body of the deceased. This resulted in an increase in procurement, especially in collaborating non-university hospitals [3]. The number of objections of the family remained extremely low, less than 10%. In Antwerp, however, the mean refusal rate was 23.7% (M. De Broe, pers. comm.). Figure 3 illustrates that the impact of the law was negligible in Antwerp, while the number of effective donors increased substantially in Leuven. This observation eliminates the effect of the publicity given to organ donation as a cause of the increase in organ procurement after the implementation of the law. These observations indicate beyond a reasonable doubt the efficiency of the Belgian presumed consent law in providing an adequate legal environment for organ procurement. As a consequence, the centre of Antwerp recently reconsidered its position and decided to make use of the flexibility permitted in the presumed consent law.

Which factors are relevant for the efficiency of a presumed consent law?

In a recent and excellent study by the King's Fund Institute in London on the means to improve the supply of donor organs, it is concluded that "There is good evidence for the effectiveness of a presumed consent legislation in other countries, although the medical profession, the transplant community and public opinion are split over the ethics of such a law and so it would be inappropriate to recommend an immediate change in the law. If such a change provoked an acrimonious public debate it could damage the reputation of, and public confidence in, the transplant technology as a whole" [2]. It is clear that acceptance by the public and the medical profession is an essential condition for successful organ procurement. Therefore it is interesting to discuss briefly the acceptance of the law in Belgium and the factors responsible.

Acceptance by the public

Before the enactment of the law, not only the medical profession but also the public were divided on the issue of presumed consent, and the subject was debated bitterly in the media. Interestingly, after enactment the controversies gradually faded out. Eight years after introduction of the law the public seems no longer interested in the issue. Three factors may have played a role in this attitude. The possibility for every citizen to easily register and to modify his will at any time, with the guarantee that his decision will be honoured, was certainly an important point. Although less than 2% of citizens have made use of this possibility, it has prevented emotional reactions by those who strongly opposed donation for religious or other reasons. The possibility for the family to object to organ removal in the absence of a registered will of the deceased prevented the risk of angry discussions over the possession of a dead body. Finally, a very important factor has been a change in the climate surrounding the decision for organ removal. In most cases, the family was relieved of the burden of responsibility for allowing the mutilation of the body of their deceased relative. It appears more easy not to oppose, than to take the responsibility for, organ donation. To understand this attitude it is important to realise the special "sacred" status of a dead body in nearly all cultures. This is reflected not only in funeral rituals, but also in most "laws prescribing the way a dead body is to be treated, ensuring its 'appropriate' and 'respecful' handling, and imposing criminal penalties when treatment fails to match our standards of decorum" [4]. On the other hand, a legal post-mortem examination, decided by an established authority, is usually accepted easily by the family, in sharp contrast to the stress of taking the responsibility for organ donation. By making organ procurement for transplantation as official as legal autopsies, the Belgian presumed consent law apparently succeeded in taking organ procurement, to some extent, out of its sacrilegious aura.

Acceptance by the medical profession

Before its adoption, the law was heavily debated and the medical profession was divided. Here also the controversies subsided, although some doctors still reject presumed consent. Two factors contributed greatly to the absence of active opposition to the law. The first is legal safety. The possibility to consult the computerised registry eliminates all discussions about the intensions of the deceased. In addition, in the absence of a will of the deceased, the initiative for objection must come from the family. This eliminates all later discussions on how and to whom the information was given. A presumed consent law, however, shifts the responsibility for the decision from the family to the doctors. This could partly explain the reluctance of some doctors. Yet, the law is flexible enough to allow all doctors to act according to their ethical principles. This was also an essential point for the acceptance. Those who are opposed can continue asking for the explicit permission of the relatives. The others can make use of the possibilities offered by the law to decrease the burden imposed by organ removal on the bereaved family.

In a situation where the interests of the patients awaiting a transplant and the family of the deceased and the community are conflicting, the Belgian presumed consent law apparently succeeded in working out a compromise acceptable to all. There is, however, much more in the transplant law than the principle of presumed consent. The final result will largely depend on the way in which these aspects are well balanced.

Acknowledgements

The author is much indebted to L. Roels, transplant coordinator, and to Prof. M. Waer for their critical review of the manuscript. He thanks the many doctors who agreed to discuss and to provide data on the procedure for organ donation in their unit, especially V. Bosteels, L. Janssens, E. Matthys, M. Segaert and Prof. Van Aken. He thanks also Prof. P. Lauwers who provided the data on the number of intensive care units.

References

1. Land W, Cohen B. Post-mortem and living organ donation in Europe: transplant laws and activities. Transplant Proc 1992; 24(5) (October): 2165–7.
2. New B, Solomon M, et al. A question of give and take – improving the supply of donor organs for transplantation. Research Report 18, ed. 25–8. London: King's Fund Institute, 1994.
3. Michielsen P. Organ shortage – what to do? Transplant Proc 1992; 24(6) (December): 2391–2.
4. Prottas JM. Buying human organs – evidence that money doesn't change everything. Transplantation 1992; 53(6): 1371–3.

6. Causes and socio-psychological dimensions in donation refusal

J. TRAEGER & J. J. COLPART

Organ transplantation is a victim of its success: there is now a crisis in the development of this activity. The numerous new achievements have raised much spectacular but, also, fragmented information by the media, leading the public to be confused and not willing to easily accept the new concepts. Moreover, the sophisticated and expansive organization which is now necessary to run the transplantation activities has made the state an obligatory ruler, leaving the professional in second place and creating a frustrated feeling among the transplant team.

One of the most evident manifestations of this crisis is the overall reduction in the number of organ transplantations in the last few years. In France, during the last three years, the number of transplants dropped 10–15%, instead of the generally growing rate of 10–15% during the preceding years.

Beside socio-psychological reasons (donation refusal, disheartened transplant teams) some objective causes are present: the number of car accidents is lower (−10%) and the numbers of head injuries leading to brain death are also fewer than before (−10%) due to more rapid and effective resuscitation techniques. The number of family donor refusals is growing, which is also proof that an uneasy feeling about transplantaion exists among the population.

What is the relative importance of donation refusal among the causes of non-explantation in brain death subjects? In France, 70% of non-explantations are due to donation refusal. Each year, 130 brain death patients are not used for transplantation activities; likewise, 130 cardiac and hepatic and 260 kidney transplantations (15% of the total kidney transplantation in France) are not performed due to donation refusal (France Transplant 1993).

Donation refusal appears to be important – it is a growing problem – and should be studied in order to find the causes, mainly socio-psychological.

In France, the opting out law (presumed consent) has been in place for almost 20 years, but this law is not really used as it was initially planned: asking permission of the family was not thought to be necessary, but further hospital regulations urge medical teams to do so. One of the most suitable

J.L. Touraine et al. (eds.), *Organ Shortage: The Solutions*, 41–47.
© 1995 *Kluwer Academic Publishers*.

Table 1. Sociological factors involved in organ donation

Categories	No.	Yes	No	+ or −
Population	5849	31%	9%	60%
Males	2950	30%	9%	61%
Females	2776	34%	7%	59%
<30	2197	31%	8%	61%
Age 30 to 45	2564	33%	9%	58%
>45*	966	32%	9%	59%
Married	3773	33%	8%	59%
Single	1970	29%	9%	62%
0 children	2186	29%	9%	62%
1 to 3 children	3130	32%	9%	59%
>3 children	123	46%	4%	50%
Executive	513	41%	8%	51%
Employee	3026	34%	7%	59%
Woreker	2139	25%	11%	64%
Commerce	2422	25%	7%	68%
Industry	675	37%	12%	51%
Healthcare	990	40%	6%	54%
Services	1760	32%	11%	57%

*Non Significant.

aspects of the law was lost and, moreover, set a useless burden and difficult decision upon the family.

An analysis of socio-psychological aspects of donation refusal can be worked out correctly only if done in two parts:

- Donation refusal by the one who thinks quietly of this problem, far from any death event
- Donation refusal by the family confronted with the drama of the unexpected next-of-kin death

Polls conducted in France and other countries show that almost 90% of the population is in favor of organ donation (89% in France, SOFRES, 1992; 72% in the USA, Gallup 1993; 64% in Belgium . . .). If further questions are asked, the positive percentage becomes lower (67% positive answer for next-of-kin, 61% for a child), showing limits of the general positive tendency for agreement.

Feelings of social and racial exclusion are very important negative factors: only 57% (instead of 72% for the general population) of U.S. citizens of Spanish origin are in favor of organ donation, only 52% of blacks are in favor, 35% of whom think that racial discrimination exists for organ allocation. The feeling of exclusion from society, the professional failure have important negative effects on the will for organ donation: "Why should I give to the Society which has not given anything to me?" (ETC Newsletter 1993).

An interesting poll in Belgium points to the paradoxical fact that M.D.S are not in favour of organ donation. This was also previously suspected in France. In Belgium, only 44% of general practitioners are in favor; 30% are against; 26% have no opinion. These rather strange answers may be due to a feeling of exclusion, contributed to by transplant teams which did not try strongly enough to inform and convince their colleagues (ETCO Newsletter 1993).

A very important inquiry has been recently published, performed among 5,800 men and women working in factories, looking for the sociological factors involved in organ donation. Table 1 shows some results of this poll. Familial status is important (the greater the number of children, the more positive the answer). Position in the social hierarchy also influences the answer (willingness to give is more frequent among the highly ranked personnel than among workers). There is probably a double explanation for this: feelings of social exclusion for some, and poor information, education, and understanding of the problem of organ donation for all (Drouet et al. 1993).

What are the grounds for organ donation refusal? A poll conducted by SOFRES among the French population in 1992 shows that 37% of the population put forward religious and moral motives. Other responses suggest body integrity is not respected (22%), fear and ignorance (10%) and uncertainty as to why they are against organ donation (26%).

These arguments must be discussed. Religious motivation? All religions have accepted explantation after brain death. Even Islamic religions are not against organ donation and Saudi Arabia is a good example of what can be achieved in Islamic countries. These positive answers are not well known by the population. A lack of information in this matter is highly unfavourable for organ donation (Grundel 1991).

What can we say of the 26% of the population that do not know anything about organ donation? They have never thought of this problem and no one has really made any effort to push them to think about it.

Twenty-two percent of the population think that body integrity is not respected, which, in a sense, is true. This strong feeling goes along with the personal, profound respect which a dead body should warrant. However, this argument is not easy to accept when it is known that more and more cremations are being performed. An inquiry in our region (Lyon) shows that more than 50% of the deceased are incinerated and this proportion is growing.

Brain death as a definition of death is not well accepted by the population in certain countries. This is the case in Japan, where 70% of polled people are against this definition of death. And the Buddhist belief, that the soul only leaves the body several days after death, does not facilitate the transplantation development in this country: only 3% of dialyzed patients are transplanted in Japan (Atsumi 1992).

In Western countries, the brain death definition of death is difficult to understand by a large proportion of the population: how is it possible that the brain is dead whereas other organs are kept alive? Ancestral fears of being buried alive do remain even in our present times. We are reminded of this by all sorts of gadgets which were used for centuries for helping the dead should they awake in the coffin: food, means of communication, ventilation tubing, etc. Even incineration was first considered as the absolute means to be sure that the dead are really dead. Such old and ancestral fears can only be eradicated from the general population with repeated information and explanations which should begin at school (Lery 1987; Pottecher 1993; Sass 1991).

When the media (newspaper and television) represents the only information on transplantation for 72% of the U.S. population, can we think that the old beliefs will disappear and that this percentage of the population has a true knowledge of organ donation? Certainly not, because newspapers and television give only quick, superficial, fragmental information; their aims are mainly scoop, sensational news, rather than true information and education (Croon 1991). Moreover, the press and television very often have given a false view of transplantation and organ donation, due to the thrilling aspects of the news. There are numerous examples of deleterious effects of such sensational information which are often presented as being usual and not exceptional: in France (Affaire D'AMIENS, de l'Hôpital Tenon) and in foreign countries (in Sweden, definition of cerebral death in 1988, first heart lung transplantation in 1990).

The absence of true information on organ donation and transplantation appears perfectly clear when you consider the results of a poll made by SOFRES in 1992, showing that 98% of the population does not know the name of the law on organ donation, the law being used for 20 years in France (Loi Caillavet, law on presumed consent). Fifty-eight percent of the population thinks that this law is for expressed consent.

If transplantation is thought to be a useful therapeutic procedure and should continue, and if organ donation must be developed, it becomes necessary to seriously inform and educate public opinion on cerebral death, to explain the meaning of organ donation, to explain what the law is for organ donation and, more generally, to give information on transplantation problems – negative and positive aspects must be openly discussed. The necessity of solidarity should be conveyed, with the notion that, nowadays, death can give rise to life.

These informative and educational activities should be driven by the state health organization with the necessary financial means, with the help of organ donor associations. Information should be primarily delivered to young populations in schools, colleges, universities and the army, and to the part of the population which has difficulties in being completely integrated and successful in society. Special efforts should be extended toward general practitioners by the transplant teams.

Family refusal for organ explantation from a brain dead patient is a totally different problem: death is present and mourning, with its intense psychological stress is here. It is a state of shock with tiredness, apathy and insomnia; thinking and decision-making are difficult. This state of transitory confusion may last hours, days or weeks. The basic problems of organ donation will certainly not be handled with calm and serenity. Therefore, the answer of the family may not exactly fit the opinions on organ donation which were reported before. Asking permission of the family under these circumstances appears as psychological aggression, which was not the initial plan of the regulation of the presumed consent law.

Numerous studies have been done by organ coordinator teams in France and other countries to better understand the factors which lead to organ donation refusal in these circumstances. First of all, the frequency of organ donation refusal is highly variable from one place to another, and in the same location it varies with time. For instance, in Brest, frequency of refusal was 5.25% in 1991, 16.25% in 1992, 9% in 1993; in Rennes frequency of refusal was 20% in 1991, 37% in 1992, 15% in 1993. These great variations should depend on the skill of the coordination team members. The psychological skill with which the request is represented to the family is certainly one of the most important factors which influences their response.

The answer depends also on the nationality of the family: 91% of Meghrebin families gave a negative answer; in Latin countries, 42% of families gave a negative answer, and for Europe as a whole a mean of 26% gave a negative answer. In France, the usual negative response is 34%.

The cause of brain death is a factor: the family more easily gives a positive answer when the brain death is caused by suicide (70%); 64% agree when it was caused by a head injury car accident; and 61% agree when brain death is due to cerebrovascular disease. The age of the brain death victim is also a factor which influences the family's answer. The younger the person is when brain death occurs, the more difficult it is to obtain a positive answer (from 18 to 25 years, 39.7% refusal), 25–45 years, 28% refusal).

Arguments given by the family agree with those found in the poll mentioned before, but with some differences. Twenty-six percent refuse with no argument – this is probably an instinctive response expressed during a stress situation – and 18% evoke the prior negative will of the dead (usually with no proof). Loss of body integrity accounts for 21% of the arguments for refusal; being against the presumed consent law is said to be the cause of refusal for 16%; and 13% refuse on religious grounds.

Social factors, some of which were presented before, also play a role: craftmen, staff members and employers give a favorable answer in 70% of the cases; farmers, 55%; workers, 47%.

As previously stated, the dramatic events of the death of a next-of-kin demand a highly qualified psychological approach of the family. This seems to be of the utmost importance. Only trained and skilled nurses and MDs, will be able to introduce a request for donation without raising resentment. The need for such training is now evident, and French, Spanish and European programs have been organized for the education of coordinator transplant teams. These sessions should be repeated yearly to avoid weariness towards a stressing psychological activity.

Does this study of socio-psychological factors involved in organ donation lead to a preference for the "opting in" (expressed consent) or "opting out" (presumed consent) law?

The opting in law seems to be less effective because only a few people make the decision in advance: in Holland, only 20% of the population has a donor card, while 52% is willing to give. Several inquiries in countries with an opting out law have shown a greater efficacy of this regulation, but drawbacks do exist. The legislation must be well established and a great deal of information should be given to avoid the frustrated feeling which may appear among those who think they have no possibility of choice (which is wrong).

The "Caillavet" law – opting out law – which was established 20 years ago in France, was in advance of its time. As it was initially conceived, without the necessity to ask permission of the family, this law considered the cadaver as belonging as much to society as to the family. When, through medical progress, death may give rise to life, why should the cadaver not be used to save the life of other members of the society?

It becomes more and more evident that the beneficial effect of organ transplantation warrants the disappearance of organ donation refusal. The study of socio-psychological factors involved in organ donation refusal shows that most could be overcome by education and factual information, not by the media but by a well-planned official campaign.

As long as it is necessary to ask family permission for explantation of organs from a brain death victim (establishment of a computerized registry of organ donation refusal could overcome this necessity), it will be necessary to work with psychologically trained nurses or MDs who are able to perform such difficult interviews.

References

Croon AC. Does media coverage of organ donation and transplantation influence attitude to organ donation. ETCO Newsletter 1991; 9(3): 16–7.

Drouet et al. France Transplant Annual Report. Paris: Hôpital St Louis, 1993.

ETCO Newsletter. A Belgian survey on attitude about organ donation. 1993; 11(1).

ETCO Newsletter. The American public's attitude toward organ donation and transplantation. 1993; 11(1): 17.

France-Transplant Annual Report. Paris: Hôpital St Louis, 1993.

Grundel J. Theological aspects of brain death with regard to the death of a person in organ replacement therapy – ethics, justic and commerce. W. Land-J.B. Dossetor Springer Verlag, Heidelberg, 1991: 244–8.

Atsumi K. Japanese view of life and organ transplantation in ethical problems in dialysis and transplantation. Dordrecht, The Netherlands: Kluwer Academic Pub., 1992: 183–8.

Lery N. L'heure de la mort in "La mort a vivre" Revue Autrement 1987; 171–8.

Pottecher T, et al. Information des familles de donneurs d'organes. Facteurs d'acceptation ou de refus. Enquête multicentrique. Ann. Fr Anesth Reanim 1993; 12: 71.

Sass HM. Philosophical arguments in accepting brain death in organ replacement therapy – Ethics, justice and commerce. W. Land-J.B. Dossetor Springer-Verlag, Heidelberg, 1991: 244–8.

7. Disappointing rate of altruism in the population

G. SCHÜTT & G. DUNCKER

In the Eurotransplant region – as well as in most European transplant organisations – the number of donated organs decreased in the last two years.

The negative trend in organ donation even increased in the first period of 1994. The decrease rate has now reached 14% compared to the same period in 1993 (January–February) [1]. Various factors were discussed that might contribute to this:

- lack of cooperation among medical professionals,
- reduced death rates in traffic accidents,
- negative media reports concerning organ donation, and
- relatives objecting to donation.

The cooperation of the medical professionals might be influenced by:
- better information about organ donation and standardized educational material;
- regulated cooperation with just one transplant center and avoidance of multiple transplant center activities in the donor hospital;
- educating medical professionals in the field of approaching the relatives regarding organ donation in a professional way – a task of the EDHEP (European Donor Hospital Education Program) program that was introduced by Eurotransplant; and
- providing a transplant law that regulates organ donation.

These facts were recognized and approached in Germany in recent years and a transplant law is currently in preparation.

The reduced death rates in traffic accidents – in Germany mainly due to laws that enforce wearing safty belts in cars and helmets when riding a motorcycle – are desirable and benefit all of us. However, in the regard of organ donation, this trend might be overcome by using more donors that die from natural death causes. This might involve the usage of older donors;

J.L. Touraine et al. (eds.), *Organ Shortage: The Solutions*, 49–52.
© 1995 *Kluwer Academic Publishers.*

Table 1. Eurotransplant donation activities

1990	2466 donors (MOD)
1991	2456 donors (MOD) steady state
1992	2223 donors (MOD) − 9.7%
1993	January–February kidney donors 483
1994	January–February kidney donors 419 − 14%

Table 2. Public attitudes toward organ donation

Polls	Consent to donate own organs	Consent to donate relatives' organs
1992 South Africa [2]	89%	76%
1991 US (Gallup) [3]	75%	60%
1993 Germany [4]	90%	80%
1991 Chile [5]	33%	–

reports in the literature about extending donor pools by the usage of older organ donors are encouraging.

Negative media reports are mainly concerned about organ trade. The selling of organs from living donors, or the trading of body parts after one's death for usage in pharmaceutical products, have been themes in the German media for the past 6 months. Sales of organs are reported from Third World countries and former East European countries. Extirpation and sales of body parts (dura mater, hypophyseal glands, corneae, etc.) without consent of the deceased or the relatives are reported from German hospitals. Due to these practices, trust for medical professionals seems to have lowered in the general population.

This lack of trust in the medical profession seems to result in less consent towards organ donation. This trend worries all who are involved with organ transplantation, but actual data regarding consent toward organ donation in families are scarce.

Publications about organ donation are mainly based on two facts: public polls and the refusal rate toward solid organ donation. Consent among the public varies from figures as high as 90% in favor of organ donation of own organs in Germany (n = 440), and to those as low as 33% among black Americans (n = 232). Large polls such as the Gallup, where a few thousand Americans were questioned, showed a 75% consent rate. The figures were lower when subjects were asked for consent in case of a relative's death, but still considerably high.

Actual consent rates from families in the case of death of a close relative are hard to obtain. According to German transplant centers, from all donors that were reported to them, consent toward organ donation was 81% in 1991 and had dropped to 75% in 1993. However, these data are questionable, because they presume the reporting of every brain dead deceased, even when a doctor at a donor hospital has already obtained family refusal before contacting a transplant center and, therefore, transplantation will most likely not be done.

Our transplant center performs transplants of all solid organs and, in addition, maintains cornea and heart-valve banks. The guidelines for cornea donation differ from those for solid organs:

- there is literally no age limit (our oldest donor was 100 years old),
- nearly all deceased are acceptable donors regardless of the cause of death (with the exception of septic patients, HIV and hepatitis infections, slow virus infections and spread malignoma), and
- enucleation can be done up to 72 hours after death.

We expected the demand for cornea donation to be met, however, even after extensive campaigns among the medical profession and general public, the rate of organ donation remained much too low. To evaluate the reasons, a prospective study was carried out in two large hospitals in Kiel: during a three-month period we followed-up on all 150 deaths that occurred in the two hospitals.

The doctors in charge of the patients before death were contacted and were asked to obtain consent for corneal donation from the families. From the 150 potential donors, 12 were judged medically unsuitable and we did not try to obtain consent (8%). In 2 cases, no relative could be identified and, in 7 cases, the relatives could not be reached in time for corneal removal, even after several tries (6%). In 10 cases, the doctor in charge refused to ask the relatives for corneal donation. The reasons were connected to the circumstances of the deaths, without closer description (6.7%).

The final result was 119 potential donors. All families were approached for consent. Corneas were obtained in 40 cases – 33%. Therefore, the refusal rate of the families was 66%. This high refusal rate – contesting a declared 90% positive attitude toward organ donation in Germany – was very surprising. The deceased were mostly elderly people (60% > 70 years old, only 1.5% under the age of 30 years), the deaths occurred after prolonged hospital stays and were not unexpected. The families were not approached immediately after death and were allowed ample time to reach a decision.

We discussed the impact of these findings on our educational program and changed the following:

- public campaigns were started, where a personal situation was emphasized, rather than the general aspects of corneal transplantation;
- radio interviews were given with the opportunity for patients to call in and discuss their own personal findings as well as objections toward organ donation with medical professionals;

– doctors were encouraged to ask their patients about their own opinion toward organ donation when admitted to the hospital – rather than approaching the families after a patient's death.

We continued the prospective study parallel to the extensive campaign. Yet, the next three-month period (207 deaths occurring in the two hospitals) still had a 70% refusal rate of the families of possible donors.

These findings indicate that the actual will to donate organs in the case of death of a close relative and the attitudes expressed in polls still differ immensely – even after transplantation af all organs now has become routine medical treatment. Germany has to continue its public campaign, the need for a transplant law is definite, and one suggestion now discussed is to routinely talk about the theme of organ donation in all schools.

References

1. Eurotransplant Newsletter 1994; 114(March).
2. Annual Report. Leiden, The Netherlands: Eurotransplant, 1992.
3. Pike R, Odell J, Kajn D. Public attitudes to organ donation in South Africa. Transplant Proc 1992; 24: 2102.
4. Sheehy E, Beasly C, Drachman J, Gortmaker S. What 6,000 Americans think about organ donation: results of a nationwide Gallup survey. Soc of Organ Sharing Vancouver 1993; Abstract.
5. Schütt G, Schroeder P. Public attitudes toward organ donation in Germany. Transplant Proc 1993; 25: 3127–28.
6. Martinez L, Vaccarezza A, Rodriguez L. Public opinion regarding organ donation in Chile. Transplant Proc 1991; 23: 2528.
7. Davidson M, Devney P. Attitudinal barriers to organ donation among black Americans. Transplant Proc 1991; 23: 2531–32.

PART TWO

Expanding the donor pool

8. Organ procurement from non-heart-beating donors

JAN-WILLEM DAEMEN, YIN MING & GAUKE KOOTSTRA

Introduction

As a reaction to the increasing discrepancy between the availability of kidneys for transplantation and the length of the waiting list, there is a renewed interest in retrieving kidneys for transplantation from the so-called Non-Heart-Beating (NHB) donor. At the University Hospital Maastricht, over a period of 10 years, 20 percent more kidneys have become available through an NHB donor program [1]. Programs have also been started in other locations, but a systemic involvement of all transplant centers has not yet been achieved. The NHB donor concept, however, is not new in Europe.

History

Before the notion of death based on neurological or brain criteria, often called "brain death", was introduced in medicine, organ retrieval was performed after cardiac arrest of the donor. All these patients suffered severe brain damage. However, through a general acceptance of the criteria of brain-death, multi-organ donation became routinely acceptable and interest in NHB donors waned. In addition, it is important to notice that the results of cadaveric kidney transplantation were improving considerably at the same time, through HLA-DR matching and the introduction of ciclosporine [2].

Several factors probably contributed to the nearly exclusive use of donors declared dead based on neurologic or brain criteria. In these cases, organs are procured while the heart is still beating – the so-called Heart-Beating (HB) donors. It is likely that the fear of transplanting an unviable organ, as might be the case from a NHB donor, made NHB donors unpopular.

Nevertheless, in Maastricht we have continued to use the NHB donor in the years 1980 to 1993, albeit for kidneys only. We continued to publish the results [3, 4] and to advocate its use. Interest is gradually increasing in Europe and the results of what is still a rather small degree of activity are being published [5, 6]. There is a range of different protocols and procedures

J.L. Touraine et al. (eds.), *Organ Shortage: The Solutions*, 55–60.
© 1995 *Kluwer Academic Publishers.*

necessitating a proper and clear definition and description of the different NHB donor categories.

Non-heart-beating donor categories

We propose the following four categories of NHB donors.

Category 1 – dead on arrival

A person is brought into the Accident and Emergency (A & E) department already declared dead outside the hospital. Neither outside nor inside the hospital will an attempt have been made to resuscitate because of the obvious senselessness of it. Examples are patients who died of trauma (a broken neck, open head injury, dead on the scene of an accident) or cardiac arrest for at least 15 minutes for whatever reason. This category – dead on arrival – is by far the largest pool of potential donors. However, it is the most difficult category as well, due to several factors.

For the transplant team the viability of the organs (only kidneys are likely to be recovered) is a major point of concern.

Access to this category of NHB donors is another factor and has several obstacles. First, the body has to be brought into the A & E department, for an in-situ-preservation procedure. This can only be done in a country with legislation based on presumed consent, or with a donor card on the dead body. When consent of the relatives is needed, the time span until this is obtained might be unbridgeable. When death is due to an unnatural cause, consent of the district attorney is also needed.

Second, information on the period of cardiac arrest has to be precise and reliable. We consider a period of 30 minutes without circulation the limit of acceptance.

Category 2 – unsuccessful resuscitation

This category considers patients who are resuscitated by an ambulance crew and brought into the A & E department where resuscitation is taken over by the hospital team. Because of the absence of success it is decided by the resuscitation team to discontinue treatment. Examples are patients with cardiac arrest after myocardial infarction at home or in the street, or a victim of a gunshot to the head, resuscitated for a time by volunteers, ambulance crew and hospital team, but ultimately, unsuccessfully.

Donors from category 2 – unsuccessful resuscitation – are currently the major source of NHB donors in our program, although the absolute numbers are still small. The difficulty in this category is determining when to discontinue resuscitation and establish death on cardiac criteria. We prefer a strict separation of the resuscitation team and procurement team. When the resuscitation team decides to stop, we prefer to abstain from any supportive handling (artificial ventilation, external cardiac massage) for five minutes before the transplant team takes over. These five minutes are intended to demonstrate to all those present in the room that there is a change from trying to save someone's life to the preservation of the kidneys for the benefit of the potential recipients. The transplant team restarts artificial ventilation and external cardiac massage. Drugs supposed to be of beneficial effect for the condition of the organs are given (for instance, heparin, regitine). This action is continued until permission for organ donation from the relatives has been granted or refused. In the last case, all action is discontinued. In case of permission for organ donation, a cooling catheter is introduced [7].

We accept donors sustaining a maximum of 30 minutes of cardiac arrest plus 2 hours of efficient resuscitation for our donor program.

Category 3 – awaiting cardiac arrest

These are hospital patients whose prognosis is certain death but for whom the diagnosis of brain death cannot be established because the criteria are not met. These patients can be ventilator-dependent or spontaneously breathing. In all cases cardio-pulmonary arrest is awaited and thereafter organs are procured.

This diverse category contains patients with severe neuro-trauma (who will not be resuscitated and do not fulfil brain death criteria) and patients with a primary brain tumour in the terminal phase of their illness. What all donors in this category have in common is that they do not fulfil the criteria of death based on *brain criteria* and the only way to procure these organs, is by changing to death based on *cardiac criteria*.

The main ethical point that arises is that the treating physician, although death of the patient is imminent, proceeds to organ donation prior to either death on brain criteria or death on cardiac criteria.

An important subgroup in this category are the patients who serve as an organ donor through the "ventilator-switch-off procedure". When this procedure is performed in the operating room (OR) and all provisions are made for a fast organ retrieval, not only kidneys but pancreas, liver and lung can be procured and successfully transplanted as well [8].

Category 4 – cardiac arrest while brain dead

All donors in this category are patients who are in the process of being diagnosed brain dead or who have already been declared brain dead and have an irreversible cardiac arrest. Organ procurement in NHB donors in category 4 – cardiac arrest while brain dead – is not always realized. This might be due to an unjustified uneasiness to warm ischemia. We would like to stress that in every potential or declared (Heart-Beating) donor, a set for introduction of the femoral cooling device should be available and ready for

58 *Jan-Willem Daemen, Yin Ming & Gauke Kootstra*

use at the bedside. Several donor procedures have been successful in spite of unexpected cardiac arrest in brain dead donors or during the process of diagnosing brain death, because of immediate performance of the in-situ-preservation procedure.

We have also noticed a special group within this category. These are patients for whom brain death has been diagnosed, but whose family cannot accept organ removal while the heart is still beating. They will only accept organ procurement after cardiac arrest. In a few cases, we have been successful through the ventilator-switch-off procedure to procure at least the kidneys in this situation.

An additional subdivision of NHB donors can be made: *controlled* versus *non-controlled*. The *controlled* subgroup contains those donors for whom cardiac arrest is awaited in the OR, after a ventilator-switch-off procedure. Conditions are so close to HB donors that in this subgroup, as mentioned before, besides kidneys other organs can be procured and successfully transplanted as well.

In-situ-preservation procedure

It is obvious that cooling of the kidneys as soon as possible after circulatory arrest is mandatory, in order to slow down metabolism and prevent the kidneys from further decay. Cooling devices, such as the Double Balloon Triple Lumen (DBTL) catheter have been developed [9]. In all categories, except cases with a ventilator-switch-off procedure in the OR, the in-situ-preservation procedure is performed using such a cooling device.

For donors in category 2 – unsuccessful resuscitation – the time after declaration of death on heart criteria until the consent for introduction of the cooling catheter is bridged through external cardiac massage and artificial ventilation. Also, heparin and phentolamine are administered intravenously. When the family arrives at the A & E department, they are approached for organ donation. In case of refusal, the above-mentioned handling is discontinued; in case of consent, the in-situ-preservation procedure is started.

Through an incision in the groin the DBTL-catheter is introduced in the femoral artery and the aorta, and external cardiac massage and artificial ventilation is discontinued. After partially inflating the abdominal balloon, the catheter is retracted until it occludes the aortal bifurcation; both balloons are then inflated fully. The position of the catheter is checked on a plain abdominal X-ray (we use radio-opaque dye for inflating the balloons). Perfusion is then started with cold histidine-tryptophan-ketoglutarate (HTK) solution at a pressure of 100 cm water; the venous out-flow is secured by inserting a urine catheter in the caval vein through a femoral phlebotomy. The perfusion continues until nephrectomy, preferably performed within 1 1/2 hours after cooling begins.

The family is given the opportunity to visit their deceased relative. This is done in the A & E department while the cooling continues. Thereafter the body is transferred to the OR.

Whenever there is consent for donation before the final cardiac arrest (category 3 – awaiting cardiac arrest – and category 4 – cardiac arrest while brain dead) or in countries with an opting-out principle for organ donation, the catheter can be introduced immediately after the patient is declared dead.

Transplantation results

We have published several analyses of the results of our NHB donor kidneys [3]. Compared with a matched HB donor group, no difference in long-term results for graft and patient survival was observed [4]. In the short-term, delayed function occurred significantly more often in the NHB donor group.

A recent analysis of all but three of our NHB donor kidneys transplanted in the Eurotransplant area included 57 NHB donor kidneys. They were compared to a group of 114 HB matched controls, collected in collaboration with the Eurotransplant data base. The groups are comparable, the main difference being the first warm ischemia time. The outcome was more delayed function in the NHB donor kidneys, but there was no difference in long-term results – up to 5 years – either in graft or patient survival. The percentage of never-functioning kidneys was 14 in the study group and 8 percent in the control group. This difference did not meet statistical significance.

Other groups in Europe using NHB donors report similar results [5, 6, 10]; short- and long-term results are as good as in HB donor kidneys, albeit a significantly higher incidence of delayed function in all programs.

Preservation

Recent experimental work revealed that preservation of ischemically damaged kidneys by continuous hypothermic perfusion is superior to preservation by simple cold storage [11]. Also, in human kidney transplants, delayed graft function was significantly lower in NHB donor kidneys preserved by machine perfusion as compared to simple cold storage [12, 13]. Therefore, today we preserve the NHB donor kidneys on a perfusion machine using UW-gluconate as the perfusion fluid. During the perfusion, a testing program is performed based on histological [14], functional [15] and biochemical parameters to try and judge the viability of these ischemically damaged kidneys.

References

1. Kootstra G, Wijnen RMH, van Hooff JP, van der Linden CJ. Twenty percent more kidneys through a non-heart-beating program. Transpl Proc 1991; 23: 910–1.
2. Thorogood J, van Houwelingen JC, van Rood JJ, Persijn GG. Time trend in annual kidney graft survival. Transplantation 1988; 46: 686–690.
3. Vromen MAM, Leunissen KML, Persijn GG, Kootstra G. Short- and long-term results with adult non-heart-beating donor kidneys. Transpl Proc 1988; 20: 743–5.
4. Wijnen RMH, Booster MH, Speatgens C, Yin M, van Hooff JP, de Boer J, Kootstra G. Long-term follow-up of transplanted non-heart-beating donor kidneys: preliminary results of a retrospective study. Transpl Proc 1993; 25: 1522–3.
5. Varty K, Veitch PS, Morgan JDT, Kehinde EO, Donnelly PK, Bell PRF. Response to organ shortage: kidney retrieval programme using non-heart beating donors. Br Med J 1994; 308: 575.
6. Schlumpf R, Candinas D, Zollinger A, Keusch G, Retsch M, Decurtins M, Largiadèr F. Kidney procurement from non-heartbeating donors: transplantation results. Transpl Int 1992; 5: S424–8.
7. Booster MH, Wijnen RMH, Vroemen JPAM, van Hooff JP, Kootstra G. In situ preservation of kidneys from non-heart-beating donors – a proposal for a standardized protocol. Transplantation 1993; 56: 613–7.
8. D'Alessandro AM, Hoffman RM, Knechtle SJ, Eckhoff D, Love R, Kalayoglu M, Sollinger HW, Belzer FO. Successful extrarenal transplantations from non-heart-beating donors. Proceedings of the 20th annual Scientific Meeting of the American Society of Transplant Surgeons; Chicago, 1994 May 18–20.
9. Garcia-Rinaldi R, Lefrak EA, Defore WW, Feldman L, Noon GP, Jachimczyk JA, De-Bakey ME. In situ preservation of cadaver kidneys for transplantation. Ann Surg 1975; 182: 576–84.
10. Castalao AM, Griñó JM, González C, Franco E, GilVernet S, Andrés E, Serón D, Torras J, Moreso F, Alsina J. Update of our experience in long-term renal function of kidneys transplanted from non-heart-beating cadaver donors. Transpl Proc 1993; 25: 1513–5.
11. Booster MH, Wijnen RMH, Yin M, Tiebosch ATM, Heineman E, Maessen JG, Buurman WA, Kurvers HAJM, Stubenitsky BM, Bonke H, Kootstra G. Enhanced resistance to the effects of normothermic ischemia in kidneys using pulsatile machine perfusion. Transplant Proc 1993; 25: 3006–11.
12. Kozaki M, Matsuno N, Tamaki T, Tamaki M, Kono K, Iti H, Uchiyama M, Tamaki I, Sakurai E. Procurement of kidney grafts from non-heart-beating donors. Transpl Proc 1991; 23: 2575–8.
13. Matsuno M, Sakurai E, Tamaki I, Uchiyama M, Kozaki K, Kozaki M. The effect of machine perfusion preservation versus cold storage on the function of kidneys from non-heart-beating donors. Transplantation 1994; 57: 293–4.
14. Yin L, Terasaki PI. A rapid quantitated viability test for transplant kidneys – ready for human trial. Clin Transplantation 1988; 2: 295–8.
15. Tesi JT, Elkhammas EA, Davies EA, Henry ML, Ferguson RM. Pulsatile kidney perfusion for evaluation of high-risk donors safely expands the donor pool. Clin Transplantation 1994; 8: 134–8.

9. Heart transplant from non-beating heart donor Past experience and report of one clinical case

G. DUREAU

History

In the past, "Cadaver Heart Transplantation" was the term applied to procedures using non-beating-heart donors.

Actually, this was the only condition considered ethically possible by some authors [1–3]. Yet, on 3 December 1987, C. Barnard performed the first human cardiac allotransplantation from a beating heart donor, thereby frustrating N.E. Shumway and R. Lower from their own "premiere", despite the fact that they had themselves invented the technique and developed the first animal models [8].

The success of Barnard's procedure was such that as many as 100 heart transplantations were done the following year throughout the world, at a time when only two teams were ready to perform cadaveric heart transplantation. However, from the very beginning, the beating heart donor procedure bore two major criticisms, which remain significant as the heart transplant program develops:

1. A brain-death definition of death still represents an obstacle in some cultures (Japan) and may be the cause of refusal in other countries. This explains why Japan is the only country to continue research in this field [6,10].
2. Limiting the pool of potential donors to brain dead subjects results in organ shortage. If research and development had been based on non-beating-heart procedures, more donors could have been expected.

Due to the fact that today 25% of patients die while on waiting lists [9], cadaveric heart transplantation is being reconsidered, accepting the increased risk for the sake of therapeutic efficacy.

J.L. Touraine et al. (eds.), Organ Shortage: The Solutions, 61–66.
© 1995 *Kluwer Academic Publishers.*

Experimental models

Several points were discovered in the sixties:

1. Successful orthotopic heart transplantation could be achieved in dogs using arrested hearts 30 minutes after the last beat when it was asphixiated (Dureau *et al.*, 1966b) and 45 minutes when it was exanguinated (Angell & Shumway, 1966).
2. Resuscitative perfusion was necessary prior to transplantation either *ex vivo* (Angell & Shumway, 1966) or *in vitro* (Dureau *et al.*, 1966a).
3. Evaluation of the resuscitated organ, carried out during isolated perfusion after recovery, was mandatory to obtain good results (Dureau *et al.*, 1966b).
4. Hypothermic storage could be combined with the resuscitative procedure for up to 24 hours (Dureau, 1970).

Clinical prospective

Isolated blood perfusion of the heart (*in vitro* or *ex vivo*) represents the major obstacle toward a clinical application of the experimental model, due to risk of infection and other complications as compared to the current procedure which condemns this or such technique to experimental and marginal attempts. On the other hand, the recipient's blood perfusion represents the best biological perfusate to resuscitate the heart, provided that the circulatory burden is released from the graft. This is the condition of the transplanted heart still under extracorporeal circulation. These considerations lead to shifting the evaluation of the graft prior to the resuscitative perfusion, representing a new proposal compared to the experimental results (Fig. 1).

Clinical case

October 1 1985, a 20 year old male, suffering from dilatative cardiomyopathy was admitted to the intensive care unit of our hospital in critical hemodynamical condition. He was immediately intubated for respiratory assistence while adrenergic support was initiated with Adrenalin ($16 \gamma/kg/mn^{-1}$), Dopamin ($3.8\gamma/kg/mn^{-1}$) and Dobutrex ($24 \gamma/kg/mn^{-1}$). The case was complicated by a staphylococcus aureus infection. A call for emergency transplantation was initiated and on the sixth day a heart from an adult male gunshot victim was proposed. By this time, the hemodynamic condition of the recipient had further deteriorated and diuresis fell under $0.5 L/day^{-1}$.

The donor was also questionable since brain death resulted from a cardiac arrest consecutive with a hemorragic shock. Resuscitated with a cardiac massage, normal pressure required $30 \gamma/kg/mn^{-1}$ of Dopamin at the time of proposal.

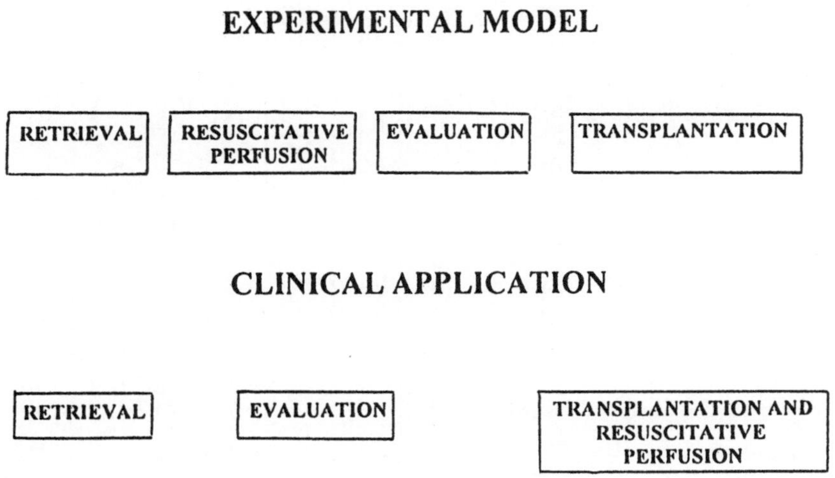

EXPERIMENTAL MODEL

RETRIEVAL	RESUSCITATIVE PERFUSION	EVALUATION	TRANSPLANTATION

CLINICAL APPLICATION

RETRIEVAL	EVALUATION	TRANSPLANTATION AND RESUSCITATIVE PERFUSION

Fig. 1. Cadaveric heart transplantation

Despite this, the heart was accepted, considering the condition of the recipient, for whom we did not dispose of mechanical circulatory assistance.

During the hasty kidney retrieval, Collins' solution was accidently infused in the donor resulting in cardiac arrest. After discussion, we decided to continue the procedure: the chest was opened and the heart was removed after 15 minutes of warm ischemia. The heart was cold cardioplegied and orthotopic heart transplantation was carried out as usual, according to Shumway's technique, except that the left ventricle was vented. Cold ischemia time was 2 hours and warm ischemia time was 45 minutes.

Reperfusion was carefully initiated by releasing the aortic clamp at very low (30 mm Hg) pressure, as experimental data has shown us the importance of this. This perfusion pressure was increased to 45 mm Hg after electrical defibrillation, which was obstained with one shock, 5 minutes after reperfusion.

Very abnormal, enlarged QRS complexes followed cardioversion. As for the experimental models, they remained abnormal up to the thirtieth minute of reperfusion, when they changed abruptly to more normal complexes. By the 45th minute, complexes had improved further, allowing normal weaning of the extra-corporeal circulation after 55 minutes of resuscitative persusion and assistance (Fig. 2).

Immediate follow-up, respiratory assistance and adrenergic post-operative support was not different from normal transplantations. Post-operative cardiac enzymes were normal and the first endomyocardial biopsy did not show evidence of necrosis or fibrosis.

At one year, isotopic ejection fraction was normal. Recently, after 9 years, it has been reevaluated (Table 1).

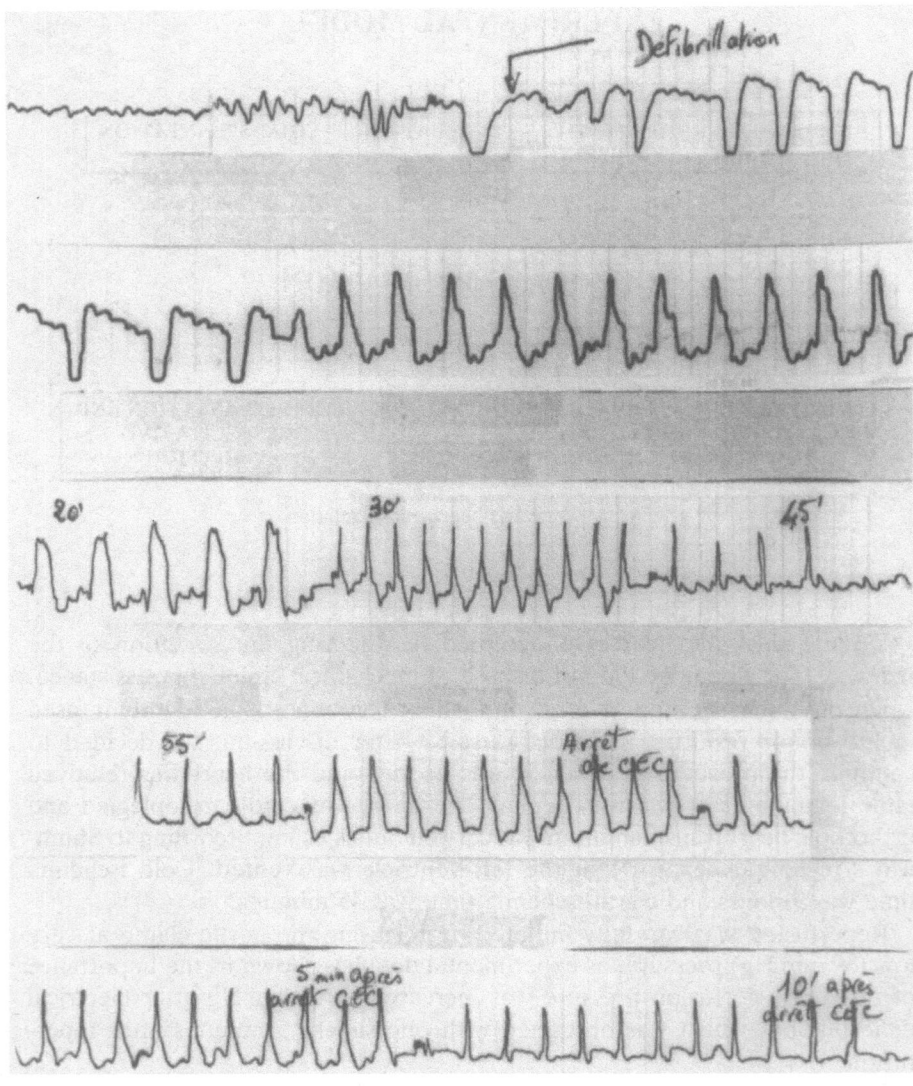

Fig. 2. E.C.G. Evolution of the resuscitative perfusion.

Discussion

The most surprising feature of this clinical case was the close reproduction of the experimental data found in the sixties regarding cadaveric resuscitation of dog and human hearts. Namely, the same drastic improvement of ECG and QRS complexes after 30–45 minutes of reperfusion.

In experimental studies we paralleled this situation with changes in the

Table 1

1987				1994			
Work load	Heart rate b min	Arterial pressure mm Hg	Left ventrical ejection fraction %	Work load	Heart rate b min	Arterial pressure mm Hg	Left ventricle ejection fraction %
0 w	77	110	54	0 w	95	109	68
30 w	90	120	65	50 w	100	135	Missing
90 w	105	160	74	80 w	118	147	70
120 w	120	170	80	110 w	136	152	76

mitochondrial aspects [4]. We could not propose an explanation for such rapid changes in the mitochondria but they were consistently found throughout the studies.

The immediate and long-term evolution clearly showed that the arrest of a heart does not prohibit its use for transplantation under favorable conditions, that is, a patient already on the operating table with a surgical team ready for intervention. It should be noted that 10–15% of donors' hearts stop during retrieval organization by the coordinator team, and this consideration could lead to a different attitude for heart retrieval, where previously only the kidneys were retrieved [7].

This case also showed the sound approach of cardiac resuscitation on the recipient, which is a better solution than isolated perfusion. Also, we require some kind of evaluation of the organ's potential viability since the cadaveric heart is grafted directly to the recipient: RMN spectrometry and vascular resistance could be helpful in assessing organ status, keeping in mind that mechanical circulatory support may be used for difficult situations.

References

1. Angell WN, Shumway NE. Resuscitative storage of the cadaver heart transplant. Surgical Forum 1966; 17: 224.
2. Dureau G. Demonstration at the 2nd CITIC, 1970. "Workshop on Conservation" Lyon CITIC 1970.
3. Dureau G, Okura T, Schilt W, Kantrowitz A. Transplantation orthotopique de coeur de cadavre chez le chien. Ann Chir Thorac et Cardiovasc 1966a; 13–14: 700–706.
4. Dureau G, Okura T, Schilt W, Kantrowitz A. Cadaver heart: evaluation of potential viability. Circulation, suppl. III, XXXIV no 4, 1966b, 91.
5. Dureau G, Schilt W, Loire R. Tolérance and resistance of myocardium to anoxia. Experimental studies. J Cardiovasc Surg 1975; 16: 261–264.
6. Hisamochi K, Morimoto T, Bando K et coll. Impact of hydroxyl radical scavenger "EPC" on cadaver heart transplantation (HT) in canine model. J Heart and Lung Transpl 1993; 12(1), part 2: S39–S110 abst.
7. Kosaki M, Matsuno N, Tanaka M et al. Procurement of kidney grafts from non-heat-beating donors. Transplantation Proceedings 1991; 23(5): 2575–2578.

8. Lower RR, Dong E, Shumway NE. Long term survival of cardiac homografts. Surgery 1965; 58: 110–119.
9. McManus RP, O'Hair DP, Beitzinger JM *et al.* Patients who die awaiting heart transplantation. J Heart Lung Transpl 1993; 12: 159–172.
10. Shirakura R, Hirose H, Nakata S *et coll.* Experimental study of 24-hour storage of arrested cadaver hearts: orthotopic canine heart transplantation. J Heart Transpl 1986; 5(5): 375.

10. Total body cooling for organ procurement

R. VALERO, M. MANYALICH, C. CABRER, L. SALVADOR &
L.C. GARCIA-FAGES

Introduction

Since the experimental and clinical studies performed by Garcia-Rinaldi et
al. [1], who successfully initiated the "in situ" preservation of kidneys by
means of cold perfusion of organs within the cadaver, the possibility of
obtaining organs from non-heart-beating donors (NHBD) has been reconsidered for transplantation purposes.

During the last few years new techniques have been developed to improve
the perfusion and posterior viability of the organs obtained from NHBD,
one of which is "total body cooling".

We present here the results of our work in this field.

Potential NHBD admitted to hospital were included in this study. NHBD
were considered those patients who suffered a cardiocirculatory arrest just
before or in the initial hours of admission to hospital. These donors have
been called "the uncontrolled NHBD" [2]. We consider "controlled NHBD"
to be those heart beating donors who suffered cardiac arrest before scheduled
organ harvesting could be performed. In our series we did not consider
patients for whom brain death had been diagnosed but for whom cardiac
arrest had to be awaited before organ harvesting commenced, due to a lack
of brain death legislation, as happens in some countries regarding NHBD.

The procedure for non-heart-beating organ extraction begins after death
is diagnosed. At this point, it is necessary to calculate accurately warm
ischemia time (WIT) from the moment of death until effective cardiopulmonary resuscitation techniques are initiated. Criteria to consider a dead patient
as a potential NHBD include – in addition to the general criteria of donor
selection – age younger than 60 years and a WIT of less than 30 minutes.
Time elapsed until the commencement of cold perfusion must be less than
120 minutes.

Initially, basic cardiopulmonary maneuvers are set in motion and the donor
is heparinized. Subsequently, vascular access is attained by surgical dissection
and cannulation of the femoral vessels, and cold perfusion is begun through
the aorta.

J.L. Touraine et al. (eds.), *Organ Shortage: The Solutions*, 67–72.

In our early cases, "in situ" perfusion was achieved by means of cold perfusion of Collins' liquid by gravity. We used a multiperforated catheter placed into the aorta, by insertion through the femoral artery. Venous drainage was made possible by a catheter in the femoral vein. A double balloon catheter is preferable for this purpose, although different kinds of catheters have also been used with good results.

During the last few years, a new technique has been developed. "Total body cooling" uses blood to perfusate the whole body. Blood is oxygenated and cooled by means of extracorporeal circulation, and posteriorly reintroduced in the donor. Koyama [3] and Gómez [4] and their colleagues used the technique of corporal hypothermia by means of cardiopulmonary bypass in non-heart-beating human kidney donors with good results. Moreover, experimental studies by Hoshino and coworkers [5] have opened the way to the procurement of livers from this type of donor using total body cooling techniques.

In later cases, we have also used total body cooling through extracorporeal circulation. Cannulation was accomplished using a 18F cannula for the femoral artery and vein. Perfusion was achieved by means of a portable device which incorporated a roller pump, a temperature exchanger, and a bubble oxygenator/container, interposed in an extracorporeal circuit filled with Ringer's lactate serum, a colloidal solution, mannitol, and sodium bicarbonate. Bypass was begun with a progressively increasing flow ($1-2$ 1 min^{-1}) and decreasing temperature (to 15 to 20°C). This device allowed the procedure to take place in an intensive care unit or in the emergency unit to which patients with cardiac arrest had been admitted. With this device, the oxygenation and cooling of all the donor's organs was possible while permission was being requested.

There are a number of advantages to core-cooling. 1) Cooling is induced progressively and smoothly, providing for homogeneous cooling of kidneys and surrounding organs and tissues [3, 5]. The fact that sufficient perfusion pressure and high flow rate can be produced by the pump is also an advantage, since low perfusion pressure and low flow rate causes vasoconstriction which leads to ischemic damage [6]. 2) Using blood as the coolant in this system confers a number of advantages over crystalloid perfusates: it is a colloid, it is an effective buffer solution, it contains substrate for tissue metabolism, and it contains physiologic free radical scavengers. It seem likely that tissues damaged due to ischemia would recover more easily if they were perfused with cold hyperoxygenated blood [3, 5, 7]. 3) More time is allowed for precise dissection [5]. 4) Although procurement of livers using in situ perfusion with a very short warm ischemia time have been described [8], perfusion of all the organs through total body cooling will allow the extraction and transplantation of other organs in the near future [5, 9]. 5) Blood is maintained inside the vessels and, if consent is not obtained, a return to the original situation is easier with this technique. 6) Lastly, although skilled technical assistance is required, the technique is relatively simple and the perfusion apparatus is portable, so the procedure is not very complicated.

There is, however, one disadvantage to core-cooling: difficulties in obtaining good venous blood return have been described when the cause of death was a politraumatism, due to the loss of vascular tree (hemothorax, aortic rupture, hemoperitoneal bleeding, . . .). This may cause ineffective extracorporeal circulation and, consequently, insufficient organ perfusion. Guidelines for this situation include increasing the volume of fluid in the oxygenator/container while checking the position and permeability of the venous line [4]. If this is not sufficient, the technique must be reconsidered and in situ perfusion may be started [8].

In situ perfusion is perhaps the most widely practiced method of preservation. It has a number of advantages. The technique is simple and involves a minimum of specialist equipment. It is rapidly executed and provides fast and efficient cooling of the kidneys. Finally, harmful blood constituents are flushed out (fibrin, complement, platelets, leukocytes).

Although Hoshino has experimentally demostrated that livers obtained through total body cooling are more viable than those obtained by in situ perfusion [5], no other controlled studies have yet been performed comparing kidney viability using these two techniques.

In our series, organs obtained from NHBD were transplanted into recipients whose characteristics and history had previously been analysed. Kidneys were transplanted to blood type-compatible and negative cross-match recipients and, in this way, we were able to reduce cold ischemia time to 6 hours in the first transplanted kidney and 12 hours in the second one. Immunosuppression treatment was given in each case, according to the protocol in use at the time of transplantation. Graft and patient survival was analysed by means of the Kaplan-Meier method.

Results

Between October 1986 and May 1994, 21 potential NHBD were included in our study, with two family refusals. Etiology of death in our series was politraumatism (11 cases), heart disease (6 cases), isolated brain injuries (3 cases, including 2 "controlled" NHBD) and stroke (1 case).

In 13 cases we used in situ perfusion through a femoral catheter by gravity. Two of these cases were controlled NHBD; four kidneys and one liver were obtained from these patients. Transplantation of the liver was possible due to a short WIT. In another case, where the patient died after unsuccessful emergency cardiac surgery, the organs were rejected following a positive Human Inmunodeficiency virus antibodies test. Of the remaining 10 donors, 15 kidneys were transplanted (4 of them in another center), one donor was rejected following bad macroscopic perfusion and another was refused by

Table 1. Characteristics of non-heart-beating donors distributed in two groups according to the method of organ perfusion: in situ perfusion or total body cooling (TBC)

Method	Number	Age	Male	Female	Transplanted kidneys	Family refusal	Clinical con- traindication
In situ	13	34.9 (8–60)	8	5	19 + 1 liver	1	2
TBC							
PLT	5	30.8 (17–46)	4	1	2	0	4
NoPLT	3	37 (28–47)	2	1	4	1	0
Total	21	34.2 (8–60)	14	7	25 + 1 liver	2	6

PLT = politraumatism; NoPLT = No politraumatism; Age in years: mean (range)

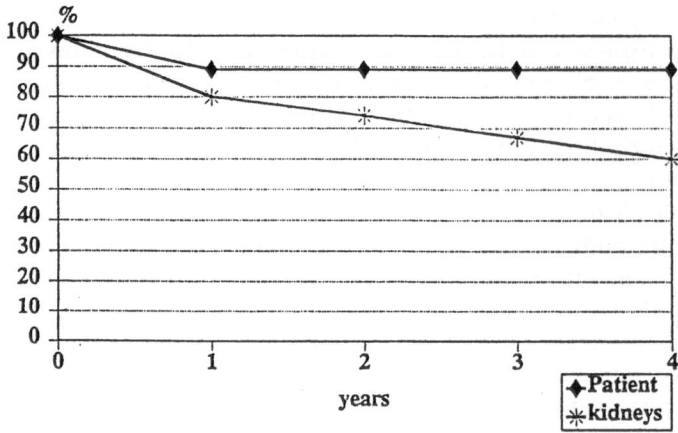

Fig. 1. Actuarial survival curve of grafts and recipients from non-heart-beating donors.

the family. One kidney was not transplanted due to recipient problems (Table 1).

The total body cooling technique was used in the remaining eight cases, which may be divided into two groups according to the etiology of death. In the first group, five donors died following politraumatism. In these cases, there were difficulties in obtaining good venous blood return to make extracorporeal circulation possible, and it was necessary to start the in situ perfusion technique. The difficulties were due to hemothorax in three cases, traumatic ventricular cardiac rupture in one case and hemoperitoneal bleeding in the remaining case. Only two kidneys from this group were suitable for transplantation. The other eight kidneys were rejected because of bad macroscopic perfusion. In the second group, we included three cases in which the cause of death was myocardial infarction (2 cases) or isolated brain injury (1 case). We had one family refusal. Extracorporeal circulation was accomplished in the two remaining donors without problems and four kidneys were obtained and later transplanted (Table 1).

In total, 25 kidneys and one liver obtained from NHBD were transplanted. The actuarial kidney survival curve shows survival rates of 80% and 60% in one- and four-year periods, respectively (Figure 1). The functioning kidneys show a plasmatic creatinine level of 1.38 ± 0.78 mg dl^{-1}. One year after transplantation, the liver is functioning correctly. The actuarial patient survival curve shows a survival rate of 89% at one year, which continues after four years.

Conclusion

Organs obtained from NHBD have shown adequate viability over long-term follow-up and must be considered a useful way of increasing the number of donors. Our results suggest that, except in those cases where a disruption of the vascular integrity is suspected (politraumatic), which could make extracorporeal circulation difficult or impossible, the technique of portable total body cooling allows the correct perfusion, oxygenation and cooling of the donor, and is likely to be the method of choice for the procurement of organs from this group of donors.

Acknowledgements

This study has been partially supported by FIS Grant no. 92/1125 and 94/1227.

References

1. Garcia-Rinaldi R, Lefrak EA, Defore WW, et al. In situ preservation of cadaver Kidneys for transplantation: laboratory observations and clinical application. Ann Surg 1975; 182(5): 576–84.
2. Kootstra G, Ruers TJM, Vroemen JPAM. The non-heart-beating donor: contribution to the organ shortage. Transplant Proc 1986; 18(5): 1410–2.
3. Koyama I, Hoshino T, Nagashima N, Adachi H, Ueda K, Omoto R. A new approach to kidney procurement from non-heart-beating donors: core cooling on cardiopulmonary bypass. Transplant Proc 1989; 21(1): 1203–5.
4. Gómez M, Alvarez J, Arias J, et al. Cardiopulmonary bypass and profound hypotermia as a means for obtaining kidney grafts from irreversible cardiac arrest donors: cooling technique. Transplant Proc 1993; 25(1): 1501–2.
5. Hoshino T, Koyama I, Nagashima N, Kadokura M, Adachi H, Ueda K, Omoto R. Liver transplantation from non-heart-beating donors by core cooling technique. Transplant Proc 1989; 21(1): 1206–8.
6. Anaise D, Yland MJ, Waltzer WC, et al. Flush Pressure requirements for optimal cadaveric donor Kidney preservation. Transplant Proc 1988; 20(5): 891–4.
7. Rijkmans BG, Buurman WA, Kootstra G. Six-day canine kidney preservation. Transplantation 1984; 37: 130–3.

8. Valero R, Manyalich M, Cabrer C, Salvador L, García-Fages LC. Organ Procurement from non-heart-beating donors by total body cooling. Transplant Proc 1993; 25(6): 3091–2.
9. Shirakura R, Kamiike W, Matsumura A, et al. Multi-organ procurement from non-heart-beating donors by use of Osaka University cocktail, Osaka Rinse Solution, and the portable cardiopulmonary bypass machine. Transplant Proc 1993; 25: 3093–4.

11. The living donor program in Scandinavia

U. BACKMAN, D. ALBRECHTSEN, H. LØKKEGAARD
& K. SAALMELA

One way of alleviating the shortage of grafts in renal transplantation is to use organs from living donors. In Scandinavia, the number of living donors greatly differs between our countries – from 3.4 per million inhabitants in Finland to 16.7 per million inhabitants in Norway. Yet, the number of cadaveric kidney transplantations does not differ much between the countries. The average in Scandinavia is 28.1 per million inhabitants, compared to Eurotransplant's 27.45 per million. Thus, the main difference in the total number of transplantations performed in Scandinavia is due to the number of transplantations from living donors. Also, the difference between the countries probably reflects the policy of each, regarding the treatment of end-stage renal failure, economical considerations and dialysis facilities. Table 1 shows the total number of transplantations performed in 1992 in Scandinavia compared with those by Eurotransplant.

With only one transplantation centre in Helsinki, Finland has the lowest number of transplantations with grafts from living donors. However, the number is still higher than in most other European countries. Only related donors are accepted in Finland [1].

Denmark and Sweden have about the same frequency of transplantations with grafts from living donors. The frequency of living related donors in the four different centers in Sweden varies between 10–25% of the total number of transplantations.

Norway also has only one transplantation centre, in Oslo. And, although the living donor transplantation policy has been rather active through the years, the national transplantation rate has been regarded as too low. To overcome this problem, Norway began transplanting kidneys from non-related living donors, usually spouses, beginning around 1985 [2].

A few non-related living donor transplantations have been performed in Denmark and Sweden, and the number is increasing (at least in Stockholm and Uppsala [3]). Until 1990, 44 patients were transplanted with non-related living donors in Norway and, in Sweden, 25 patients in Stockholm-Uppsala. The results regarding graft survival are excellent and comparable to that of

J.L. Touraine et al. (eds.), *Organ Shortage: The Solutions*, 73–76.

Table 1. Solid organ transplantation activities 1992

	Population (million)	Cadaveric kidney tx		Living donor kidney tx		Total kidney tx	
		Total	Per million people	Total	Per million people	Total	Per million people
Finland	5.0	142	28.4	17	3.4	159	31.8
Sweden	8.6	229	26.6	88	10.2	317	36.9
Norway	4.3	222	28.3	72	16.7	200	46.5
Denmark	5.2	155	29.8	44	8.5	199	38.3
Scandia Trans	23.1	648	28.1	221	9.6	875	37.9
Eurotrans	112.8	3101	27.5	140	1.2	3241	28.7

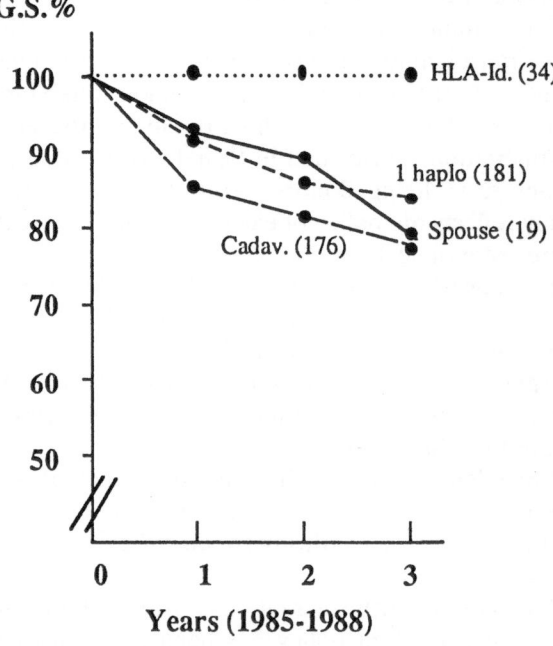

Fig. 1. Graft survival in Norway (patients < 55 years).

HLA-one haplotype-matched transplantations (Figures 1 and 2). No serious complications were seen in any of the donors.

Renal function of the grafts has been good. Results from Sweden show that 6 months after transplantation the serum creatinine was 136 μmol l^{-1} compared to 175 μmol l^{-1} for recipients of cadaveric grafts [4].

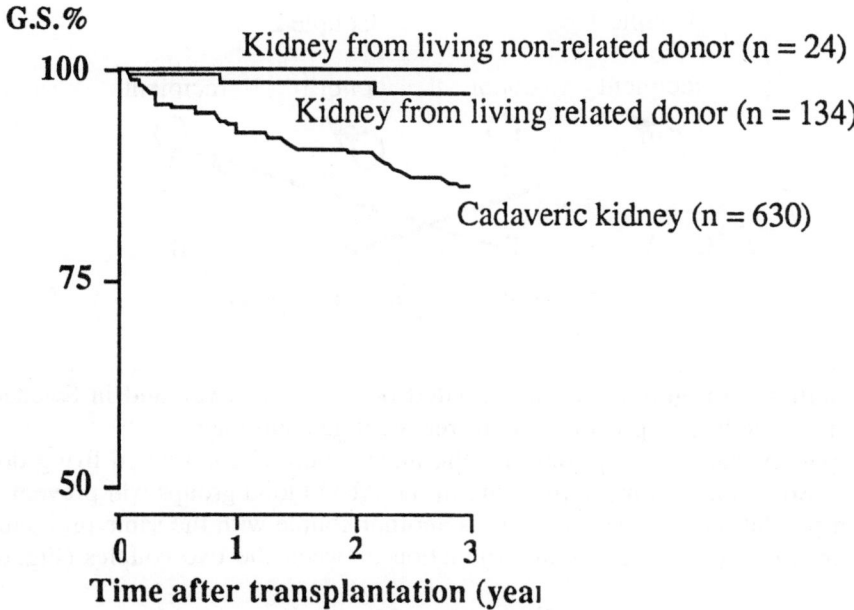

Fig. 2. Actuarial graft survival in Sweden.

Immunosuppressive treatment

Each country in Scandinavia has its own regimen for immunosuppressive treatment. Finland has the most specified program with different protocols depending on the HLA-matching grade. For HLA-identical siblings, the routine program consists of the conventional treatment, azathioprine and prednisolone. For related, haplo HLA-one-type matched transplants, the patients are given pretransplant treatment consisting of DST (donor-specific transfusion) of 200 ml of fresh whole blood on three separate occasions within a two-week interval. From the day of the first transfusion the patients are also given coverage with azathioprine. After transplantation, treatment is the same as for identical siblings [1].

In Norway and Sweden, the immunosuppressive regimen is the same, irrespective of the HLA-matching grade and, principally, also the same as for patients receiving cadaveric grafts. A short pretransplant treatment is given over two days with Cyclosporin A and prednisolone, which are the only drugs given after transplantation.

For the future, with a continued shortage of cadaveric grafts and an increasing need for kidney transplantations, there will be a greater demand for donation from living donors. Despite efforts to expand the supply of grafts from both cadaveric donors and living related donors, it has been impossible to avoid long waiting times in dialysis. The success of trans-

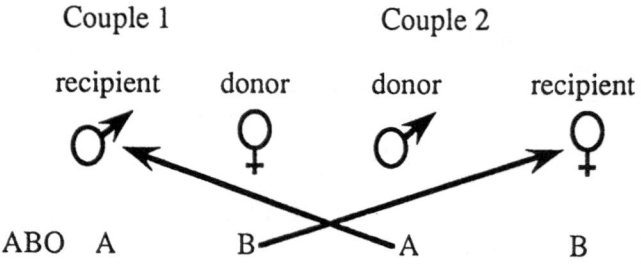

Fig. 3. Cross-donation between two couples.

plantation with grafts from non-related donors in Norway and in Sweden seems to indicate a possible way to reduce organ shortage.

Spouses will probably comprise the main group of non-related living donors. Sometimes an incompatibility in the ABO blood groups will prevent a transplantation; however, if there is another couple with the same problem, the possibility exists for a cross-donation between the two couples (Figure 3).

From an ethical point of view there should be no problems regarding transplantation from non-related living donors, as the decision is made completely voluntarily and, also, since a spouse might be more motivated to donate a kidney than, for example, a sibling. However, one should probably hesitate when there is a so-called friend willing to donate a kidney, as economical considerations might be involved in such a case.

References

1. Albrechtsen D, Sødal G, Jakobsen A, Brekke I, Bentdal Ø, Berg KJ, Fauchald P, Pfeffer P, Taiseth Leivestad T, Flatmark A. Kidney transplantation from a spouse: an alternative to years of dialysis waiting for a graft that may never turn up? Transpl Proc 1990; 22: 1435.
2. Eklund B, Ahonen J, Saalmela K, Höckerstedt K, Isoniemi H, Koskimies S. Donor-specific transfusions in HLA-one haplotype matched kidney transplantation. Transpl Proc 1990; 22: 151.
3. Dansk Nefrologisk Selskab: Landsregister for patienter i aktiv behandling for kronisk nyresvigt 1994.
4. Brattström C, Wilczek H, Pettersson E, Claesson K, Wadström J, Backman U, Groth C-G. Utmärkta resultat vid transplantation med njurar från maka/make. Läkartidningen 1994 (in press).

12. Pancreas transplants from living related donors

RAINER W.G. GRUESSNER, JOHN S. NAJARIAN,
ANGELIKA C. GRUESSNER & DAVID E.R. SUTHERLAND

Introduction

Living related donors (LRDs) were first used for kidney transplantation [1]. The consistently high patient and graft survival rates of LRD kidney transplants have led to their increasing popularity in the United States, accounting for up to 50% of all kidney transplants at some centers. The pancreas was the first extrarenal solid organ in which successful LRD transplants were done [2]. Over the last 5 years, the use of LRDs has received increasing attention for liver [3], lung [4], and intestinal [5] transplantation.

In general, the rationale to perform transplants from LRDs rather than cadaver donors (CADs) is two-fold. First, for kidney and liver transplants, there is a shortage of CADs. However, the number of pancreas transplants now being done is less than the number of CADs available; if matching is ignored, there is currently no shortage of pancreases. Second, technically successful LRD transplants are consistently associated with higher graft survival rates due to a lower incidence of rejection, compared with CAD transplants; this is true of pancreas as well as kidney transplants [6]. Rejection remains the Achilles' heel of pancreas transplantation, accounting for up to 30% of graft losses within the first year [7]. But, as we have previously reported, the incidence of graft loss from rejection is significantly lower with LRD than with CAD pancreas transplants [8].

According to the International Pancreas Transplant Registry (IPTR), the number of pancreas transplants worldwide has consistently increased over the last 20 years; patient and graft survival rates have significantly improved with both LRD and CAD transplants, due to better immunosuppression and organ preservation as well as refinement of surgical techniques [7]. An increasing willingness to biopsy the pancreas (either cystoscopically or percutaneously) [9, 10] has improved our ability to diagnose and treat rejection early, avoiding anti-rejection treatment when not indicated.

The main reason that LRD pancreas transplants have not become as popular as LRD kidney transplants is a higher technical failure rate. In contrast to kidney transplants, the technical failure rate has remained higher

J.L. Touraine et al. (eds.), *Organ Shortage: The Solutions*, 77–83.

for LRD than for CAD pancreas transplants: only a segment of the pancreas is transplanted, and the vessels used for engraftment (splenic artery and vein) are small in diameter and short. Thus, LRD pancreas transplants are more prone to arterial and venous thrombosis than LRD kidney transplants. At first glance, this high technical failure rate might seem to diminish our incentive to use LRDs. However, the technical failure rate is lower in LRD pancreas transplants than the immunologic failure rate (i.e. graft loss from rejection) in CAD transplants [11]. Therefore, for technically successful pancreas transplants, the probability of long-term success is significantly better with an LRD than a CAD allograft. Another reason in favor of LRD pancreas transplants is that they may be the only option for highly sensitized patients and for those requiring minimal immunosuppression.

Until February 1994, LRD pancreas transplants have been done either for nonuremic patients (PTA, pancreas transplant alone) or for patients who had received a previous kidney transplant (PAK, pancreas after kidney transplant). We have recently done 2 simultaneous LRD pancreas-kidney transplants, demonstrating that this is a safe, successful approach for uremic patients with insulin-dependent diabetes mellitus. Compared with sequential transplants (PAK), simultaneous pancreas-kidney transplants require only one procedure and the physical consequences are no different for the LRD.

The University of Minnesota began to use LRDs for pancreas transplants in the 1970s [2, 8]. We previously reported our experience with LRD pancreas transplants, including our observations in recipients of grafts from nondiabetic identical twin donors. We showed that diabetes recurred in the isografts of 3 twins transplanted without prophylactic immunosuppression [12, 13]. In subsequent twin transplants, we used low-dose immunosuppression and demonstrated that disease recurrence can be prevented [14]. This paper updates our experience with LRD pancreas transplants.

Materials and methods

Between June 1, 1978 and May 31, 1993, a total of 607 pancreas transplants were done at the University of Minnesota: 525 (82%) from CADs, 82 (14%) from LRDs (81 genetic relatives, 1 spouse). Of the 81 genetic relatives, 10 (12%) were identical twins (9 sisters, 1 brother), 32 (40%) were HLA-identical siblings (19 sisters, 13 brothers), and 39 (48%) were mismatched relatives (20 siblings – 13 sisters, 7 brothers; 18 parents – 13 mothers, 5 fathers; 1 male cousin). One patient received a living unrelated pancreas transplant from his spouse who had previously donated her kidney to him.

Of the 82 LRD pancreas transplant recipients, 49 (60%) had a PTA. Of these 49 PTA recipients, 9 (18%) later received a kidney: 3 from the same LRD as the previous pancreas, 6 from a different donor (3 from another LRD, 3 from a CAD). Of the 82 LRD recipients, 31 (38%) had a PAK transplant: 24 from the same donor (16 siblings, 8 parents), 7 from different

UNIVERSITY OF MINNESOTA 7/78-6/94

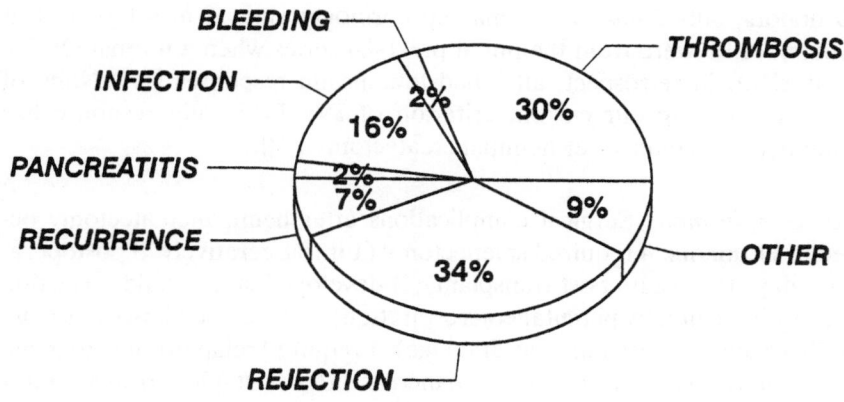

Fig. 1. Causes of LRD pancreas graft loss.

donors (2 siblings, 4 parents, 1 spouse). There were 2 (2%) SPK recipients: kidney and pancreas allografts were from the mother in one case, from the sister in the other.

Fourteen recipients of the primary LRD pancreas transplants underwent 22 retransplants (3 from another LRD and 19 from a CAD); 5 patients underwent one retransplant, 7 underwent two, and 1 underwent three.

Exocrine pancreas secretions were managed with enteric drainage in 55 (67%) transplants, bladder drainage in 14 (17%) (ductocystostomy in 10, ductoureterostomy in 4), duct injection in 8 (10%), and open duct drainage in 5 (6%). The surgical techniques have previously been described [15].

Of the 82 LRD pancreas transplants, 27 (33%) failed for technical reasons (16 of 49 PTA, 11 of 31 PAK): 16 from thrombosis, 9 from infection, 1 from pancreatitis, and 1 from bleeding. The rate of thrombosis has been higher, compared with our CAD pancreas transplants [15]. Causes of graft loss are shown in Figure 1.

Donor criteria All LRDs met the following criteria: at the time of donation they were at least 10 years older than the age of onset of diabetes in the recipient (and the onset of diabetes in the recipient must have been at least 10 years pretransplant); in addition, for sibling donors, no family members other than the recipient were diabetic. When these two criteria pertain, donors are at no greater risk to become diabetic than the general population, even if they are HLA identical with the recipient [16]. All potential LRDs undergo a thorough endocrine workup to determine their suitability. Metabolic criteria have changed over the years: initially (until 1984), only a normal oral glucose tolerance test (OGTT) was required preoperatively. But in 1984,

an intravenous glucose tolerance test (IVGTT) was added; only individuals
with a post-IV glucose stimulatory first phase insulin level above the 30th
percentile of the normal range are now accepted as donors [17]. Of the 82
LRD donors, only 3 have not remained normoglycemic (2 at <1 year, 1 at
>4 years). All 3 were from the initial pre-1984 series when a normal OGTT
was sufficient; in retrospect, all 3 had low insulin responses [17]. None of
the donors meeting our current criterion of IVGTT insulin response has
become hyperglycemic after hemipancreatectomy [18].

Donor complications Surgical complications after hemipancreatectomy occurred in 11 donors: 4 required splenectomy (1 intraoperatively, 3 postopera-
tively 2 days to 4 years post-transplant); 3 developed sterile fluid collection
(successfully treated by percutaneous aspiration); 2 developed abscesses (successfully treated by percutaneous drainage); 1 required relaparotomy to ligate
the duct at the cut surface of the pancreas after a staple closure; and 1
required relaparotomy to retrieve a sponge.

Statistical analysis Patient and graft survival rates were calculated according
to Kaplan-Meier. Grafts were defined as functioning if the recipient was
insulin-independent.

Results

Patient survival rates at 1 and 5 years post-transplant were 93% and 90%
(Figure 2). For all transplants, the graft survival rate was 51% at 1 year. For
technically successful transplants only, graft survival rates at 1 and 5 years
were 68% and 50%. A comparison of LRD versus CAD transplants for PTA
and PAK categories showed no difference between groups in overall graft
survival rates; when only technically successful transplants were included in
the analysis, patient and graft survival rates were significantly better for
LRD than for CAD transplants for both PTA and PAK categories. The
immunologic advantage of LRD transplants was apparent: only 13% of LRD
allograft recipients lost their graft from chronic rejection versus 41% of
CAD recipients (PTA and PAK categories). LRD recipients were able to
maintain stable, long-term graft function: 15 (18%) have had functioning
grafts for more than 5 years. Of these recipients, 9 had a PTA (1 from an
identical twin, 5 from HLA-identical siblings, and 3 from mismatched relatives, with 2 receiving subsequent kidneys from the same donor), and 6 had
a PAK transplant (5 HLA-identical siblings, 1 mismatched relative); 12 of
the pancreas grafts were enteric-drained (9 PTA, 3 PAK), 2 bladder-drained
(both PAK), and 1 duct-injected (PAK).
    LRD transplants can be done for all recipient categories. We have recently
done the first 2 successful LRD simultaneous pancreas-kidney transplants.

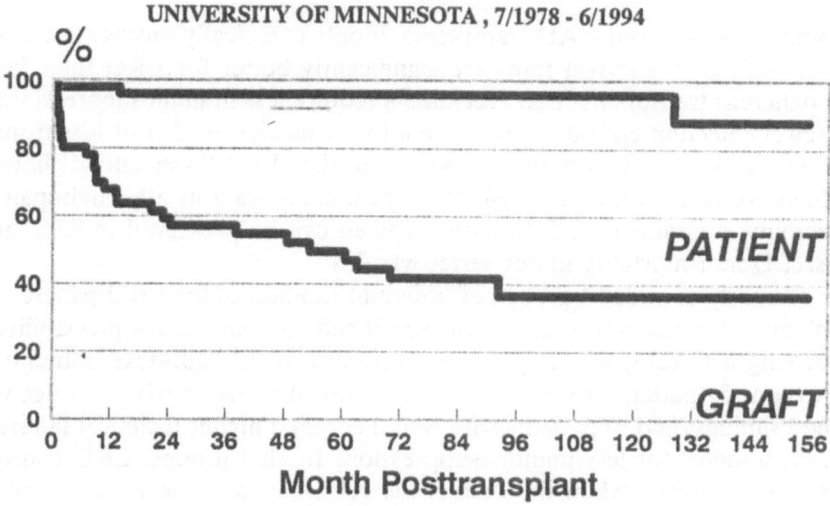

Fig. 2. Graft and patient survival of technically successful LRD pancreas transplants.

Both donors and both recipients are doing well. This approach may become more frequent.

Our experience with 7 identical twin transplants was previously reported [12, 14]. In the absence of immunosuppression, the first 3 recipients were susceptible to isletitis and disease recurrence. All 3 became hyperglycemic 6 to 12 weeks post-transplant [12]. Twins #2 and #3 received Minnesota antilymphocyte globulin (ALG) and azathioprine after graft biopsies showed isletitis and selective cell destruction [13], but their grafts were not salvageable. Twin #4 received azathioprine prophylactically and was normoglycemic for 3 years. Hyperglycemia then occurred with selective cell destruction, per graft biopsy; the patient initially responded to ALG and cyclosporine, but resumed insulin 5 years post-transplant. Twins #5, #6, and #7 have received immunosuppression with cyclosporine and azathioprine; all 3 are currently (June 1994) normoglycemic at 3.75 to 7 years post-transplant. Twin #5 had pancreas biopsies at 1 and 5 years post-transplant that showed normal islets. Twin #6 had elevated glucose levels at 6 months post-transplant and was successfully treated with ALG after a graft biopsy showed mild isletitis; a biopsy 2 years later showed no isletitis. Twin #7 had normal islets, per biopsy 2 years post-transplant.

Discussion

Our experience with LRD pancreas transplants shows that their morbidity and mortality are minimal for both donors and recipients. Patient survival rates are 90% at 1 and 5 years post-transplant. Overall graft survival rates are comparable with our CAD transplants; if only technically successful cases are included, graft survival rates are significantly better for LRD than for CAD pancreas transplants. LRD recipients require less immunosuppression, have fewer rejection episodes, and have a lower incidence of graft loss from rejection. All of our donors since 1984 (when the IVGTT was added) have remained normoglycemic. The risk of surgical complications after hemipancreatectomy is minimal, and the donor spleen can be preserved in 95% of all cases. Donor mortality in our series was 0%.

We currently consider 4 groups of potential candidates for LRD pancreas transplants: 1) patients who are highly sensitized and have a low probability of receiving a CAD graft; 2) patients who must avoid high-dose immunosuppression; 3) patients with nondiabetic identical twins or with 6-antigen-matched siblings; and 4) patients who would accept a higher technical failure rate as a tradeoff for less immunosuppression. In all 4 groups, LRD transplants are done only when the donor, the recipient, and the entire family understands advantages and disadvantages of both procedures.

LRD pancreas transplants can be safely done in all recipient categories. Results for PTA and PAK recipients are well documented. A longer follow-up of our 2 most recently transplanted SPK recipients may demonstrate that this is an additional alternative for a small subgroup of uremic patients with insulin-dependent diabetes mellitus.

Our experience with pancreas transplants from identical twin donors has shown that disease recurrence with subsequent graft loss occurs only in the absence of immunosuppression. With adequate immunosuppression, recurrence of diabetes can be prevented. This observation provides strong evidence of an autoimmune etiology of diabetes.

Based on our patient and graft survival rates, we believe that LRD pancreas transplants should be applied more liberally in the future to advance the field of endocrine replacement therapy for diabetes mellitus.

References

1. Murray JE, Merrill JP, Harrison JH. Renal homotransplantation in identical twins. Surg Forum 1955; 6: 432–436.
2. Sutherland DER, Goetz FC, Najarian JS. Living-related donor segmental pancreatectomy for transplantation. Transplant Proc 1980; 12: 19–25.
3. Broelsch CE, Lloyd DM. Living related donors for liver transplants. Adv Surg 1993; 26: 209–31.
4. Starnes VA, Lewiston NJ, Luikart H, Theodore J, Stinson EB, Shumway NE. Current trends in lung transplantation: Lobar transplantation and expanded use of single lungs [discussion]. J Thorac Cardiovasc Surg 1992; 104: 1060–5.
5. Deltz E, Schroeder P, Gundlach M, Hansmann ML, Leimenstoll G. Successful clinical small-bowel transplantation. Transplant Proc 1990; 22: 2501.
6. Sutherland DER, Goetz FC, Gillingham K, Moudry-Munns KC, Najarian JS. Medical risks and benefit of pancreas transplants from living related donors. In: Land W, Dossetor JB,

editors. Organ replacement therapy: ethics, justice and commerce. Berlin: Springer Verlag, 1991; 93–101.
7. Sutherland DER, Moudry-Munns K, Gruessner A. Pancreas transplant results in United Network for Organ Sharing (UNOS) United States of America (USA) Registry with a comparison to non-USA Data in the International Registry. In: Terasaki, I, Cecka, JM, editors. Clinical Transplants Los Angeles: UCLA Tissue Typing Laboratory, 1994: 47–69.
8. Sutherland DER, Goetz FC, Najarian JS. Pancreas transplants from related donors. Transplantation 1984; 38: 625–33.
9. Casanova D, Gruessner RWG, Brayman K, Jessurun J, Dunn D, Xenos E, Sutherland DER. A retrospective analysis of the role of pancreatic biopsy (open and transcystoscopic technique) in the management of solitary pancreas transplants. Transplant Proc 1993; 25: 1192–3.
10. Jones JW, Nakhleh RE, Casanova D, Sutherland DER, Gruessner RWG. Cystoscopic transduodenal pancreas transplant biopsy: a new needle. Transplant Proc 1994; 26: 527–8.
11. Sutherland DER, Goetz FC, Najarian JS. Experience with single pancreas transplantation compared with pancreas transplantation after a kidney transplantation; and with transplantation with pancreas grafts from living related compared with cadaveric donors. In: Groth CG, editor. Pancreatic Transplantation. London: Grune and Stratton Ltd., 1988: 175–89.
12. Sutherland DER, Sibley RK, Xu XZ, et al. Twin-to-twin pancreas transplantation: reversal and reenactment of the pathogenesis of type I diabetes. Trans Assoc Amer Physicians 1984; 97: 80–7.
13. Sibley RK, Sutherland DER, Goetz FC, Michael AF. Recurrent diabetes mellitus in the pancreas iso- and sllograft: a light and electron microscopic and immunohistochemical analysis of four cases. Lab Invest 1985; 53: 132–44.
14. Sutherland DER, Goetz FC, Sibley RK. Recurrence of disease in pancreas transplants. Diabetes 1989; 38: 85–7.
15. Sutherland DER, Dunn DL, Goetz FC, Kennedy W, Ramsay RC, Steffes MW, Mauer SM, Gruessner RWG, Moudry-Munns KC, Morel P, Viste A, Robertson RP, Najarian JS. A ten-year experience with 290 pancreas transplants at a single institution. Ann Surg 1989; 210: 274–85.
16. Barbosa JJ, King R, Goetz FC. Histocompatibility antigens in familiers with juvenile insulin dependent diabetes mellitus. J Clin Invest 1977; 60: 989–90.
17. Kendall DM, Sutherland DER, Goetz FC, Najarian JS. Metabolic effect of hemipancreatectomy in living related pancreas transplant donors: preoperative prediction of postoperative oral glucose tolerance. Diabetes 1989; 38: 101–3.
18. Seaquist ER, Robertson RP. Effects of hemipancreatectomy on pancreatic alpha and beta cell function in healthy human donors. J Clin Invest 1992; 89: 1761–6.

13. Expanding the donor supply by using high risk donors: the use of pulsatile kidney perfusion for evaluation of high risk kidney donors

RAYMOND J. TESI, ELMAHDI A. ELKHAMMAS,
ELIZABETH A. DAVIES, MITCHELL L. HENRY & RONALD
M. FERGUSON

Introduction

Access to transplantation is limited by a lack of donor organs. This problem is common for all solid organs, but the largest number of patients affected are those awaiting renal transplants. There are two options for bringing the supply of kidneys for transplant into balance with the need. We can increase the number of kidneys available for transplant – increase supply; or we can limit access to renal transplantation – decrease demand.

Decreasing the demand for renal transplantation is not palatable to many health care professionals. Recent management strategies have focused on expanding access to renal transplantation [1], not limiting access. The costs of dialysis also exceed transplantation in many studies [2]. Increasing the supply has been difficult, but several options exist: increased living donation, changes in consent laws, incentives for organ donation, the use of non-heart-beating donors and expanding the criteria for acceptable cadaveric donors. The last method, utilizing the "high risk" donor, is one of the easiest to implement. Paradoxically, attempts to increase organ supply need to balance the numerical increases with clinical outcome due to financial and immunologic penalty of a failed transplant [3].

Traditional cadaveric donor evaluation has focused on a combination of demographic and medical parameters to determine if an organ was to be used. The use of often incomplete medical histories and demographic data may not be the most accurate way to assess donor organ quality. The use of pulsatile perfusion for kidney preservation provides an opportunity to quantitatively evaluate the suitability of a renal allograft for transplantation.

We have reviewed 87 kidneys from 59 donors to determine if the pump parameters are more useful than donor medical history, and demographic and laboratory characteristics in predicting the functioning of a cadaveric kidney (CAD) in a group of "high risk" donors. "High risk" donors are considered kidneys from donors who are aged ≥ 60 or have a history of hypertension (HTN), or are kidneys not used at other centers because of donor characteristics (IMPORT).

J.L. Touraine et al. (eds.), Organ Shortage: The Solutions, 85–92.
© 1995 *Kluwer Academic Publishers.*

Materials and methods

Eighty-seven kidneys were obtained from 59 consecutive donors ≥ 40 years of age during a 34–month period. Local donor management and organ procurement procedures have been previously reported [4, 5]. Briefly, aggressive donor hydration and optimization of hemodynamic parameters and urine output are undertaken before the donor is taken to the OR. Intraoperatively, donors are aggressively hydrated and receive mannitol 50–100 g and methylprednisolone 500 mg. En bloc cold perfusion with iced lactated Ringers solution with verapamil 10 mg l^{-1} is performed to eliminate warm ischemia time. Kidneys are removed en bloc and transferred to a Mox100 perfusion machine (Waters Inc, Rochester, MN) for pulsatile perfusion and preservation using Belzer2 perfusate. Imported kidneys are secondarily perfused from the time of arrival at our institution until transplant, as previously reported [6].

Pump pressures were adjusted to maintain a systolic pressure ≤ 40 mmHg (never exceeding 50 mmHg). In response to pressure and FLOW parameters, pharmacological adjustment of perfusate was performed: 1) osmolality was adjusted to 310–330 osm kg^{-1} with mannitol; 2) pH was adjusted to 7.45–7.5 using $NaHCO_3$ and CO_2 gas; 3) a vasodilator (usually verapamil) was added to the perfusate to optimize perfusion parameters and minimize renal resistance (RR). RR was calculated as: mean perfusion pressure (mmHg) / flow (ml min^{-1}). Kidneys were not used if calculated $RR \geq 0.4$ or FLOW < 70 ml min^{-1}. The FLOW and RR values reported were last value obtained before transplant or discard of the organ.

Donor information was obtained from the donor sheets. Donor risk groups were defined by donor age, the presence of HTN, and source (LOCAL vs. IMPORT). Old donors (OLDDON) were ≥ 60 years old (yo). The younger donors (YOUNGDON) included consecutive donors age 40–59. The current use of antihypertensive drugs was considered evidence of significant hypertension in the donor.

Recipients received sequential quadruple immunosuppression with triple therapy maintenance immunosuppression with azathioprine, prednisone and cyclosporine as has been previously reported [7]. Recipient outcome parameters included: 1) patient and graft survival; 2) ATN as defined by the need for *any* dialysis post-transplant; 3) 72–hour urine output; 4) length of hospital stay; and 5) Day 10, 30, 60, 90 and current serum Cr values.

Statistical analysis was performed using parametric techniques for two-tailed T-tests and χ^2 analysis with $p < 0.05$ considered significant. The Kaplan-Meier estimate and Cox analysis were performed using BMDP software.

Results

Eighty-seven kidneys from 59 donors were evaluated. Mean donor age was 57 years old (yo) and donors were in the hospital a median of 2 days before

Table 1. Twelve of 82 locally evaluated kidneys were discarded for failing to meet minimal perfusion criteria (RR $\leqslant 0.4$ and FLOW $\geqslant 70$ ml min^{-1}).

Risk group	TX	Discard
Old donor	33	12
Young donor	37	0
No HTN	22	7
HTN	33	5
LOCAL	36	4
IMPORT	34	8

All 12 discarded kidneys were from donors aged $\geqslant 60$ ($p = 0.002$). A history of HTN and donor source (LOCAL vs. IMPORT) did not affect the discard rate.

Table 2. The pump parameters of renal resistance (RR) and FLOW on the 69 kidneys transplanted at our center stratified by risk group.

	LOCAL	IMPORT	HTN	NO HTN	YOUNGDON	OLDDON
RR	0.3240	0.3192	0.3270	0.3345	0.2956	0.3485
FLOW	108	102	102	105	112	98

Donor source (LOCAL vs. IMPORT) or the presence of HTN in the donor did not affect perfusion parameters. Donor age $\geqslant 60$ had a negative effect on perfusion parameters with an increased RR and decreased flow. $p = 0.0033$ YOUNGDON vs. OLDDON.

organ procurement. The most common cause of death was intracerebral hemorrhage and the average serum Cr at procurement was 1.2 mg dl^{-1}. Thirty-seven kidneys were from YOUNGDON and 50 were from OLDDON with an average age of 48 yo and 64 yo, respectively. The presence of HTN could be determined in 72 of the kidneys. HTN was present in 39 of the kidneys and was more common in IMPORT than LOCAL kidneys ($p = 0.0473$), but not more common in OLDDON. Five kidneys were exported to other centers (one kidney was discarded and one kidney required dialysis) and were excluded from subsequent analysis. Eighty-two kidneys were transplanted locally and were available for evaluation in this study.

Total preservation time of the 82 kidneys evaluated at our center averaged 22.6 hours (h) (range: 14–47 h). LOCAL kidney preservation time averaged 14.6 h, all as pulsatile preservation. IMPORT kidneys had significantly longer preservation time (28.5 h; $p < 0.0001$) due to an average of 14.3 h cold preservation and 14.2 h pump preservation. The average FLOW of the kidneys during perfusion was 98 ml min^{-1} (range: 40–150 ml min^{-1}) with a RR = 0.334 (range: 0.162–0.57). Twelve kidneys were discarded for failure to meet minimal pump perfusion parameters. Average RR and FLOW of discarded kidneys was 0.4 and 62 ml min^{-1}, respectively. These parameters were significantly lower ($p < 0.001$) than for the transplanted kidneys (RR = 0.32; FLOW = 105 ml min^{-1}). All discarded kidneys were from OLDDON ($p = 0.002$). A history of HTN or the origin of the kidney (LOCAL vs. IMPORT) were not important risk factors for discard (Table 1).

Table 3. Six of 69 locally transplanted kidneys developed ATN.

	No dialysis	Dialysis
N	63	6
Donor age	55	62
Pump time (h)	14.9	13.3
Preserve time	22.6	25.5
FLOW (ml min^{-1})	106	98
Renal res.	0.32	0.36
Recipient age	50	54
% IMPORT	44	83

Donor age, preservation time, and perfusion parameters of RR and FLOW did not predict the need for dialysis. The percentage of IMPORTS in the no ATN group was one half that of the ATN group, but this failed to reach statistical significance ($p = 0.1632$).

Sixty-nine kidneys were transplanted at our center. FLOW and RR were compared in the kidneys by risk group (OLDDON vs. YOUNGDON, no HTN vs. HTN, IMPORT vs. LOCAL). FLOW was significantly lower and RR was significantly higher in OLDDON compared to YOUNGDON ($p < 0.01$). A history of HTN or the source of the kidney had no effect on RR or FLOW (Table 2). ATN developed in 6 kidneys transplanted at our center (8.7%). Five of the 6 kidneys were IMPORTs with an average of 14 h of cold storage. Pump parameters failed to predict ATN in this selected group of organs (Table 3). A multivariate analysis of the risk of needing dialysis using donor and preservation variables of transplanted kidneys found IMPORT as the only independent variable in predicting ATN (relative risk = 8.6).

Hospital course was compared in the 69 recipients transplanted at our center. All recipients were primary transplants. Recipient age of OLDDON kidneys was significantly greater than YOUNGDON organs (57 yo vs. 44 yo, respectively; $p < 0.0001$). Renal function in both groups was acceptable. Median 72 h urine output was 14.3 l, median hospital stay was 10 days and Day 10 serum Cr averaged 2.0 mg dl^{-1}. Recipients of OLDDON organs had a lower Day 30 Cr (1.6 mg dl^{-1} vs. 2.4 mg dl^{-1}; $p = 0.0058$). Recipients of organs from donors with HTN had higher Day 10 Cr than donors without HTN (3.0 vs. 1.7; $p = 0.0125$), but Day 30 Cr was equivalent. IMPORTs had lower 72 h urine output than LOCAL (17.8 l vs. 12.5 l; $p = 0.0084$). None of these differences complicated patient management.

Uncensored graft survival of 69 kidneys transplanted at our center were 89% and 82% at 12 and 24 months, respectively. Graft survival was worse in the IMPORT vs. EXPORT kidneys (81% vs. 95% at 12 months; $p = 0.0105$). Donor age or the presence of HTN did not affect graft survival (data not shown). Cox survival analysis using donor risk group and patient outcome as variables found that IMPORT was the only independent variable for uncensored graft loss (relative risk = 5.7).

Discussion

The demand for solid organ transplantation has exceeded the supply of available donor organs. The use of the "marginal donor" is one strategy for expanding the donor pool [8]. CAD kidney donor evaluation incorporates a number of demographic and medical variables to evaluate donor acceptability. Factors which have a known effect on renal function (i.e., older age, hypertension, and diabetes) are considered to be relative contraindications for donor use. The impact of donor age on CAD kidney outcome is the subject of controversy [8, 9], and many centers are reluctant to use these kidneys for transplant. The combination of an elderly donor and HTN appears to increase the incidence of delayed graft function [10] which has been shown to compromise one-year graft survival [11, 12].

Pulsatile preservation has been the source of considerable controversy. Two recent trials have suggested no benefit from pulsatile perfusion [13, 14], but both used antiquated preservation solutions [4]. The excellent results of cold storage with UW solution [10] has tempered the enthusiasm for the more costly and laborious pulsatile preservation. More recently, a multi-center database has suggested no advantage of pulsatile preservation over cold storage with UW solution, despite a decreased incidence of delayed graft function with pump preservation [15]. This conclusion is contrary to previous reports from the same authors [16, 17].

We propose that the use of subjective variables of donor demographics (e.g., age, sex, race, etc.), medical history (e.g., h/o HTN, h/o cardiac arrest, etc.) and current medical condition (e.g., current serum Cr, use of pressors, etc.) fail to accurately evaluate the suitability of the kidneys for transplant. We utilized the pump parameters while the organs were undergoing pulsatile perfusion to determine suitability for transplant. The excellent preservation of the organs combined with active manipulation (pharmacologic) of the perfusate to optimize the perfusion characteristics of the organ while on the pump provides quantitative data which can be used to determine the suitability of an organ for transplant with a low ATN rate. Over 1400 kidneys have undergone pulsatile preservation at our program since 1982 with an ATN rate of <5%.

These data support the accuracy of perfusion characteristics in predicting a good early kidney function. Only 6 of the 69 CAD kidneys transplanted at our center required dialysis (8.6%). The low ATN rate occurred despite an unfavorable mix of donor characteristics. All donors were aged ≥42 and 48% were aged ≥60. IMPORT kidneys comprised 48% of the total. All IMPORT kidneys were received through UNOS because the procuring center did not feel the kidney was suitable for transplant, due to concerns about donor characteristics; that is, these kidneys would have been discarded at the original center. (None of the organs were received for 6–antigen match recipients.) Sixty percent of donors had a history of HTN. The use of pump parameters of RR < 0.4 and FLOW ≥ 70 ml min^{-1} have allowed successful use of these organs with an ATN rate below the national average (21%) for kidneys stored ≤24 h – the best risk group [17].

Six kidneys transplanted at our center developed ATN; five of these were IMPORTs. A multivariate analysis demonstrated that IMPORT was the only independent variable predicting the need for dialysis (relative risk = 8.6). IMPORT kidneys have three important differences when compared to LOCAL kidneys: 1) pre-procurement donor resuscitation is often less aggressive than our local procurement protocol (i.e. higher serum Na, more pressor use); 2) all IMPORTs have a significant amount of simple cold storage (avg. = 14.2 h); 3) IMPORTs have a longer overall preservation time (avg. = 28 h). The multivariate analysis suggests that undefined donor factors and not preservation time (cold or total time) are more important in predicting ATN. Unfortunately, no pump parameter was able to predict the development of ATN in kidneys that were considered acceptable for transplant.

Two-year graft survival for the overall series exceeds 82%. The use of pump parameters as selection criteria for kidneys to transplant has eliminated the penalty associated with the use of organs from older donors [17]. We could not demonstrate a difference in graft survival based on donor age (p = 0.2711). This difference may be a function of selective use of organs from older donors (majority of discarded organs were from the donors age ≥60) or due to the small sample size. The single independent risk factor for graft loss in our data was the receipt of an IMPORT kidney for transplant (relative risk = 5.7). The UNOS database suggests that there is no penalty in the transplant of shared organs [17]. We have two possible explanations for this difference. The selection criteria we use (pump parameters) allows for a substantially lower ATN rate than the UNOS standard. Secondly, the exclusion of shared 6–antigen match kidneys removes a pool of organs with universally superior outcome that may have been obscuring the negative impact of shared less than 6–antigen match kidneys.

We have failed to clearly demonstrate that the kidneys discarded because of failure to meet minimal pump parameters would not have worked. Only a randomized trial would clearly determine this. We are unwilling to perform this due to the cost of a failed kidney transplant and consequences of DGF on long-term graft survival [3]. A regression analysis of the 82 kidneys evaluated suggested that donor age ≥60 was the independent variable in predicting discard (relative risk = 2.5; data not shown). We propose that the low ATN rate in this group of kidneys from suboptimal donors (often from organs deemed unacceptable by the local transplant center) validates the use of pump parameters to select kidneys for transplantation. The use of these selection criteria allows us to choose which organs to transplant and prevents us from transplanting organs that will not work. The cut-off points for acceptable RR and FLOW are based on data previously reported [18] and substantial unreported experience.

In conclusion, the use of pulsatile preservation with active pharmacological modification of the perfusate to optimize the pump parameters of RR and FLOW has allowed the use of kidneys from marginal donors with a low ATN rate. This has allowed our center to safely expand the use of marginal donors without compromising outcome. Surprisingly, these data also suggest a significant penalty for the use of non-6-antigen match shared kidneys. IMPORT organs had a higher rate of ATN and a worse graft survival that was independent of preservation time. This implies that programs to increase organ sharing may result in decreased graft survival because of increases in ATN. We believe that the use of quantitative values of organ quality (FLOW and RR) are superior to subjective measures of donor suitability (especially the presence of HTN and donor age) in predicting organ quality. This approach will be particularly important as attempts are made to expand the donor pool with "non-heart-beating donor" programs.

References

1. Tesi RJ, Elkhammas EA, Davies EA, Henry ML, Ferguson RM. Renal transplantation in older people. Lancet 1994; 343: 461.
2. Karlberg I. Cost analysis of alternative treatments in end-stage renal disease. Transplant Proc 1992; 24: 335.
3. Rosenthal JT, Danovitch GM, Wilkinson A, Ettenger RB. The high cost of delayed graft function in cadaveric renal transplantation. Transplantation 1991; 51: 1115.
4. Henry ML, Sommer BG, Ferguson RM. Improved immediate function of renal allografts with belzer perfusate. Transplantation 1988; 45: 73.
5. Tesi RJ, Elkhammas EA, Davies EA, Henry ML, Ferguson RM. Pulsatile kidney perfusion for preservation and evaluation: use of high-risk kidney donors to expand the donor pool. Transplant Proc 1993; 25: 3099.
6. Henry ML, Sommer BG, Tesi RJ, Ferguson RM. Improved immediate renal allograft function after initial simple cold storage. Transplant Proc 1990; 22: 388.
7. Sommer BG, Henry ML, Ferguson RM. Sequential antilymphoblast globulin and cyclosporine for renal transplantation. Transplantation 1987; 43: 85.
8. Alexander JW, Vaughn WK. The use of "marginal" donors for organ transplantation: the influence of donor age on outcome. Transplantation 1991; 51: 135.
9. Yuge J, Cecka JM. Sex and age effects in renal transplantation. Clin Transplantation 1991; 257–67.
10. Ploeg RJ, Van Bockel JH, Langendijk PTH, et al. Effect of preservation solution on results of cadaveric kidney transplantation. Lancet 1992; 340: 129.
11. Sanfilippo F, Vaughn WK, Spees EK, Lucas BA. The detrimental effects of delayed graft function in cadaver donor renal transplantation. Transplantation 1984; 38: 643.
12. Halloran PF, Aprile MA, Farewell V, et al. Early function as the principal correlate of graft survival. Transplantation 1988; 46: 223.
13. Merion RM, Oh HK, Port FK, Toledo-Pereyra LH, Turcotte JG. A prospective controlled trial of cold-storage versus machine-perfusion preservation in cadaveric renal transplantation. Transplantation 1990; 50: 230.
14. Halloran P, Aprile M. A randomized prospective trial of cold storage versus pulsatile perfusion for cadaver kidney preservation. Transplantation 1987; 43: 827.
15. Koyama H, Cecka JM, Terasaki PI. A comparison of cadaver donor kidney storage methods: pump perfusion and cold storage solutions. Clin Transplantation 1993; 7: 199.

16. Lim EC, Terasaki PI. Early Graft Function. In: Terasaki P, Cecka JM, editors. Clinical Transplants 1991. Los Angeles, CA: UCLA Tissue Typing Laboratory, 1992: 401.
17. Zhou Y-C, Cecka JM. Preservation. In: Terasaki P, Cecka J, editors. Clinical Transplants 1992. Los Angeles, CA: UCLA Tissue Typing Laboratory, 1993: 384.
18. Henry ML, Sommer BG, Ferguson RM. Renal blood flow and intrarenal resistance predict immediate renal allograft function. Transplant Proc 1986; 18: 557.

14. Relative effect of HLA matching and cold ischemia time

JOYCE YUGE & PAUL I. TERASAKI

Introduction

One of the principal arguments against the use of HLA matching in renal transplantation is that, in most cases, cold ischemia time would be increased while a well-matched recipient is located and the kidney is shipped [1]. It has even been suggested that by shortening the cold ischemia time HLA typing can be eliminated [2]. Despite this argument, there is strong evidence that well-matched transplants overcome any detrimental effects of increased cold ischemia time [3–6]. The *relative* effect of HLA matching and cold ischemia time on transplant outcome is examined here.

Patients and methods

For this study, 31,144 first cadaver donor transplants reported to the UNOS Scientific Renal Transplant Registry from 1988 through 1993 were analyzed.

Results

The results obtained are given in the following figures and legends.

Figure 1. The clear effect of HLA ABDR mismatching is evident. The highest graft survival rates are achieved with 0 ABDR mismatched transplants, followed by the other mismatch grades in sequence. The 88% one-year survival of 0 mismatched cadaver donor transplants is comparable to that of parental donor transplants. At three years, there is an 18% difference in survival between 0 and 6 mismatched groups (82% vs. 64%).

Figure 2. The highest graft survival rate at one year is seen with a CIT of 6–12 hours (84%). Interestingly, transplants with the shortest CIT studied (1–6 hours) did not have the best graft survival as a result of a possible center effect. At three years, the difference between the highest and lowest

J.L. Touraine et al. (eds.), *Organ Shortage: The Solutions*, 93–97.

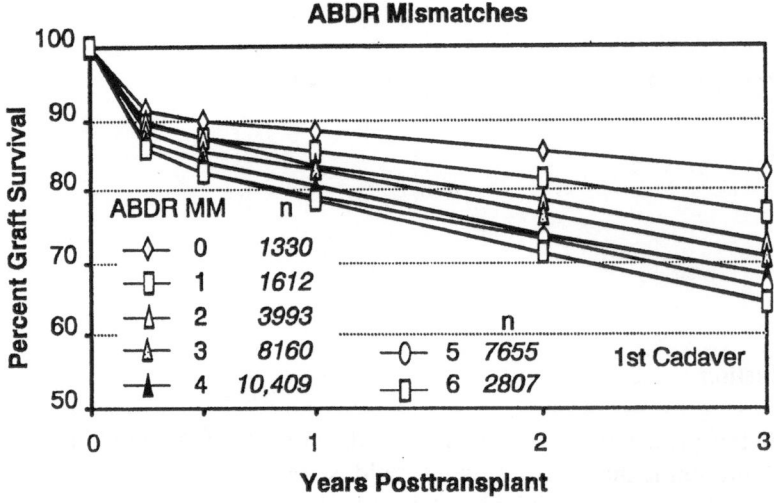

Fig. 1. HLA matching.

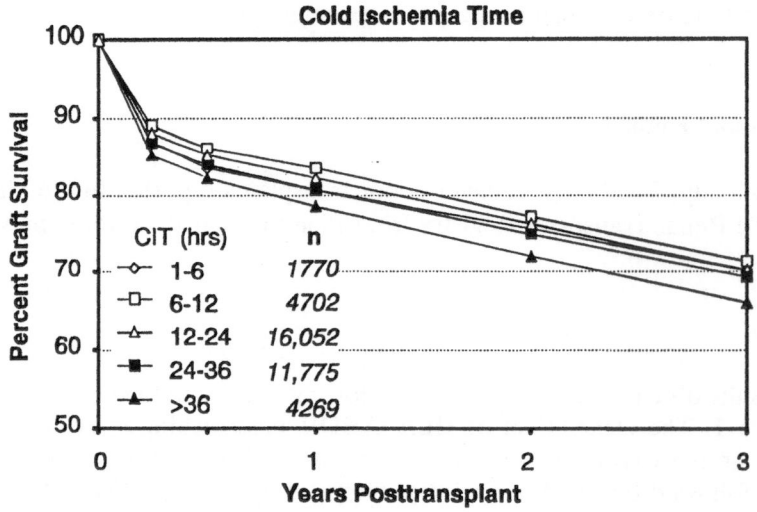

Fig. 2. Cold ischemia time (CIT).

survival rate was 5%. However, if the low 66% survival for a CIT greater than 36 hours is excluded, the difference becomes only 3%.

Figure 3. It is clear that at 3 years, 0, 1, and 2 ABDR mismatched transplants had a higher one-year graft survival rate than transplants with the shortest cold ischemia times. There was an 11% difference between graft

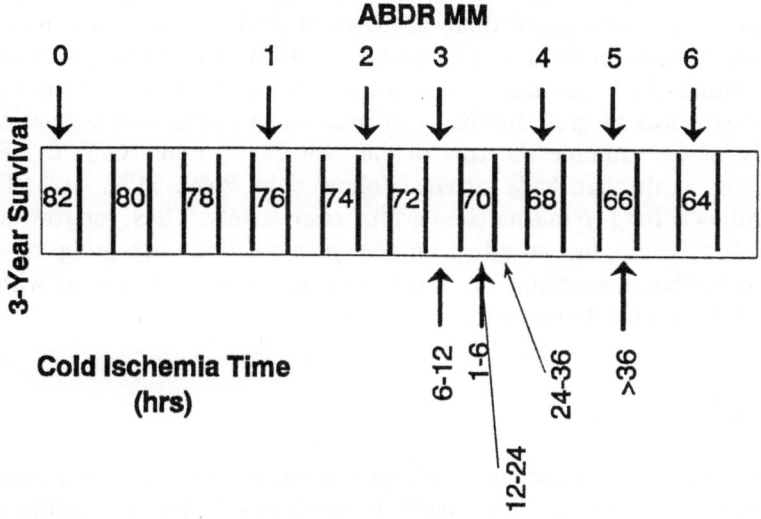

Fig. 3. Relative effects of HLA matching and CIT when examined as univariates.

3-YEAR GRAFT SURVIVAL

CIT (hrs)	ABDR MM						
	0	1	2	3	4	5	6
1-6	(69)	(80)	77	70	67	71	69
6-12	(78)	83	79	[75]	[70]	[68]	60
12-24	80	78	[74]	[72]	[69]	[66]	[67]
24-36	84	76	[71]	[71]	[69]	[65]	64
>36	84	77	68	67	[66]	62	62

◯ N < 100   ▢ N > 1000

Fig. 4. Relationship between HLA matching and CIT.

survival of 0 ABDR mismatched transplants and the shortest CIT (82% vs. 70%). The highest 3-year graft survival that could be obtained was 71% with a CIT of 6–12 hours. However, this was below that of 0 and 1 and 2 mismatched transplants. The advantage of HLA matching was obvious.

Figure 4. Zero ABDR mismatched transplants were able to overcome the detrimental effects of long cold ischemia time as shown in the first column. Even transplants with more than 36 hours of cold ischemia time had a 3-year graft survival of 84% if they had a 0 ABDR mismatched transplant. With 36 hours of CIT, as is apparent from examination of the row, there was a progressive loss in graft survival with increasing degrees of mismatching. Similarly, if we examine the row of data for 24–36 hours CIT, 0 ABDR mismatched grafts had 84% survival followed by 76%, 71%, 71%, 69%, 65%, and 64% for 1–6 mismatched grafts, respectively. Thus, the rows show that HLA matching has an effect on transplants within each group of CIT. On the other hand, examination of the columns shows that patients with the shortest CIT did not have the best survival.

Discussion

With respect to the question of whether reduction of CIT can provide a better means of selecting transplants as compared to HLA matching, this study comes to the opposite conclusion of Aswad et al. [2].

The results of this analysis showed that regardless of the length of cold ischemia time, 0 ABDR mismatched transplants had the highest graft survival rates at one and three years. The degree of HLA matching influenced graft survival to a much higher degree than cold ischemia time. The survival rates decreased as the number of mismatched groups increased as seen with the three-year graft survival results (Figure 3).

Even if CIT were to be reduced to under 6 hours, the 3-year graft survival rate was only equivalent to 3 ABDR mismatched transplants. The marked superiority of the 0 ABDR mismatched graft to short CIT is shown in Figures 3 and 4.

We conclude that CIT should be kept below 36 hours with current kidney storage fluids. If improved methods are developed, longer cold ischemia times could be considered. Obviously HLA matching improves graft survival, and should be used regardless of the cold ischemia time. Even in kidneys stored more than 36 hours, the graft survival was greatly influenced by the HLA match (Figure 4).

Summary

At 3 years, there was an 18% difference in graft survival between the best and worst HLA matched transplants, whereas for cold ischemia time, the difference between the 1–6 hr CIT and >36 hr CIT was only 5%. Moreover, at 3 years, the 0 ABDR mismatched transplants had an 11% higher graft survival than the 1–6 hr CIT kidneys.

Zero ABDR mismatched transplants had the highest 3-year graft survival regardless of the CIT. Even kidneys with >36 hr CIT with 0 ABDR mismatches had an 84% 3-year graft survival. Also, a 1 ABDR mismatched transplant with >36 hr CIT was superior to >3 ABDR mismatched kidneys with short CIT. We conclude that it is worthwhile to ship 0 ABDR kidneys, even if long CIT is necessary.

References

1. Hunsicker LG, Held PJ. The role of HLA matching for cadaveric renal transplants in the cyclosporine era. Semin Nephrology 1992; 12(4): 293–303.
2. Aswad S, Mann SL, Khetan U, et al. Omit HLA matching to attain shorter cold ischemia time? Transplant Proc 1993; 25: 3053–5.
3. Iwaki Y, Cicciarelli J, Aswad S, et al. Cold ischemia time and MHC Class II matching in renal transplants. Transplant Proc 1992; 24: 2456–7.
4. Zhou YC, Cecka JM. Preservation. In: Terasaki PI and Cecka JM, editors. Clinical Transplants 1992. Los Angeles, CA: UCLA Tissue Typing Laboratory, 1993: 383.
5. Cicciarelli J, Iwaki Y, Mendez R, et al. Effects of cold ischemia time on cadaver renal allografts. Transplant Proc 1993; 25: 1543–6.
6. Zhou YC, Cecka JM. Effect of HLA matching on renal transplant survival. In: Terasaki PI and Cecka JM, editors. Clinical Transplants 1993. Los Angeles, CA: UCLA Tissue Typing Laboratory, 1994: 499.

15. Are kidneys of very young donors suitable for transplantation?

P. COCHAT, L. DUBOURG, A. HADJ-AÏSSA, M. DAWAHRA,
M.H. SAÏD & L. DAVID

Introduction

In the early stages of kidney transplantation, very young cadaver donors –
including newborns – were used. Even anencephalic infants were considered
as possible organ donors, however organ harvesting was impossible until
brain-stem activity ceased. Under such conditions, organ procurement is
not allowed by current law. Moreover, prenatal diagnosis of such a lethal
malformation is now easily accomplished with ultrasound examination [1].

In the French experience, one third of pediatric cadaver donors are under
2 years of age, probably because of the high mortality rate in this age group
and because most of these patients are referred to university pediatric centres
[2]. However, very young donors have been progressively abandoned in most
centres, due to poor results [3]. Considering the critical lack of donors
for kidney transplantation, it is becoming increasingly important that all
potentially successful donor organs be used and, on this basis, the special
features of renal transplantation from very young donors are reviewed.

This strategy provides two main advantages – i.e. a low risk of transmitted
viral disease and a low risk of native arteriosclerosis – and two major inconveniences – i.e. a high risk of vascular thrombosis/stenosis and a theoretical
risk of acquired glomerulosclerosis because of hyperfiltration.

Graft survival

Most studies on the effect of donor age on graft survival come from pediatric
series, since young cadaver donors are mainly used for patients under the
age of 18. In all series, kidneys from donors under 5 years of age have a
lower survival rate [4–6]. In a report of 787 cadaver donor renal transplants
in children from the North American Pediatric Renal Transplant Cooperative
Study (NAPRTCS), 25% were under 6 years of age but it has been shown
that the ideal donor age was 20–25 years [4]. The risk of graft loss from a
neonate donor was 2.7-fold that of the ideal donor; vascular thrombosis,

primary non-function and other technical problems account for 9.9% of graft failure when the donor is less than 5 years of age, compared to 4.4% when the donor is 10 to 39 years old [4].

In a study of 37 kidneys donated from anencephalic infants, only 11 transplants were successful [7]. In another series from Gagnadoux et al. [5], the 2–year-graft survival was 58% when the donor was under 5 years of age versus 77% when older donors were used ($p < 0.001$); in these patients, vascular thrombosis was the cause of 40% of graft failure with "small" kidneys versus 9% with kidneys from older donors ($p < 0.001$). There was no significant difference in the rate of graft loss or thrombosis between donors under 2 years of age and those 2 to 5 years of age [5]. This excess graft loss appeared to occur within the first 3 months post-transplantation [3, 4, 8].

The relationship between the recipient age and graft survival is controversial: some authors have shown that it has no influence [4] whereas others have found a lower graft survival in recipients younger than 5 years of age [3, 5].

Urological complications

The urological complication rate in kidneys from donors 0–2 years of age is higher than with kidneys from adult donors, and consists mainly of ureteral fistulas [9].

Long-term consequences

It has been shown that the transplant kidney is capable of compensatory renal growth [10]. However, kidneys of very young children might be susceptible to focal glomerulosclerosis due to the small nephron mass, leading to hyperfiltration and overload nephropathy [11, 12]. This has been retrospectively studied by Hayes et al. who showed that, in adult recipients from donors aged less than 6 years, glomerulosclerosis was more frequent than in the control group (donors aged 7 or more) [12]. In addition, protein excretion and serum creatinine were significantly higher than in control patients at 13 ± 6 months post-transplant (1.60 ± 0.37 vs. 0.49 ± 0.15 g 24 h^{-1} and 173 ± 10 vs. 145 ± 8 µmol L^{-1}, $p < 0.03$ and $p < 0.01$, respectively).

On the other hand, it has been shown that the small size of the graft in pediatric cadaver recipients has no deleterious effect, since GFR improves more rapidly in those patients and reaches adjusted GFR comparable to patients who received a graft from cadaver donors of larger size [13].

The risk of arterial hypertension secondary to transplant artery stenosis is increased if very young donors are used and its treatment, either by percutaneous or by surgical procedure, is difficult.

Management of transplant patients with kidneys from young donors

Even if the risk of early graft loss and long-term complications is increased, kidneys from young donors may work in a large number of patients, so that it is difficult to refuse them routinely.

The optimal use of these organs first includes a good matching and a short ischaemia time. Moreover, recipients should be selected in an age range of 5 to 12 years, since the young age of the recipient (i.e. under 5 years) might have deleterious effects and, on the other hand, it may be argued that it is unreasonable to use a small renal mass for a large adult recipient [8, 11].

There have been several reports on the appropriate procedures to be used for transplantation of kidneys from very young donors. In order to minimize ureteral and vascular damage, attention must be paid to careful harvesting [9]. The en-bloc technique allows good results with donors less than 1 year of age despite a significant risk of thrombosis [14].

The overall risk of vascular thrombosis should be lowered by maintaining stable haemodynamic conditions at the early postoperative period. The prophylactic use of a low molecular weight heparin has significantly decreased the frequency of such thromboses. If the donor is less than 5 years of age, it seems appropriate to begin this treatment before surgery (for example nadroparine, 50 IU anti-Xa kg^{-1} 24 h^{-1}, i.e. 0.05 ml 10 kg^{-1} day^{-1}).

Conclusion

The rapidly widening gap between the number of patients awaiting kidney transplants and the availability of donor organs has prompted many centres to reevaluate kidney transplantation from pediatric donors. There have been a few reports of successful transplantation of kidneys from young donors [15]; on the other hand, because of the high risk of graft failure, some authors have advised against the use of kidneys from donors under 6 years of age [3]. Data obtained from large series suggest that 4 to 6 years is the "safe age" above which graft survival can be expected to be consistently good [5, 6, 12, 16]. However, the use of donors less than 5 years of age should be revisited on the basis of adapted strategies (low molecular weight heparin, en-bloc technique, etc.) in order to improve organ harvesting.

References

1. Hewmon DA, Capron AM, Peacock WJ, Schulman BL. The use of anencephalic infants as organ sources. J Am Med Assoc 1989; 261: 1773–81.
2. Floret D. Prélèvements d'organes en pédiatrie. Pédiatrie 1993; 48(suppl 1): 15s–17s.
3. Ruder H, Schaefer F, Gretz N, et al. Donor kidneys of infants and very young children are unacceptable for transplantation. Lancet 1989; ii: 168.
4. Harmon WE, Alexander SR, Tejani A, et al. The effect of donor age on graft survival in

pediatric cadaver renal transplant recipients: a report of the North American Pediatric Renal Transplant Cooperative Study. Transplantation 1992; 57: 232–7.

5. Gagnadoux MF, Niaudet P, Broyer M. Non-immunological risk factors in pediatric renal transplantation. Pediatr Nephrol 1993; 7: 89–95.

6. Ettenger RB. Improving the utilization of cadaver kidneys in children. Kidney Int 1993; 44(suppl 43): S99–S103.

7. The Medical Task Force on Anencephaly. The infant with anencephaly. N Engl J Med 1990; 332: 669–72.

8. Harmon WE, Jabs K. Special issues in pediatric renal transplantation. Semin Nephrol 1992; 12: 353–63.

9. Hayes JM, Novick AC, Streem SB, et al. The use of single pediatric cadaver kidneys for transplantation. Transplantation 1988; 45: 106–10.

10. Provoost AP, de Keijzer MH, Kort WJ, et al. The influence of the recipient upon renal function after isogeneic kidney transplantation in the rat. Transplantation 1984; 37: 55–62.

11. Leunissen KML, Kootstra G, Bosman FT, van Hoof JP. Focal glomerulosclerosis in neonatal kidney grafts. Lancet 1987; ii: 1019–20.

12. Hayes JM, Steinmuller DR, Streem SB, Novick AC. The development of proteinuria and focal-segmental glomerulosclerosis in recipients of pediatric donor kidneys. Transplantation 1991; 52: 813–7.

13. Dubourg L. Evolution de la fonction rénale après transplantation de rein chez l'enfant. Medicine Thesis, Lyon, 1994.

14. Ratner LE, Flye MW. Successful transplantation of cadaveric en-bloc paired pediatric kidneys into adult recipients. Transplantation 1991; 51: 273–5.

15. Hudnall CH, Hodge EE, Centeno AS, et al. Evaluation of pediatric cadaver kidneys transplanted into adult recipients receiving cyclosporine. J Urol 1989; 142: 1181–5.

16. So SKS, Gillingham K, Cook M, et al. The use of cadaver kidneys for transplantation in young children. Transplantation 1990; 50: 979–83.

16. Organ procurement from cadaveric children

H. NIVET, CH. CHELIAKINE, S. BENOIT, G. DESCHÊNES,
Y. LEBRANCHU & THE TEAMS OF HÔPITAL G. DE
CLOCHEVILLE

Remarkable progress in organ transplantation has led to a dramatic rise in the demand for organs both in adults and children. All pediatric intensive care units (PICUs) are involved in harvesting organs, nevertheless, organs are collected from a limited number of potential donors. This situation is more a problem of organisation, willingness and ethics than one of techniques.

The number of transplantations decreased in France from 1991 to 1993. This decrease demonstrates the fragility of a situation that needs parental consent and is, therefore, dependent on the opinion of the general population.

The questions concerning organ procurement from cadaveric children are:

- Are organ numbers sufficient for pediatric requirements?
- Are organs from cadaveric children usable for adults?
- What are the current problems for harvesting organs from brain dead children?

Are organ numbers sufficient for pediatric requirements?

In France, the 190 children transplanted in 1993 represent 5.97% of the total transplantations (France Transplant 1993a; Rapport France Transplant 1993). Organs from 73 brain dead children were harvested, representing 7.5% of the total number of brain dead victims from whom organs were harvested. Although 190 children were operated on for transplantation, 222 organs were transplanted since some children were grafted twice in the same year. The numbers of organs transplanted in children were: 94 kidneys, 93 livers, 23 hearts, 8 lungs and 4 hearts and lungs.

The percentages of children transplanted (France Transplant 1993b) in the first 12 months after being placed on a waiting list were: hearts, 100%; kidneys, 86%; lungs, 83%; livers, 80%; and hearts and lungs, 67%. Comparison with adult data (Figure 1) shows earlier transplantation of hearts and

J.L. Touraine et al. (eds.), *Organ Shortage: The Solutions*, 103–109.

Percentages

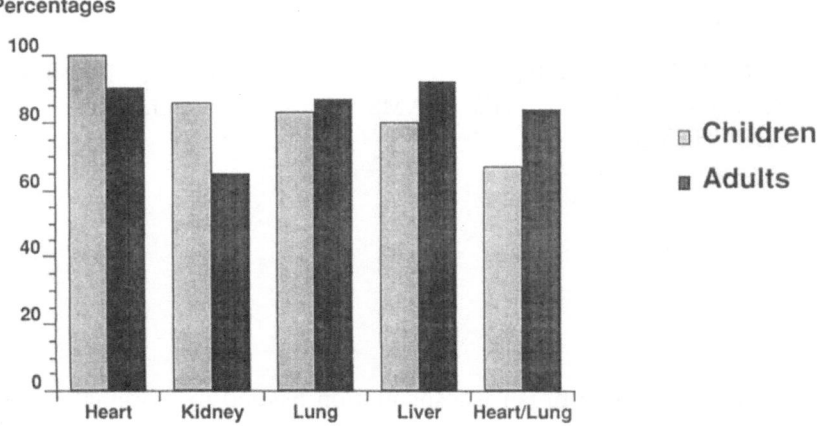

Fig. 1. Adults and children transplanted over a period of 12 months (France Transplant data 1993).

kidneys than lungs, livers, and hearts/lungs. The organs harvested from the 73 brain dead children were sufficient for hearts and kidneys but inadequate for liver, lung and heart/lung transplantations because of the need for appropriate size organs.

Are organs from cadaveric children usable for adults?

Organs from children are used in most countries first for other children and then for adults if there are no child recipients. However, some brain dead children are not harvested for livers, hearts or lungs because there is no appropriate recipient on the harvesting day. Most often organ size is given as the reason.

Transplantation of children's organs into adult recipients works as long as the size is concordant (Gruessner et al. 1990; Spees et al. 1990; Tellis et al. 1990). There is no consensus about small pediatric cadaver kidneys transplanted both in adults and children, but some results are encouraging (Merkel and Matalon 1990). Progress is needed because kidneys harvested from infants aged less than 2 years are often refused by transplantation units. Thoracic organs must be of an adequate size, but livers from young children can be used in adults if the liver weight is over 300 g. Pediatric livers weighing less than 300 g could be used as temporary auxiliary organs in cases of fulminant hepatitis.

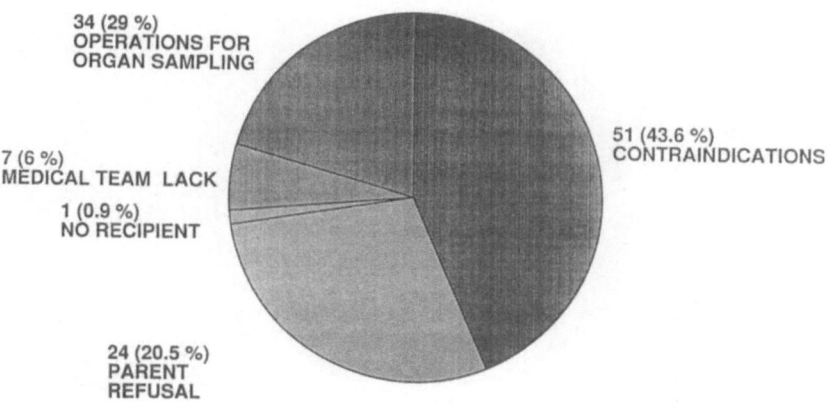

34 (29 %)
OPERATIONS FOR
ORGAN SAMPLING

7 (6 %)
MEDICAL TEAM LACK

1 (0.9 %)
NO RECIPIENT

51 (43.6 %)
CONTRAINDICATIONS

24 (20.5 %)
PARENT
REFUSAL

Fig. 2. 117 Brain dead children from 1980 to 1993 (Pediatric Intensive Care Unit, Tours, France).

What are the current problems for harvesting organs from brain dead children?

All PICUs are potentially able to provide organs for harvesting. Children's hospitals without PICUs could send brain dead children to a PICU for organ retrieval.

The definition of brain death raises some specific problems in pediatrics. Anencephalic newborns, for whom there is no unanimity regarding organ harvesting, are not harvested in France. A further problem is the electroencephalogram, which is flat in certain conditions in newborns. Later reactivity leads to a more difficult diagnosis of brain death at this age (Alvarez et al. 1988). In addition, birth accidents at delivery sometimes lead to the destruction of cortex with an undamaged brain stem leading to a vegetative state. No country allows organ retrieval in this situation.

Selection of brain dead children for organ retrieval is no longer a problem since the contraindications have been well defined. The skills and knowledge required for participation in harvesting organs are well known and regularly published (Cheliakine et al. 1992; Nivet 1989).

Parental consent is one of the main obstacles. The highly emotional circumstances under which such requests are made make it very difficult for both families and staff to communicate about donation (Nivet et al. 1988). In France, medical staff in the intensive care unit involved in the care of brain dead patients must be different from staff dealing with the transplantation.

Administration is now well established in many countries but the law must be strictly applied.

Ethical and policy issues have been established by the Council of National and International Transplantation Societies, who have published guidelines

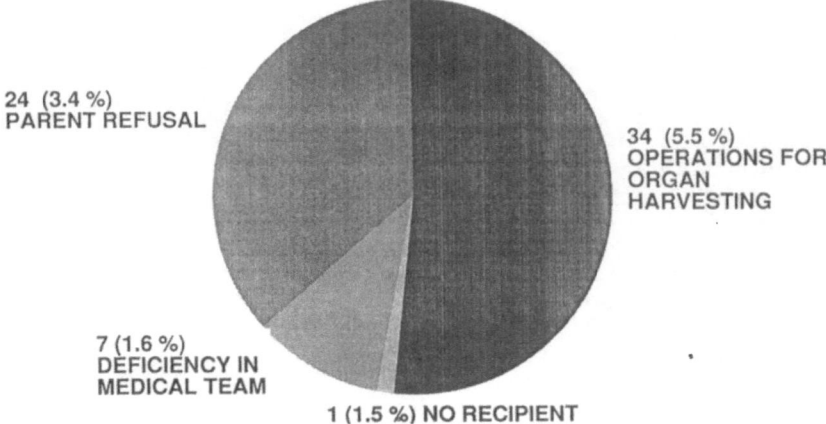

Fig. 3. 66 Brain dead children without contraindications for organ harvesting from 1980 to 1993 (Pediatric Intensive Care Unit, Tours, France).

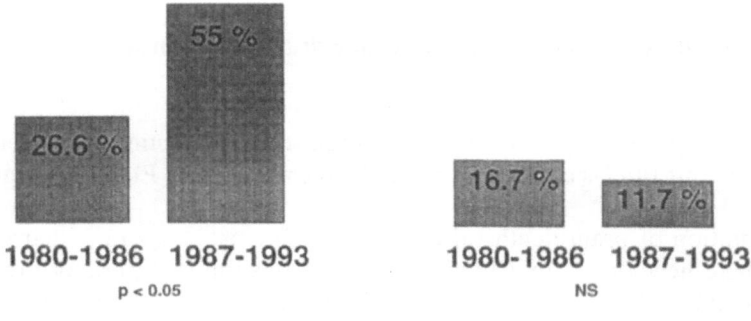

Fig. 4. Evolution of parental refusal and motivation of medical team in the PICU of Tours (France).

for cadaver organ distribution, generally with a priority for children as organ recipients.

The experience of the Universitary Hospital of Tours (France) has emphasized the problems in an area covering 2 million people. From 1980 to 1993, 117 brain dead children were admitted (Figure 2). There were 43.6% with contraindications for organ retrieval, 20.5% with parents' refusal, 6% who were not harvested because of a deficiency of the medical team, 0.9% (representing one child) had no recipient (AB blood group) and 29% were operated on for organ harvesting. During this period there were enough organs for actual recipients in the region; there were 34 donors for the 55 kidneys, 4 livers, and 5 hearts grafted.

Studying the same series of brain dead children, but without the contra-

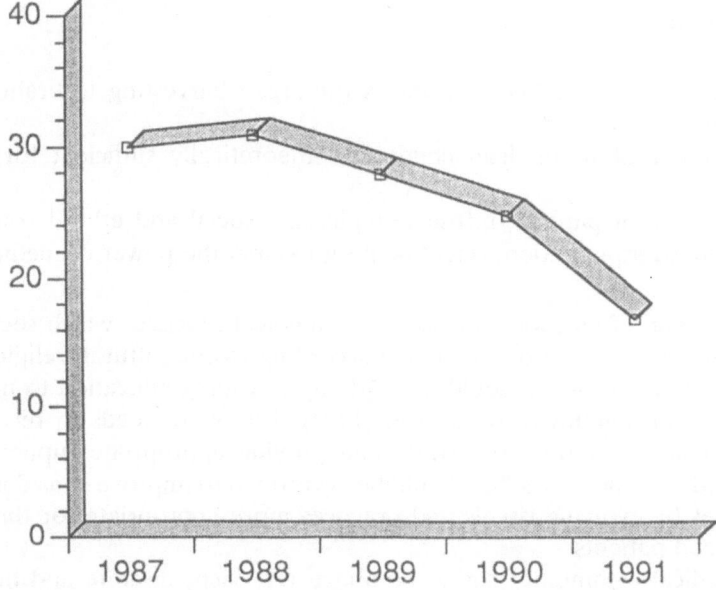

Fig. 5. Pediatric intensive care units (PICU) supplying data concerning deceased children for a multicenter investigation (Foret D, Lyon, 1993).

indications (Figure 3) is a better way to study the true obstacles. In fact, when we organized organ retrieval in 51.5% of brain dead children without contraindications, medical team deficiency was the obstacle in 10.6% and parents' refusal in 36.4%. This, of course, is the major obstacle for organ harvesting.

The trend is not optimistic, since parents' refusals increased from 26.6% to 55% from 1980 to 1986, compared with 1987 to 1993 (Figure 4).

In the same period, "deficiency of medical team" decreased from 16.7% to 11.7%. Medical teams must remain motivated. The heavy workload in PICUs limits the time available for non-urgent activities. The decrease in the number of answers to a multicenter investigation (Floret 1993) concerning deceased children demonstrated this fact (Figure 5).

The dramatic increase in parental refusal is the main problem. It is difficult to list all the reasons, but we can speculate on:

– multiorgan removal, which is a mutilating procedure;
– reports of organ trafficking in the world (Pinero 1992);
– confusion with AIDS and legal action concerning blood;
– action against physicians concerning transplantation;
– media and advertising which emphazise all these points;
– and, finally, a lack of confidence in medicine and doctors.

In conclusion:

- There are no real medical obstacles for organ harvesting in brain dead children.
- The number of brain dead children is theoretically sufficient for child recipients.
- The increase in parents' refusals emphasizes social and ethical concerns regarding transplantation, scientific progress and the power of medicine.

In fact, none of us chose this aspect of medical practice, which seems to violate a general respect of the person according to our cultural, religious or moral traditions. Progress could be made by providing education to nurses, physicians and families (Morris et al. 1992). Everyone needs to recognize the legitimacy of emotional distress and provide appropriate support, for himself and for others. Studies should be performed to improve consideration for families by evolving rituals and practices more appropriate for this new class of dead patients.

The medical community has to be above reproach, discrete and humble to recover the confidence of families.

Acknowledgements

We thank D. Raine for assistance in editing the English.

References

1. Alvarez L, Moshe S, Belman A, Maylal J, Mesnverk T, Keilson M. EEG and brain death determination in children. Neurology 1988; 38: 227–30.
2. Cheliakine Ch, Suc AL, Godde F, Nivet H. Réanimation de l'enfant en état de mort cérébrale. In: Nivet H, editor. Les prélèvements d'organes pour la transplantation. Paris: Doin Ed, 1992: 7–94.
3. Floret D. Prélèvements d'organes en pédiatrie. Pédiatrie 1993; 48(suppl 1): 15s–7s.
4. France Transplant. Paris: Hôpital Saint Louis, chiffres 1993a: 11.
5. France Transplant (Pédiatrie et évolution des greffes). Paris: Hôpital Saint Louis, chiffres 1993b.
6. Gruessner RWG, Matas AJ, Dunn DL, Kiovera G, Payne WD, Sutherland DER, Najarian JS. A comparison of pediatric versus adult cadaver donor kidneys for transplantation. Transplant Proc 1990; 20: 361–2.
7. Merkel FK, Matalon TAS. An en bloc method for use of small pediatric cadaver kidneys in adult recipients. Transplant Proc 1990; 20: 405–6.
8. Morris JA, Wilcox TR, Frist WH. Pediatric organ donation: the paradox of organ shortage despite the remarkable willingness of families to donate. Pediatrics 1992; 89: 411–5.
9. Nivet H. Harvesting organs for pediatric transplantation. Intensive Care Med 1989; 15.
10. Nivet H, Saliba E, Lacombe A, Nashishibi M, Lebranchu Y, Laugier J. Les prélèvements d'organes chez l'enfant. Arch Fr Pediatr 1988; 45: 699–702.

11. Pinero M. Enlèvements d'enfants et trafic d'organes. Le Monde Diplomatique 1992(août): 16–7.
12. Rapport France Transplant. Paris: Hôpital St Louis, 1993: 9.
13. Spees EK, Orlowski JP, Kam I, Karrer F, Dunn SM. Are pediatric donors well utilized? Transplant Proc 1990; 20: 359–60.
14. Tellis WA, Greenstein SM, Schechner RS, Glicklich. Pediatric donors: still successful in adults. Transplant Proc 1990; 20: 363–4.

17. Influence of donor age on the result of heart transplantation

G. DUREAU, J.P. GARE, M. CHUZEL, O. JEGADEN,
J.F. OBADIA, J.F. CHASSIGNOLLE & P. MIKAELOFF

Introduction

In the pioneering era of heart transplantation, an age limit of 50 years was established for the recipient of a heart transplant. This was mainly due to the weight of the steroids in conventional immunosuppressive therapy. The introduction of Cyclosporin allowed the extension of this selection criteria and several authors (Carrier et al. 1986; Miller et al. 1988; Frazier et al. 1988) have reported satisfactory results in patients over 55 years of age; they found identical survival rates, reduced rejection rates (Renlund et al. 1987) and identical rates of infection.

Therefore, an increasing percentage of "old" recipients are accepted on waiting lists, resulting in prolonged delays before transplantation. By lengthening this waiting period, as many as 20 to 25% of patients die prior to transplantation (McManus et al. 1993), decreasing the therapeutic efficacy of transplantation in a population who require it.

This evolution in the recipient's age was not paralleled with an evolution in the donor's age. Primary failure of the graft still represents a major cause of death in heart transplant patients (Kaye 1933) and long-term survival is compromised by a coronaropathy, which is traditionally linked with age. Thus, the tendency was to favor young hearts for transplantation, the ideal procedure using a donor younger than the recipient.

In an attempt to overcome organ shortage, some authors (Menkis et al. 1991) suggest accepting older hearts. Others (Mulvagh et al. 1989; Reichart 1992; Renlund et al. 1987; Schuler et al. 1989) did not find differences in function or development of coronaropathy when aged donors are used. Meanwhile, other centers continue to consider 45 years the maximum age for a donor, thus limiting their acceptance policy to cope with the needs of younger recipients.

If we are not reluctant in grafting an organ equal in age to the age of the patient, the question arises whether or not it would be better to use a younger heart. Conversely, it may appear unethical to transplant a heart older than the patient's original one.

J.L. Touraine et al. (eds.), *Organ Shortage: The Solutions*, 111–119.
© 1995 *Kluwer Academic Publishers*.

Table 1. Characteristics of the population

	No.	SD
Total transplantations	275	
Recipient gender (M/F)	236/39	
Recipient age (mean)	51.8	10.9
Donor gender (M/F)	193/82	
Donor age (mean)	34.6	11.8
Ischemic time (mean) (in minutes)	246.7	105.1
	No.	%
Preoperative diagnosis		
Ischemic heart disease	91	33.1
Cardiomyopathy	119	43.3
Valvular heart disease	32	11.6
Others	12	4.4
Retransplantation	21	7.6

To answer these questions, we retrospectively analysed the results of heart transplantation in our group from 1988, when we started using older donors, up to 1993, comparing immediate and long-term results when young donors and old donors were used. As old donors were mainly used in young recipients in emergency situations, the influence of this parameter was also quoted in order to avoid a bias in our study.

Patients

Recipients

Between January 1988 and December 1993, 275 orthotopic heart transplantations were performed in our institution, in 254 patients with 21 retransplantations. There were 236 (85.8%) males and 39 females, aged 13.5 to 68.5 years (mean 51.8 ± 10.9 years) (Table 1). Of these, 71 (25.8%) patients were 60 years of age or older ("old recipient"), and 204 (74.2%) were aged 13.5 to 60 ("young recipient"). The breakdown of recipients' ages is shown in Table 2.

Emergency status of the recipient, defined by dependence on adrenergic support or mechanical ventilatory-circulatory assistance, occurred in 53 patients (19%).

The main indications for heart transplantation were end-stage ischemic heart disease in 91 patients, dilated cardiomyopathy in 119 patients, valvular disease in 32, other causes in 12, and retransplantations in 21 patients.

Table 2. Recipient's age

Age in years	Number	Percent
0–10	0	0
10–20	4	1.4
20–30	9	3.3
30–40	31	11.3
40–50	50	18.2
50–60	110	40.0
60–70	71	25.8

Table 3. Donor's age

Age in years	Number	Percent
0–10	0	0
10–20	31	11.6
20–30	65	24.5
30–40	73	27.2
40–50	65	24.2
50–60	31	11.6
60–70	3	1.1

Table 4. Number of patients in groups

Groups	No. of patients	Percent
Group I: young donors/young recipients	173	62.9
Group II: young donors/old recipients	41	14.9
Group III: old donors/young recipients	31	11.3
Group IV: old donors/old recipients	30	10.9

Donors

There were 275 donors – 193 male, 82 female – aged 13 to 68 years (means 34.6 ± 11.8). The breakdown of donors' ages is shown in Table 3. Sixty-one were older then 45 years ("old donors") and 207 were considered "young donors".

Donor-recipient matching

The donor-recipient matching was divided into four groups (Table 4).

– Group I: young donors/young recipients
– Group II: young donors/old recipients
– Group III: old donors/young recipients
– Group IV: old donors/old recipients

Table 5. Gender, weight and adrenergic support for the 4 groups

| Groups | Gender | | Weight (Kg) | | |
	Recipient	Donor	Recipient	Donor	Adrenergic support (%)
Group I	86.1	79.2	68.3	67.9	8.7
Group II	87.8	56.4	68.2	66.7	4.9
Group III	87.1	58.1	70.0	68.3	12.9
Group IV	80.0	56.4	68.4	68.4	3.3
	NS	$p = 0.001$	NS	NS	NS

All transplantations were done in isogroup ABO according to "France Transplant" regulations.

Methods

Clinical status at the time of transplantation, degree of emergency, pulmonary resistances, ischemic time, occurrence of myocardial infarction or graft lost, and one-year and five-year survival were studied. We studied the survival rate of the graft because of inclusion of patients who underwent retransplantation. All patients were transplanted according to Shumway's technique (Lower et al. 1965) and received the same triple immunosuppressive therapy.

Statistical analysis

Data are expressed as mean values ± standard deviation. Differences in continuous variables were compared using χ^2 tests (Fisher exact test if necessary). Actuarial survival curves were calculated by life-table method and compared by log-rank test. Values of less then 0.05 were considered significant.

Results

The recipient's gender, weight of the recipient and donor, the donor's adrenergic support, pulmonary vascular resistances, and ischemic time appeared equally divided among the 4 groups. Recipient's emergency status, indication for transplantation and donor gender were statistically different, with more ischemic disease in old recipients and more male donors in group I (young donor/young recipient) (Tables 5–7).

The overall survival rate was 70% at one year and, at 5 years, was approaching 60% (Figure 1). One- and five-year survival rates were not statistically different for young and old recipients (Figure 2) nor for young and old

Table 6. Emergency status, pulmonary resistances and ischemic time for the 4 groups

Groups	Emergency status (%)	Pulmonary resistances dyns/cm^{-5}/sec	Ischemic time (min)
Group I	19.9	228.1	235.6
Group II	7.9	216.8	280.0
Group III	35.5	227.6	240.5
Group IV	20.0	230.5	271.0
	$p = 0.04$	NS	NS

Table 7. Primary heart disease

Groups	Dilatative cardiomyopathy (%)	Ischemic heart disease (%)	Valvular (%)	Retransplant (%)
Group I	48.0	26.6	9.2	11.0
Group II	39.0	43.9	12.2	4.9
Group III	35.5	35.5	19.4	0
Group IV	30.0	53.3	16.7	0

$p = 0.003$ for all categories.

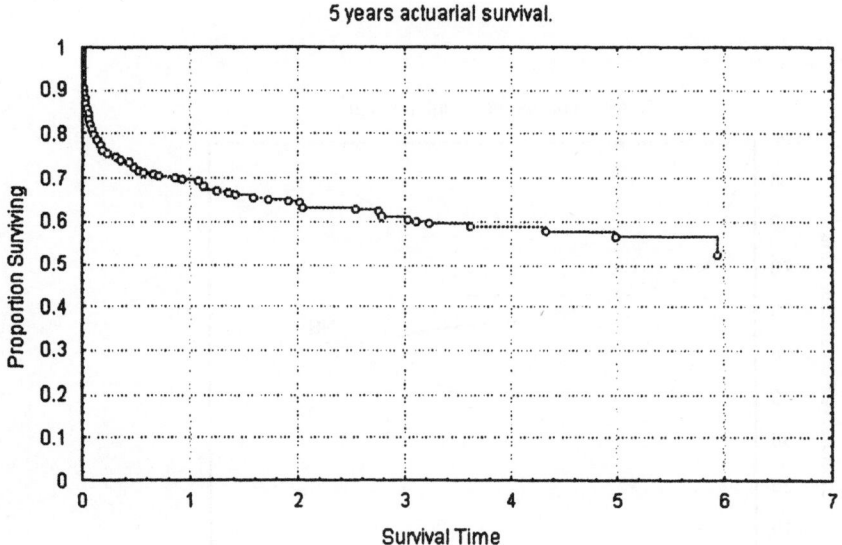

Fig. 1. Five years acuarial survival.

donors (Figure 3). Survival was not statistically different for initial pathology. However, there was a highly significant decrease in survival in the population transplanted in emergency situations (Figure 4).

When considering age-mismatched transplantation, there is a 10% de-

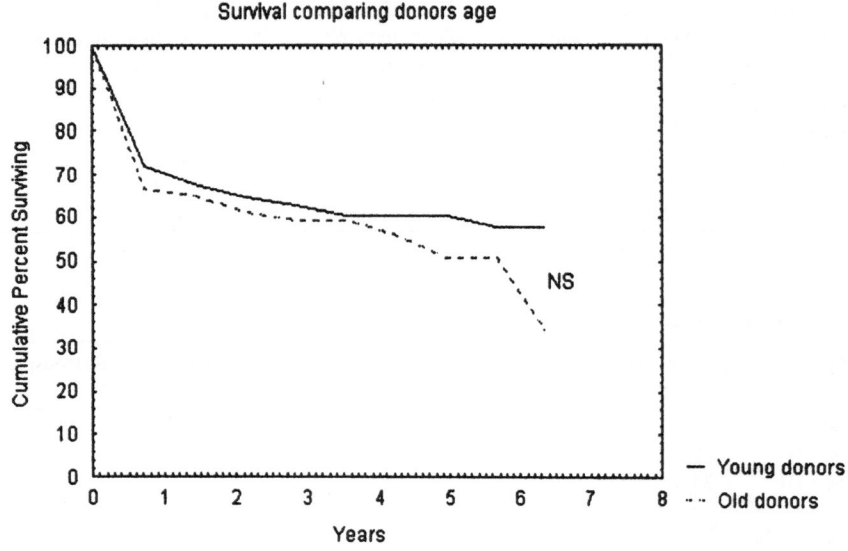

Fig. 2. Survival comparing donor age.

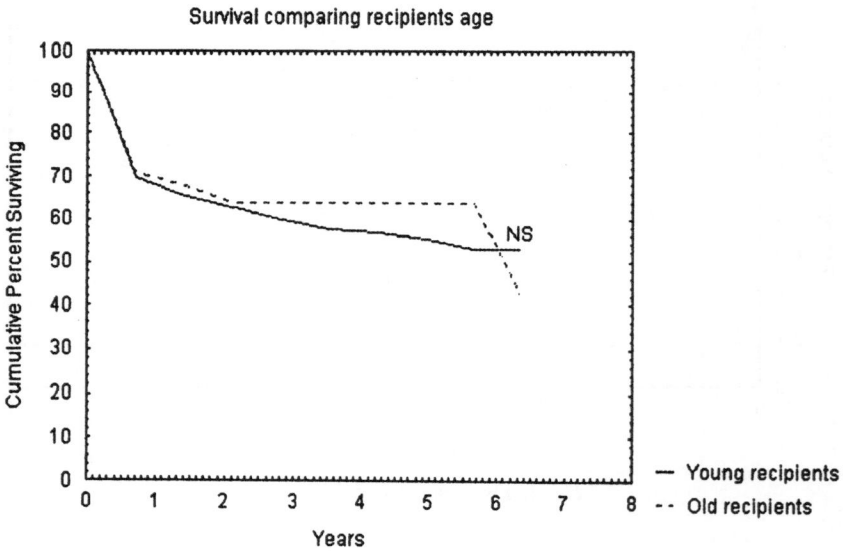

Fig. 3. Survival comparing recipient age.

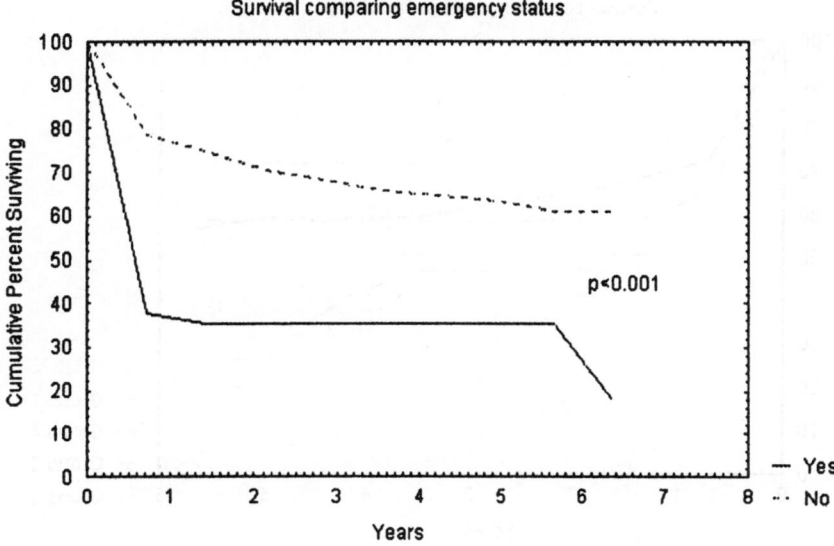

Fig. 4. Survival comparing emergency status.

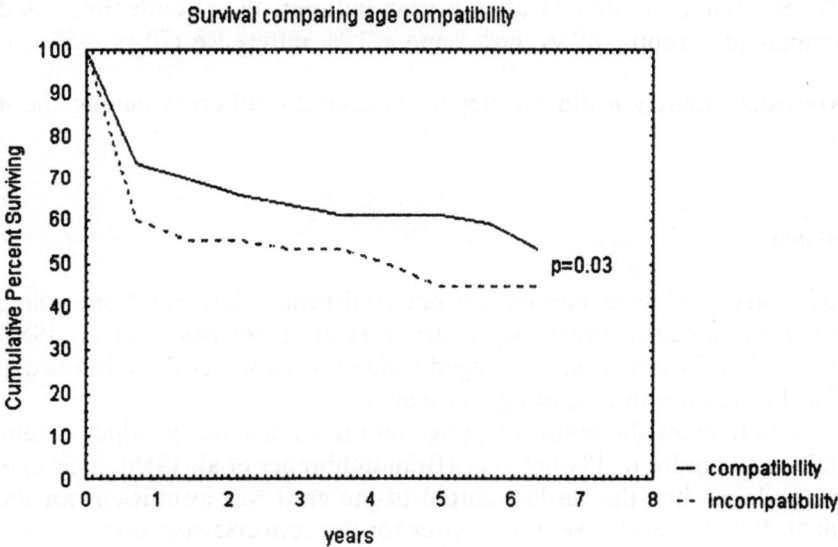

Fig. 5. Survival comparing age compatibility.

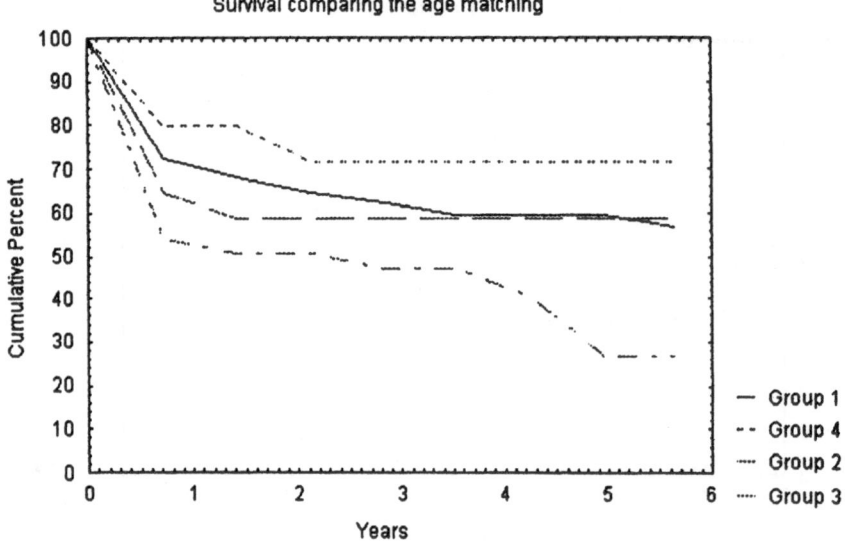

Fig. 6. Survival comparing age matching.

crease in the survival rate ($p < 0.05$) at 1 and 5 years (Figure 5). Split analysis of the 4 groups (Figure 6) confirmed this notion of age "compatibility" with a 25% difference in survival at one year between the "compatible" and "incompatible" groups (85 vs. 60%) and a 35% difference (70 vs. 45%) at 5 years.

Myocardial infarction did not appear statistically different among the 4 groups.

Discussion

Survival curves of aged donors are not statistically different from young donors and, as shown previously (Carrier et al. 1986; Miller et al. 1988; Frazier et al. 1988), for young and aged recipients. However there is a strong statistical difference in case of age mismatch.

We already know the influence of age on the cardiac index, which results in a fall on the order of 1% per year (Brandfonbrener et al. 1955). This may explain failure when the cardiac output of the graft was insufficient for the recipient, but the results were not better for the converse situation.

We may explain this paradox by considering the results of oversized hearts in pediatric transplantation, which result in hypertension, coma and general convulsion (Reichart 1992). We experienced 5 cerebral hemorrhages in our experience among the population of elderly recipients transplanted with young hearts and, also, hypertension was often difficult to control.

It should be emphasized that the best survival curve was obtained with young donors/young recipients followed by old donors/old recipients.

These results validate the concept of age compatibility in the matching of donor and recipient. They support heart transplantation in elderly patients with a normal life expectancy, using older donors, thereby sparing the younger heart for younger recipients.

References

1. Brandfonbrener M, Landowne M, Shock NN. Changes in cardiac output with age. Circulation 1955; 12: 557.
2. Carrier M, Emery RW, Riley JE, Levinson MM, Copeland JC. Cardiac transplantation in patients over 50 years of age. J Amer Coll Cardiol 1986; 8: 285–8.
3. Frazier OH, Macris PL, Duncan JM, Vanburen CT, Cooley DA. Cardiac transplantation in patients over 60 years of age. Thorac Surg 1988; 45: 129–32.
4. Kaye M. The registry of the International Society for Heart and Lung transplantations: tenth official report. J Heart Lung Transplant 1993; 12: 541–8.
5. Lower RR, Dong E, Shumway NE. Long-term survival of cardiac homografts. 1965; 58: 110–9.
6. McManus RP, O'Hair DP, Beitzinger JM, et al. Patients who die awaiting heart transplantation. J Heart Lung Transplant 1993; 12: 159–72.
7. Menkis AH, Novick JR, Kostuk WJ, et al. Successful use of the "unacceptable" heart donor. J Heart Surg Transplant 1991; 10: 28–32.
8. Miller LW, Vitale-Noedel N, Pennington DG, Mc Bride L, Kanter KR. Heart transplantation in patients over age 55 years. J Heart Transplant 1988; 7: 254–7.
9. Mulvagh SL, Thornton B, Frazier H. The older cardiac transplant donor: relation to graft function and recipients survival longer than 6 years. Circulation 1989; 80(suppl III): 126–32.
10. Reichart B. Size matching in heart transplantation. J Heart Lung Transplant 1992; 11(suppl): 199–202.
11. Renlund DG, Gilbert EM, O'CONNEL JB, et al. Age associated decline in cardiac allograft rejection. Amer J Med 1987; 83: 391–8.
12. Schuler S, Warnecke H, Loebe M, et al. Extended donor age in cardiac transplantation. Circulation 1989; 80(suppl III): 133–9.

18. Results of kidney transplantation using high risk donors

D. CANTAROVICH, M. GIRAL, M. HOURMANT, J. DANTAL,
G. BLANCHO, G. KARAM, J.N. LE SANT, P. DAGUIN &
J. P. SOULILLOU

Introduction

The limiting factor in renal transplantation today is the availability of organs. One way to increase the number of available organs is through the utilisation of "high risk" donors, for example, donors over 60 years old. In this report, we analyzed our single center experience with transplant kidneys from donors over 60 years old. The aim of the study was to evaluate the influence of donor age on the short- and long-term outcome of cadaveric kidney transplantation.

Patients and methods

Between July 1987 and May 1993, 34 kidneys from 25 cadaver donors over 60 years of age (4% of total kidneys transplanted) and 806 from cadaver donors less than 60 years of age were transplanted at our unit. The 25 elderly donors were Caucasian, 18 were men and 7 were women, their mean age was 63.4 years old (60 to 69), and 7 (28%) were over 65 years. Eleven kidneys were locally harvested and 14 were imported. The mean serum creatinine and blood urea before harvesting was 111 μmol l^{-1} (67–284) and 7.5 mmol l^{-1} (3–20), respectively. The mean last hour urine output was 233 ml (0–1000). Dopamine was given in 92% of cases and 28% of donors experienced a hemodynamic shock before harvesting. When technically and "practically" possible, a core renal biopsy was done at the time of harvesting. Kidneys with severe histological arteries lesions (malignant nephroangiosclerosis) were excluded for transplantation. Causes of brain death were CVA in 60% of cases, trauma in 32% and suicide in 8%.

In order to compare transplant survival and function, 90 kidneys from donors aged 50–59 years, 161 from 40–49, 206 from 30–39, 193 from 20–29, 109 from 10–19 and 47<10 years, transplanted during the same timer period, were analyzed and used as controls.

The mean age of the 34 recipients of elderly kidneys was 49.6 years (20–

J.L. Touraine et al. (eds.), Organ Shortage: The Solutions, 121–126.

67); 21 were over 50 years and 9 over 60 years. There were all Caucasian (22 men and 12 women). Retransplantation accounted for 5 cases and 82% of patients were on dialaysis at the time of transplantation. Causes of end-stage chronic renal failure were chronic glomerulonephritis in 12 cases, polysystic disease in 8, interstitial nephritis in 5, diabetes in 1, hypertension in 1, urological in 3 and unknown in 4.

All patients received cyclosporine (CsA) as maintenance immunosuppression (4.9 mg kg^{-1} day^{-1} at 3 months, 4.6 mg kg^{-1} day^{-1} at 6 months and 4.1 mg kg^{-1} day^{-1} at 1 year). In the majority of cases, ATG in association with azathioprine (Aza) and steroids were given before starting CsA. After the second postoperative month, steroids were discontinued and patients remained under CsA and Aza. Acute rejection episodes were treated with high doses of steroids (5, 5, 4, 3 and 2 mg kg^{-1} day^{-1} for consecutive days).

The mean cold ischemic time (CIT) was 36.4 hours (19–47). In 12% of cases, CIT was less than 24 hours, in 23% between 24 and 36 hours, and in 65% greater than 36 hours. Euro-Collins solution was used in 38% of cases, UW in 24% and UW-modified in 38%. Vascular anastomosis were done in 43.7 minutes (25–66).

Results

The incidence of delayed graft function was significantly higher in the group of recipients transplanted with elderly kidneys (>60 years). Post-transplant dialysis was required in 53% of cases (3.3 dialysis per patient). Hospitalisation time ranged from 10 to 90 days (mean 25). Three patients (37, 49 and 60 years-old, respectively) died (all with functional grafts) because of B-cell lymphoma (month 5), pneumonia (month 2) and ischemic colitis (month 5). The 60-month actuarial patient survival rate was 92% (Figure 1). In addition, 7 grafts were lost because of non-functional graft (1), vein thrombosis (1), rejections (4) and ureteral fistula (1). The 60-month actuarial graft survival rate was 70% (Figure 1).

The actuarial patient and graft survival rates, according to donor age, are illustrated in Figures 2 and 3. No statistical difference was observed in patient survival regarding donor age. In contrast, the lower graft survival was observed in patients transplanted with elderly (>60 years) and younger (<10 years) kidneys. At 60 months, however, the differences did not achieve statistical significance.

Regarding serum creatinine levels, the highest values were observed in recipients of elderly and younger kidneys (Table 1). However, serum creatinine and 24-hour creatinine clearance remained stable throughout follow-up in the elderly donor group (Table 2). Although one-year serum creatinine level did not differ between patients with and without ATN (Table 3), a statistically significant lower serum creatinine level was observed among patients with a CIT <24 hours (Table 4). The percentage of graft loss was

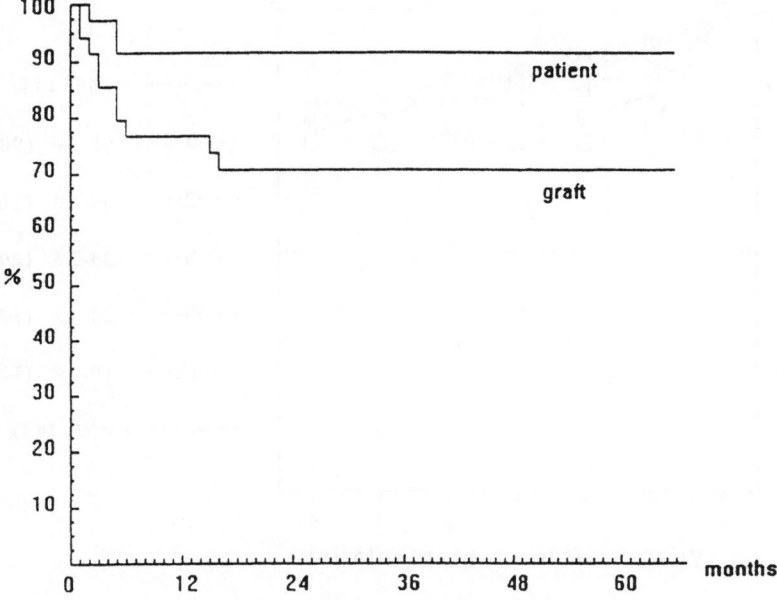

Fig. 1. Kaplan Meier patient and graft survival rates [donor age: 60 years and older].

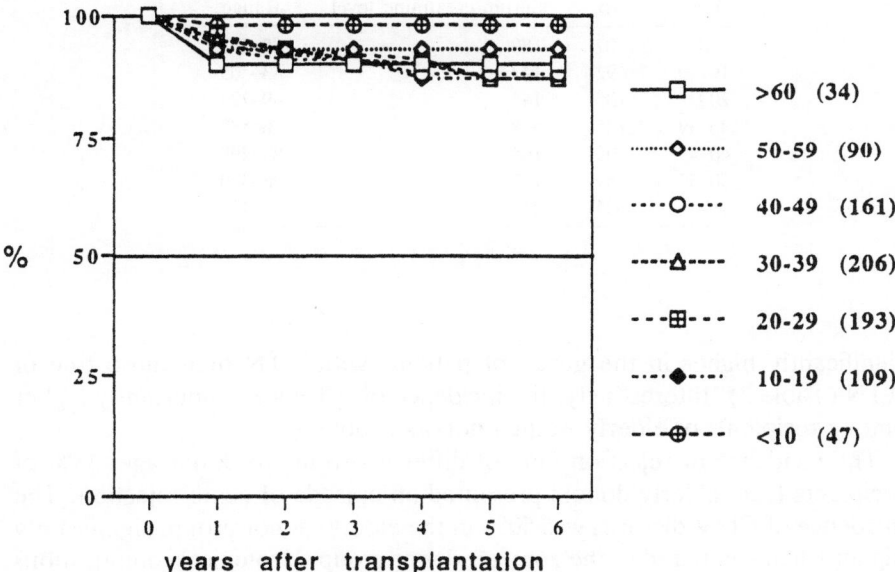

Fig. 2. Patient survival according to donor's age.

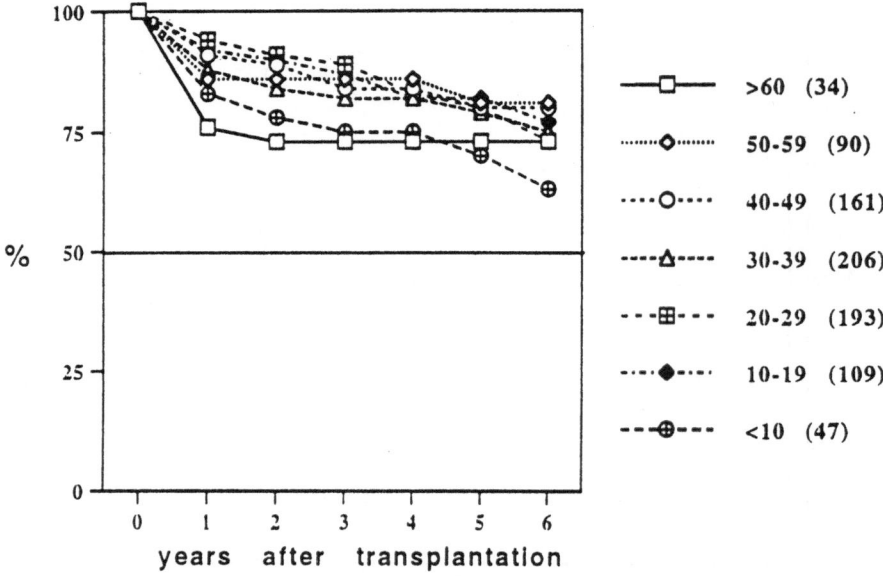

Fig. 3. Graft survival according to donor's age.

Table 1. One-year serum creatinine level according to donor age

Age	No.	Serum creatinine level	Range
<10	22	180	85–557
10–19	92	147	83–405
20–29	135	143	69–724
30–39	135	158	76–532
40–49	95	164	84–498
50–59	59	187	98–320
>60	24	211	83–414

significantly higher in the group of patients with ATN than those free of ATN (Table 3). Interestingly, the incidence of ATN was significantly higher among recipients of elderly women donors (Table 3).

The incidence of rejection did not differ according to donor age: 35% of recipients from elderly donors presented an episode of acute rejection. The incidence of CMV diseases was 50% in the elderly donor group, significantly higher when compared to the younger donor group. Urological complications were more numerous in the elderly donor group: 23.5% of patients required additional surgery because of ureteral fistulas. Finally, the incidence of hypertension and proteinuria did not differ according to donor age categories.

Table 2. Serum creatinine level (mmol l^{-1}) and 24-hour creatinine clearance (ml min^{-1})

Month	Creatinine	Clearance
3	198	42
6	200	41.6
12	211	41.5

Results are not statistically significant.

Table 3. ATN versus no ATN groups

	ATN	No ATN	X^2
Number	18	16	ns
Graft loss*	7	3	0.01
Rejection	8	4	ns
Creatinine (μmol/L)	242	199	ns
CMV	9	8	ns
Urinary fistula	4	4	ns
ATG duration	16	12	ns
Woman donor*	7	2	0.05
Man donor	11	14	ns
Woman recipient	6	6	ns
Man recipient	12	10	ns
Woman to man	5	2	ns
Woman to woman	2	0	

*Significantly higher among patients with ATN.

Table 4. 3-month serum creatinine level and cold ischemic time

CIT (hrs)	<24	24–36	>36
Creatinine*	153	204	203

*mmol l^{-1}; <24 vs. 24–36 and >36 $p<0.05$.

Table 5 shows the prevalence of hypertension and 24-hour proteinuria among the elderly donor group.

Discussion and conclusion

There have been several reports on older donor kidneys, and their utility for kidney transplant candidates. In 1981 JH Hong concluded: kidneys retrieved from the first and sixth or higher decades of donors fared significantly worse. In 1989, KML Leunissen concluded: one has to be aware of an exaggerated CsA toxicity in the older donor age group and in older patients treated with CsA. In 1990, KV Rao concluded: recipients of cadaver kidneys from older

Table 5. Incidence of hypertension and proteinuria

Month	Hypertension (%)	Proteinuria (%)	
		($>0.5 \, \mathrm{g \, d^{-1}}$)	($>1 \, \mathrm{g \, d^{-1}}$)
3	43	39	11
6	36	18	3.6
12	36	28	14

donors (>50 years) have lower graft survival and reduced post-transplant renal function. In 1991, P. Donnelly concluded: older donors are a valuable resource, but best used for older recipients. In 1992, S. Aswad concluded: older donors (>60 years) can be transplanted with excellent results. In the same year, JD Pirsh concluded: although donor age did not influence long-term graft survival, the use of younger and older kidneys was associated with slightly poorer graft survival. In 1993, A. Vianello concluded: kidneys from donors over 50 may be used, but they should probably be given to patients with a life expectation of no more than 10–15 years. Finally, L. Roels concluded in 1994; age itself should not be the sole criterion for exclusion of a potential kidney donor. Routine biopsy and age-corrected GFR assessments should be systematically done.

Our results showed that kidneys from donors over 60 years of age are not necessarily at greater risk, compared with the control groups. Donor kidneys should be considered on an individual basis. Age itself should not be the sole criteria for exclusion of a potential kidney donor. Whether older kidneys should be transplanted preferentially in older recipients its not clear. In our series, 23 and 11 of the recipients from elderly donors had, respectively, >5 or <5-year-old difference with their donor. The incidence of rejection and graft loss was similar in these two groups. In addition, when donor/recipient age difference was greater than 30 years (6 patients), again the incidence of rejection did not differ (33.3%) and 2 grafts were lost because of urinary fistula and acute rejection.

Efforts should be made to reduce post-transplant ATN. Graft loss was much more frequent in patients with, than without ATN. Long CIT seems to influence ATN. From the 18 patients with ATN, 13 were transplanted with more than 36 hours of CIT and 5 with less than 36 hours ($p < 0.007$). In addition, significantly better serum creatinine level was observed in patients transplanted with less than 24 hours of CIT. To improve results, it could be suggested to reduce the CIT to less than 24 hours when a elderly kidney is available. Furthermore, efforts should also be made to prevent ATN, especially when a female kidney donor over 60 years of age is accepted for transplantation.

19. Anesthesia and resuscitation of the genetically related living donor in liver transplantation

D. GILLE, O. BOILLOT, M. C. GRABER, P. SAGNARD, C. BAUDE, B. CHABROL, C. KOPP, D. LONG, B. DELAFOSSE & G. BAGOU

Introduction

In view of recent results, liver transplantation has become a therapeutic method proposed for an increasing number of adult and children patients affected with lethal liver disease. Consequently, there is a discrepancy between the availability of grafts from cadaveric donors and the number of waiting recipients, many of whom are at high risk of impending death, especially children.

Despite development of various technical solutions designed to increase the number of grafts available for children (such as size reduction of split adult cadaveric livers), a relatively high shortage of available organs still existed. As early as 1989 (in Brazil and Australia), this situation led to the use of livers from genetically related living donors. Due to the very low surgical risk during hepatectomy performed on non-cirrhotic livers, the concept of harvesting partial liver grafts from liver donors gained approval from several medical ethics committees. This procedure has been performed in our transplantation unit since 1992.

We describe here the anesthetic procedure used in our hospital, as well as the pre-, intra- and postoperative management, offering optimal physical and psychological safety.

Methodology

Selection of genetically-related donors

When parents request the transplant team to perform a liver transplantation on their child, using the liver from a living donor, the feasibility of the procedure should be established after a thorough medical and psychological evaluation of the donor. Pre-anesthetic patient assessment should include all the criteria required prior to any hepatic surgery: personal history, clinical examination, non-invasive exploration of hepatic, renal, cardiac and pulmon-

J.L. Touraine et al. (eds.), *Organ Shortage: The Solutions*, 127–131.
© 1995 *Kluwer Academic Publishers.*

ary functions, and biological parameters. Some additional particular data may be taken into account to protect the donor from predictable operative and postoperative complications.

To be selected, a donor should be free of any physical or psychic ailments, i.e. rated ASA 1, according to the classification of the American Society of Anesthesiologists. We think that obesity and heavy smoking are high-risk factors, since they are known sources of postoperative complications such as infections and respiratory and thromboembolic complications. Regarding female donors, we make sure they are not pregnant and that they do not take estrogen-progestogen drugs; if they do, we discontinue the procedure.

Donor management

Donor management and the anesthetic technique chosen are determined by the need for optimal safety and depend on the nature of the surgery performed: left lateral segmentectomy or left hepatectomy, which is carried out without clamping the hepatic pedicle, is a procedure with a limited, though not negligible risk of bleeding.

The risk of viral disease transmission associated with exogenous transfusions is avoided by the use of methods combining normal blood volume hemodilution with two methods of autologous transfusion: autotransfusion planned 3 weeks to one month before surgery – including collection of packed RBCs, fresh frozen plasma and platelet concentrates – and intraoperative autotransfusion using a "Cell Saver" system.

Prevention of the thromboembolic risk is initiated twelve hours before surgery by the administration of a suitable minimum dose of low molecular weight heparin and the treatment is then protracted for a month. Screening tests for venous thromboses, based on the level variation of d-dimers (biological markers of coagulation), make it possible to control the degree of decoagulation and prompt the clinician when he should to perform specific investigations for incipient thromboses.

Short prophylactic antibiotic therapy is included in the protocol.

When deemed necessary, vaccination against hepatitis B is performed.

Anxiolytic and amnestic premedication, combining benzodiazepine with hydroxyzine at suitable doses, is administered orally during the evening of the day before surgery and, again, two hours before patient installation in the operating suite.

Anesthetic technique

The usual method for liver surgery, general anesthesia, is also the method of choice in this particular procedure where organ removal is limited either to one lobe (segments II and III) or to left hepatectomy (trisegmentectomy: II, III and IV). This anesthesia is both deep and easy to control, and offers the patient maximum comfort.

Hepatic surgery requires the use of powerful analgesics, capable of suppressing both pain and the main nociceptive reactions caused by the manipulation of the liver and abdominal viscera, and ensuring relaxation of abdominal muscles, diaphragm and viscera. Quality of surgery, patient safety and postoperative outlook will depend on these two prerequisites.

The technique of general anesthesia we use is called "balanced anesthesia", for it combines various pharmacological agents – hypnotic, curare, analgesic – to meet the requirements of this type of surgery.

The choice of anesthetic agents is subject to certain conditions. To preserve the donor's hepatic function and the quality of the graft, the choice of volatile or intravenous anesthetics must imperatively meet three criteria: absence of hepatotoxicity, low hepatic metabolism and maintenance of blood flow-rate in the arterial and portal system, with respect to reciprocal arterial and portal flow-rates. Narcosis is usually induced with a rapid action hypnotic such as pentothal or etomidate, and protracted by isoflurane, a volatile halogenated agent which does not alter hepatic blood flow, respects the regulation of arterial and portal hepatic flow-rates, and has very little hepatotoxicity owing to its low hepatic metabolism.

Analgesia is obtained with the use of a potent, highly lipid-soluble morphinic drug such as fentanyl or sulfentanyl, the kinetics of which are controlled by redistribution phenomena, which is to be taken into account during recovery from anesthesia. Atracurarium is the muscle relaxant of choice, since it is not metabolized in the liver and its elimination time is rapid.

Monitoring

Intraoperative monitoring methods meet the mandatory safety standards adopted by the Société Française d'Anesthésie Réanimation and the Word Federation of Societies of Anesthesiologists. Protection of airways by orotracheal tubing and peroperative assisted ventilation are essential. Invasive cardiovascular monitoring methods are limited to continuous blood pressure monitoring by catheterism of the radial artery and central venous pressure by internal jugular catheterism. Indeed, the hemodynamic impact of left lateral segmentectomy or left hepatectomy is negligible, since this type of surgery does not consist of liver vascular exclusion. Hemodynamic stability must be obtained by adequate vascular filling, merely guided by continuous arterial blood pressure and measurement of central venous pressure, maintained between 6 and 7 cm H_2O^{-1}, to preserve the liver from any congestive episode, which would be deleterious to the liver function and a source of hemorrhage.

During hepatic arterial dissection (left hepatic artery), we administer PGE1 prostaglandins at a dosage (500 µg 24 hrs^{-1}) to protect hepatic arterial vascularization from spasmodic vasomotor disorders and to protect hepatic arterial circulation from any thrombogenic element.

Vascular filling and blood volume expansion are obtained on the basis of water and electrolyte requirements using Ringer's lactate, artificial solutes (starch), free from allergizing effect. Hematocrit monitoring is essential and the hematocrit is maintained at levels of 30–35%. The blood returning from the cell Saver is transfused together with the harvested RBCs. The units of fresh frozen plasma and platelet concentrates are transfused at the time of hemostasis.

Postoperative period

During the immediate postoperative period, patients are monitored in the intestive care unit for the first 24 hours. Invasive monitoring systems are removed as early as possible and their maintenance is limited to the postanaesthetic recovery phase.

Postoperative assisted ventilation is not indicated and may be a source complications. Postoperative analgesia is required; the patient receives morphinic drug injection through a programmed delivery system. Short-time parenteral feeding and water-electrolyte delivery are maintained until resumption of complete oral nutrition. Clinical, paraclinical and biological monitoring, particularly for hepatic data, are performed as usual during hepatic surgery follow-up, and usual and suitable therapeutics are prescribed.

Conclusion

Donor safety is the essential goal. With thorough pre- and intraoperative methodology, pediatric liver transplantation from a genetically-related living donor and required by the parents, should be a reliable technical choice. It should be performed by a team of highly qualified and experienced operators in the field of liver surgery and liver transplantation to secure optimal donor safety.

References

1. Bismuth H, Houssin D. Reduced size orthotopic liver grafts in hepatic transplantation in children. Surgery 1984; 95: 367–70.
2. Houssin D, Couinaud C, Boillot O, et al. Controlled hepatic bipartition for transplantation in children. Br J. Surg 1991; 78: 802–4.
3. Boillot O. Reduction du greffon hépatique en transplantation pédiatrique: intérêt, technique et résultats. Pediatrie 1991; 46: 351–6.
4. Houssin D, Soubrane O, Boillot O, et al. Orthotopic liver transplantation using a reduced-size graft: an ideal compromise in pediatrics? Surgery 1992; 111: 532–42.
5. Houssin D, Couinaud C, Boillot O, et al. Controlled hepatic bipartition for transplantation in children. Br J. Surg 1991; 78: 802–4.
6. Houssin D, Boillot O, Soubrane O, et al. Controlled liver splitting for transplantation in two recipients: technique, results and perspectives. Br J. Surg 1993; 80: 75–80.

7. Raia S, Nery JR, Mies. Liver transplantation from live donors. Letters to the Editor: The Lancet, August 26, 1989.
8. Broelsch CE, Whitington PF, Emond JC, et al. Liver transplantation in children from living related donors. Surgical techniques and results. Ann Surg 1991; 214: 428–39.
9. Boillot O. Transplantation hépatique pédiatrique. Aspects actuels et perspectives. Médecine infantile 1992; 4: 285–95.
10. Boillot O, Dawahra M, Porcheron J, et al. Pediatric liver transplantation from living related donor. Transplant Proc 1993.
11. Singer PA, et al. Ethics of liver transplantation with living donor. N Engl J Med 1989; 321: 620–2.
12. Lery N. Droit éthique de la santé: l'expérience d'une consultion. Med et hyg 1990.
13. Sann L, et al. Ethical considerations on hepatic transplantation from living related donors. J. Pediatrie 1993; 48: 435–45.
14. Boillot O, Dawahra M, Porcheron J, Houssin D, et al. Transplantation hépatique pédiatrique et donneur vivant apparenté. Considérations techniques et éthiques. Ann Chir 1993; 47: 577–85.
15. Liehn, et al. Risk of living related donors for liver transplantation. Proceedings of the 7th Liver Intensive Care Group of Europe; 1994 April 15–16.
16. Boillot O, Elchardus JM, Gille D. Facteurs décisionnels et prise en charge familiale en transplantation hépatique pédiatrique a partir de donneur vivant apparenté. Journées Francophones de pathologie digestives. Paris 19–23 mars 1993. Communicatione orale.
17. Gilman S. Anesthesia and the liver. In: Barash PG, Cullen BF, Stoelung RK, editors. Clinical Anesthesia. Philadelphia: Lippincott, 1133–62.
18. Mervyn Maze et al. Anesthesia for patentis with liver disease. Anesthesia edited by Ronald D. Miller, M.D. Vol 3: 1665–80.
19. Goldfarb G. Influence of anaesthetic drug on hepatic blood flow. Ann Fr Anesth Réa 1987; 6: 498–506.
20. Goldfarb, et al. Comparative effects of halothane and isoflurane anesthesia on the ultrastructure of human hepatic cells. Analg 1989; 69: 491–5.
21. Russel E, et al. Effects of anaesthetic agents and abdominal surgery on hepatic blood flow. Hepatology 1991; 14(6): 1161–6.
22. Delva E, Barberousse JP, et al. Hemodynamic and biochimical monitoring during major liver resection with use of hepatic vascular exclusion. Surgery March 1984: 309–18.
23. Delva E, Camus Y, et al. Vasculars occlusions for liver resections: Operative management and tolerance to hepatic ischemia – 142 cases. Ann Surgery Febr 1989.
24. Gaveli A, et al. Risk factors associated with hepatectomy results of a multivariate analysis of 113 cases. Ann Chir 1993; 47: 586–91.

PART THREE

Optimization of organ procurement

20. Potential donors and brain death epidemiology in the region of Madrid

ALBINO NAVARRO

Introduction

The major obstacle to organ transplantation today is the limited organ supply. It is estimated that only 1–4% of the total number of people dying in hospitals and about 10% of those dying in Intensive Care Units (ICUs) die in the situation known as "brain death" [1–5], and that of these percentages, only 15–67% become organ donors [2–7].

In 1990, a Regional Coordination Center was set up in our area and a dependent network of Transplant Coordinators Teams (TCTs), composed of doctors and nurses, was established in the 14 public hospitals of the region. The precise composition of our TCTs, their objectives and our Regional Coordination system have already been published [8]. These teams are the cornerstones of the National Organization for Transplantation in Spain, and the system adopted in Madrid is now common to all Spanish regions [9].

The first aim of the TCTs is donor detection and organ procurement. A year after the creation of our Regional Center, we undertook a study to evaluate the epidemiology of brain deaths in our region. Our second aim was to assess donor detection, the reasons for refusing donation, and organ procurement. The results should enable us to evaluate the regional activity regarding donor detection, as well as the particular detection activity for each of the 14 hospitals. The results should also enable us to adapt the composition of our TCTs, and appraise their objectives.

Materials and methods

The Region of Madrid in central Spain has a total population of 4,845,851 inhabitants and is served by 14 hospitals with 12,500 beds, 300 of which are ICU beds. In every hospital, there is a TCT composed of a doctor dedicated part-time to coordination and, in some, one or more nurses for the same purpose [8, 9]. Since 1991, these hospitals have taken part in a multicenter prospective study registering all patients with clinical neurological diagnosis

J.L. Touraine et al. (eds.), Organ Shortage: The Solutions, 135–142.
© 1995 Kluwer Academic Publishers.

of brain death (BD) [10]. The data collected include hospital, date, sex, age, blood group, cause of BD, and organs retrieved. We also recorded monthly the number of deaths in each ICU, in each hospital, and in the region. We considered the BD patients as potential donors (PDs), and as effective donors (EDs) when the organ extraction was performed. When another organ was retrieved together with the kidneys (liver, heart or lungs), we considered them to be multiorganic donors (MODs). The results obtained during the first year have been previously published [11, 12]. In this paper, we present the two-year results of our BD study. We also present data about donation, organ procurement, and transplantation carried out in the Madrid region during the past 4 years.

In Spain, in order to legally declare a patient brain dead, a complete neurological examination is needed, along with an EEG of half an hour. Furthermore, this must be repeated twice within an interval of at least 6 hours between each examination. This is why we will speak of a first and second EEG in this article.

Results

Epidemiology of cerebral death

During the period of the study we detected 541 BD patients: 273 the first year and 268 the second year, which means that the incidence during the two years was very similar. We recorded 344 males (64%) and 197 females (36%). The proportion remained the same during the two years of the study. The most frequent diagnoses were: 234 cases of craneal trauma (43%), 227 cerebrovascular strokes (CVA) (42%), 52 cases of cerebral anoxia (10%), 18 brain tumours (3%), and 10 other different causes (2%) (Figure 1). The diagnosis distribution was similar for the two years, except that the leading diagnosis of the first year was CVA.

The average age was 38.5 ± 19 years (mean ± SD), with a bimodal distribution of the two main diagnosis groups (Figure 2): the trauma group (30.6 ± 17 years) and the group of cerebrovascular strokes (47 ± 16 years). The gender distribution was also different: 72% males vs. 28% females in the trauma group, and 59% males vs. 41% females in the group of cerebrovascular strokes.

Of the total number of BD cases, 278 (51%) were ED, exactly half of them (139) each year, representing 28.7 donors per million population (pmp) yearly.

The reasons for non-extraction were: medical contraindications in 107 cases (20%), cardiac arrest during maintenance on 47 occasions (9%), family refusal in 99 cases (18%), and other causes in 10 cases (3%). The most frequent medical contraindications were sepsis (38 cases) and multiorgan failure (21 cases); 13 cases were anti-HIV positive or high risk, 11 cases had

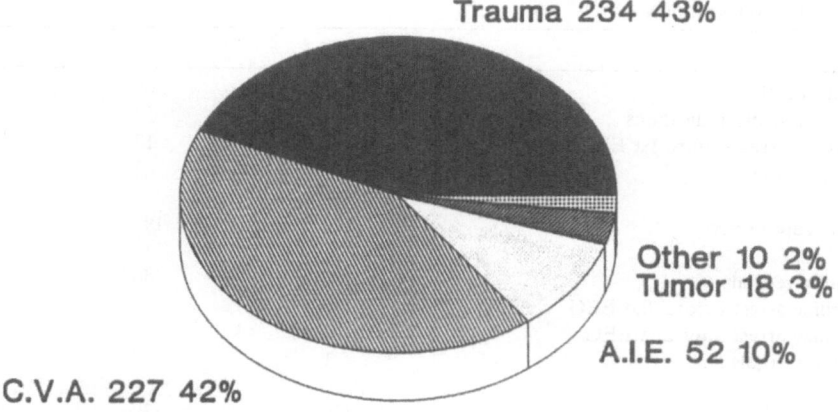

Fig. 1. Reasons for BDs among the 541 cases recorded in the Madrid region in 1991 and 1992.

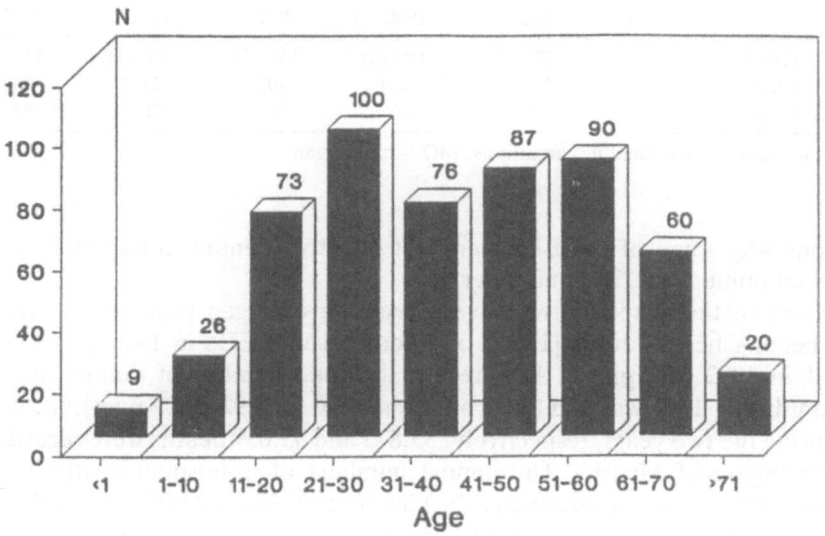

Fig. 2. Age distribution of the BD cases.

severe hypertension, tumours were found in 10, old age was cited for 7, and other causes were stated in 7 cases. Regarding family refusals, although they account for 18% of BDs, they represent 25% of cases in which family consent was requested. Due to the previously cited contraindications, some families did not need to be referred to.

Table 1 shows the donation flows of 1991 and 1992, and sums up the

Table 1. Donation flow

	1991	1992
Brain deaths	273	268
Medical contraindications	54	53
Cardiac arrest before 1st EEG	14	17
Other causes	6	1
Adequate donors	199	197
Family refusals	49	50
Cardiac arrest before 2nd EEG	6	4
Cardiac arrest after 2nd EEG	4	2
Judge refusals	1	2
Effective donors	139	139

CVA: CerebroVascular Accident; AIE: Anoxic Ischemic Encephalopathy.

Table 2. Donor procurement in the region of Madrid

	1989	1990	1991	1992	1993
Donors (No.)	97 (1)	146 (5)	146 (7)	140 (1)	129
Donors (pmp)	20	30.1	30.1	28.9	26.6
MO donors (%)	35	57	70	78	82

Asystolic donors mentioned in parenthesis; MO = multiorgan.

reasons why some of the BDs were not effective donors, thus resulting in the final number of 139 donors per year.

In one of the hospitals, we have a program of organ procurement from non-beating heart donors [13], 7 of whom became EDs in 1991 (1.4 pmp) and 1 in 1992 (0.2 pmp). As a result, the total number of donors in our region during 1991 was 146 (30.1 pmp) and 140 in 1992 (28.9 pmp).

During the two years, respectively, 35,873 and 35,039 deaths were recorded in the region of Madrid. The annual numbers of in-hospital deaths were 14,042 and 13,784 (respectively, 39.1%, and 39,3%), 2,008 and 1,980 of which occurred in ICUs (nearly 6% of total deaths and 14.3% of in-hospital ones).

Considering this data, the BD incidence in our region remained unchanged during the two years: 0.76% of all deaths, 1.94% of in-hospital deaths, and 13.6% of all ICUs deaths.

Organ donation

In 1989, before the Regional Coordination and the TCTs of Madrid were set up, 97 donors were registered, 35% of them being MOD. Table 2 shows the total number of donors, the rate pmp, and the rate of multiorgan extrac-

Table 3. Organ procurement in the region of Madrid

	1989		1990		1991		1992		1993	
	No.	pmp	No.	pmp	No.	pmp	No.	pmp	No.	pmp
Kidney	194	40	291	60	292	60	280	57.8	257	53
Liver	34	7	83	11.7	103	21.2	109	22.5	105	21.7
Heart	18	3.7	50	10.3	55	11.3	53	10.9	46	9.5
Lungs			1	0.2	3	0.6	3	0.6	6	1.2

Table 4. Organ transplantation in the region of Madrid

	1989		1990		1991		1992		1993	
	No.	pmp	No.	pmp	No.	pmp	No.	pmp	No.	pmp
Kidney	213	43.9	290	59.9	305	62.9	304	62.8	287	59.2
Liver	81	16.7	134	27.6	156	32.2	158	32.4	163	33.4
Heart	45	9.3	70	14.4	93	19.2	105	21.7	110	22.7
Lung			1	0.2	2	0.4	2	0.4	4	0.8

tions during the 4 years that followed the creation of the new structure. The average rate of these 4 years reached 29 donors pmp, per year, with a progressive upturn in multiorgan extractions, which reached 82% in 1993.

Table 3 shows the total number of retrieved organs during the past 5 years and the rate pmp. Table 4 presents the number of solid organs transplanted in the Madrid region over the same period, and the rate pmp.

Discussion

To establish the potential availability of cadaver organs for transplantation in a region it is necessary to answer two questions [14]:

1. How many patients who die in a hospital are potential donors because they are brain dead?
2. Why do some brain dead patients not provide organs?

Our study shows that approximately 2% of people dying in a hospital and approximately 14% of those dying in an ICU are brain dead. The real incidence of BD in ICUs recorded in our study is identical to that calculated in a British multicenter study: 13.6% [4], which makes us think that this figure could be used as a standard. BD detection is the first step in the donation-transplantation procedure. Therefore, we believe that defining target figures is crucial. After noticing that we had maintained a stable figure during two consecutive years and that our incidence was similar to that of the British study, we decided to use the following data as the aim for detection in all our hospitals: 2% of people dying in hospitals and 14% of those dying in ICUs.

The reasons for non-procurement of organs from brain dead patients in our series are consistent with other studies: mainly, medical contraindications (16–20% of the cases) and family refusals (18–30%). These two reasons and others mostly explain why only half of BDs become EDs [1, 2, 4]. The general analysis of why they do not become EDs is crucial to make the right decisions and improve results. Hence, we must control the evolution of medical contraindications over time, to know what can be done to prevent them (i.e. infections). We must also be aware of the number of family refusals to improve our educational activities regarding public opinion and approaches used by TCTs to ask for consent. Similarly, it is essential to compare the regional donation flow with that of each hospital (Table 1) to assess individual output, and this means the activity of each TCT existing in our centers. This method already enabled us to identify problems in some centers (lack of detection, family refusals higher than the average, etc.) and to take the necessary actions to remedy them. We believe that keeping records of BDs is fundamental for the self-control of every center of organ procurement, and we recommend such registers for each hospital, region, and nation.

In 1993, after analyzing the records of our hospitals, the region of Madrid restructured some TCTs and, thanks to that method, the results achieved were really hopeful.

Brain death records are also very interesting in defining the kinds of donors we deal with. Two main groups have been observed:

– a craneal trauma group, in which we noticed a majority of young people and a male-female rate of 4:1
– a cerebral hemorrage group of older patients, in which the male-female rate is similar

The structural change and the creation of TCTs in Madrid enabled an increase in the number of donors since 1990, mostly due to the higher detection of donors deceased because of cerebral hemorrhages. Hence, it is foremost to inform all health specialists of this change in donors' characteristics in order to improve detection. Such an observation is all the more important since the progressive decline of road accidents in western countries, and particularly in Spain, makes cerebral hemorrhages the first cause of death generating donation. As a matter of fact, the donation data of the Madrid region in 1993 revealed that only 30% of donors had died because of road accidents (i.e. 8 donors pmp per year), which proves that high donation rates are not due to an upsurge of traffic insecurity, but other factors.

The high rate of EDs in our region (on average, 29 donors pmp during the last 4 years) may mean that we have an adequate transplant organization and that the work of TCTs is very efficient. Nevertheless, our data suggest that the number of EDs could still be increased if medical contraindications or cardiac arrest during maintenance could be reduced and, also, if we could trim family refusals with educational programs.

The level of organ procurement and multiorganic extractions is also satisfactory, and we believe this is due to the efficient work done by TCTs, whose main aim is to detect potential donors and turn them into EDs. Therefore, we think that establishing this kind of structure in other regions and nations would be promising.

Transplantation is the final result of TCTs' activity. In the region of Madrid, we currently have 14 hospitals, 7 of which perform transplantation. They comprise 7 teams of renal transplantation for adults and 2 for children, 4 programs of heart transplantation, 4 of liver transplantation for adults and 2 for children, and one of lung transplantation. Table 4 summarizes the transplantation data of all these centers. The high rate of kidney, liver and heart transplantations pmp compares favourably with the data of other regions and countries, and represents the final step of donor detection and organ procurement. Therefore, the final results on transplantation by a structure devoted to donor detection seem to be better than those reached by other structures essentially devoted to transplantation or organ exchange.

Acknowledgements

The author wishes to thank all the TCT members of the hospitals of Madrid for their work and dedication to complete the brain death registers. The design of the BD investigation was performed in collaboration with Dr. Escalante and Dr. Andrés. I would like to especially acknowledge Mercedes Pascual and Gema Marmisa, TCT nurses, for their work processing and elaborating the data.

References

1. Espinel E, Deulofeu R, Sabater R, Mañalich M, Domingo P, Rué M. The capacity for organ generation of hospitals in Catalonia, Spain: a multicentre study. Transplant Proc 1989: 21: 1419–21.
2. Aranzabal J, Perdigo L. Organ procurement organization in the Basque Autonomous Community: present achievement and future prospects. Transplant Proc 1990: 22: 335.
3. Gilmore A. Procuring donor organs: firm but friendly encouragement requiered. Can Med Assoc J 1986: 134: 932–7.
4. Gore SM, Cable DJ, Holland AJ. Organ donation from intensive care units in England and Wales: two year confidential audit of deaths in intensive care. BMJ 1992: 304: 349–55.
5. Salish MAM, Harvey I, Frankel S, et al. Potential availability of cadaver organs for transplantation BMJ 1991; 302: 1053–5.
6. Bart KJ, Macon EJ, Humphries AL, et al. Increasing the supply of cadaveric organs for transplantation. Transplantation 1981; 31: 383–7.

7. Tolle SW, Bennt WM, Hickman DH, Benson JA. Responsibilities of primary physicians in organ donation. Ann Intern Med 1987; 106: 740–4.
8. Navarro A. Modelo de Coordinación Autonómica. Rev Esp Trasplantes 1993; 2: 67–72.
9. Matesanz R. Organ Procurement in Spain: the importance of a transplant coordinating network. Transplant Proc 1993; 25: 3132–5.
10. Guidelines for the determination of death. Report of the medical consultants on the diagnosis of death to the President's Commission for the Study of Ethical Problems in Medicine and Biomedical and Behavioral Research. JAMA 1981; 246: 2184–6.
11. Navarro A, Escalante JL, et al. Detection of donors and organs procurements in the autonomous community of Madrid. Intensive Care Med 1992; 18(suppl 2): S83.
12. Navarro A, Escalante JL, Andrés A, et al. Donor detection and organ procurement in the Madrid region. Transplant Proc 1993: 25: 3130–1.
13. Gómez M, Alvarez J, Arias J, et al. Cardiopulmonary bypass and profound hypothermia as a means for obtaining kidney grafts from irreversible cardiac arrest donors cooling technique. Transplant Proc 1993; 25: 1501–2.
14. Gentleman D, Easton J, Jennett B. Brain death and organ donation in a neurosurgical unit: audit of recent practice. BMJ 1990: 301: 1203–6.

21. Logistics and management for improvement of multiorgan procurement from potential brain dead donors

J.J. COLPART, M. BRET, B. CORONEL, D. DOREZ,
A. MERCATELLO, B. BOUTTIN, G. SAURY
& J.F. MOSKOVTCHENKO

Statistical considerations

Is organ shortage a permanent condition in western European countries? With efficient organization in each country, 1993 European Transplant Coordinators Organization (ETCO) statistics expect 10,000 additional potential organs.

In 1993, the number of used donors was 27.2 per million people (pmp) for Austria and 4.4 pmp for Greece. The western European mean was 14.7 pmp (Figure 1). In 1993, the percentage of multiorgan procurement activity was 80% for France, 58.4% for Germany and 52.8% for the Netherlands (Figure 2). The number of all organs procured in 1993 was 88 pmp in Austria, 39.1 pmp in Germany and 10.9 pmp in Greece. The European mean was 44.8 pmp (Figure 3).

French statistics show 3 main causes of non-available organs (Figure 4):

1. Decreasing numbers of I.C.U. failures
2. creasing refusals by the general public
3. donor medical background, which cannot be changed apart from very good health education

Therefore, it is only useful to act on I.C.U. management and refusals.

I.C.U. management

Brain dead donor management is dependent on brain death patho- physiology.

Previous central nervous system lesions

In a typical traffic accident, the brain is propelled forward against the anterior wall of the brain pan. This produces one edematous contusion area (Figure

J.L. Touraine et al. (eds.), Organ Shortage: The Solutions, 143–159.

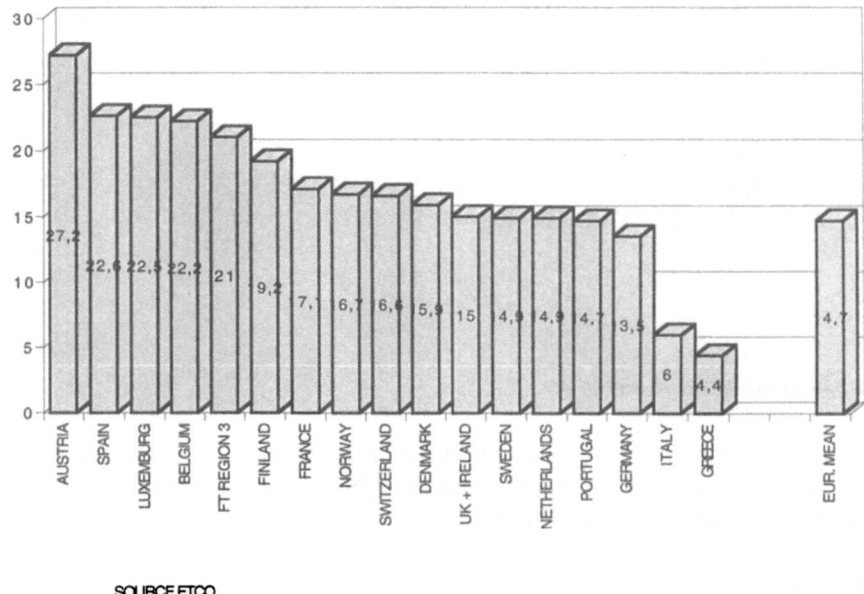

Fig. 1. Cadaveric donors (pmp) 1993.

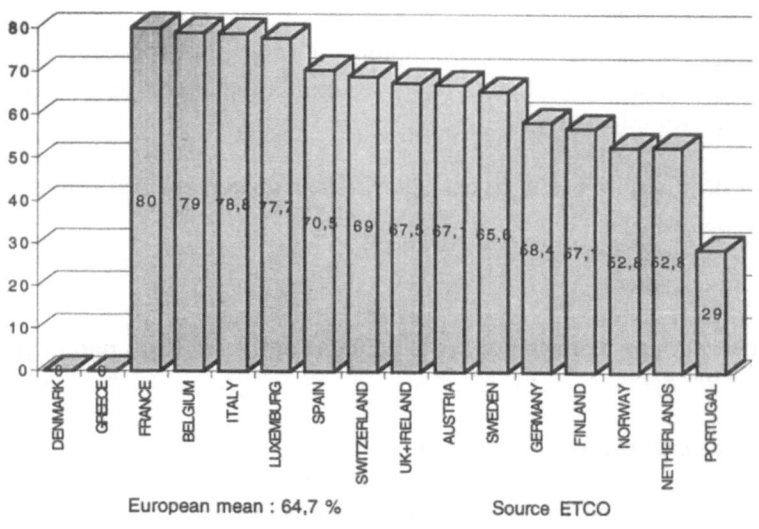

European mean : 64,7 %   Source ETCO

Fig. 2. Multiorgan donation (%) in Europe 1993.

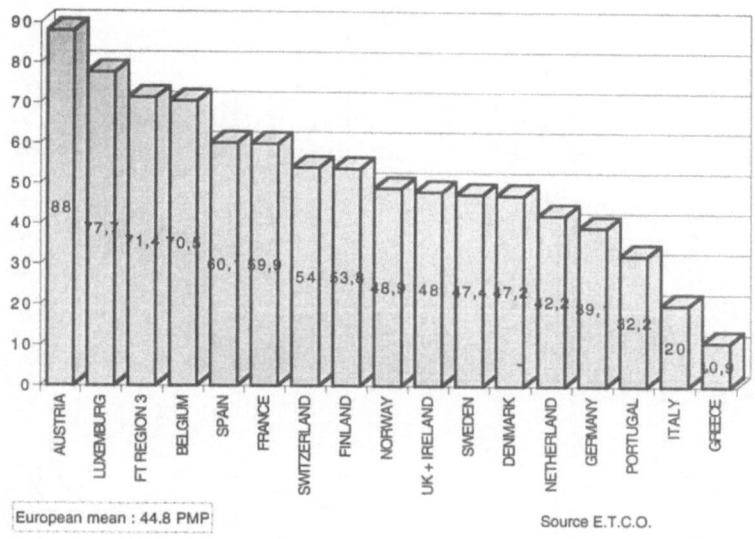

Fig. 3. All organ procurement (pmp) in Europe 1993.

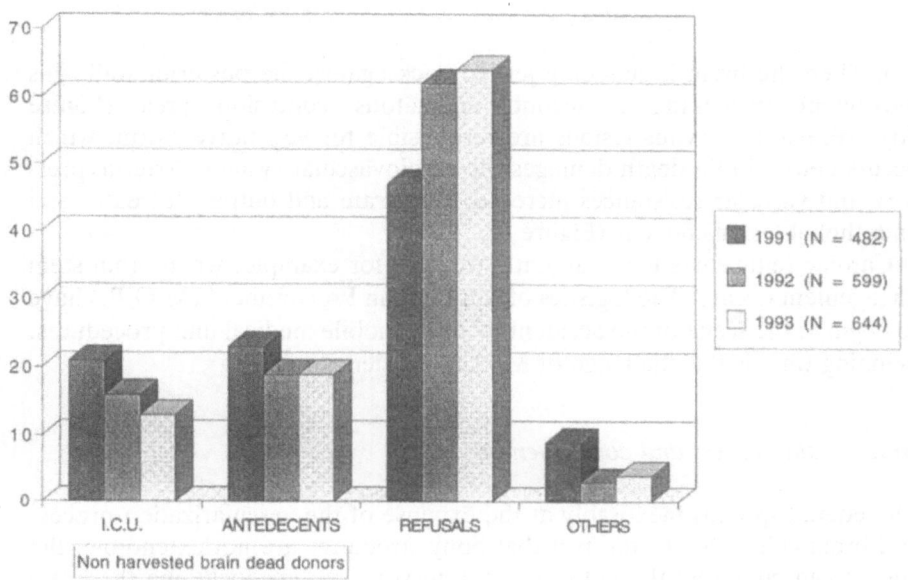

Fig. 4. French non-organ harvesting causes.

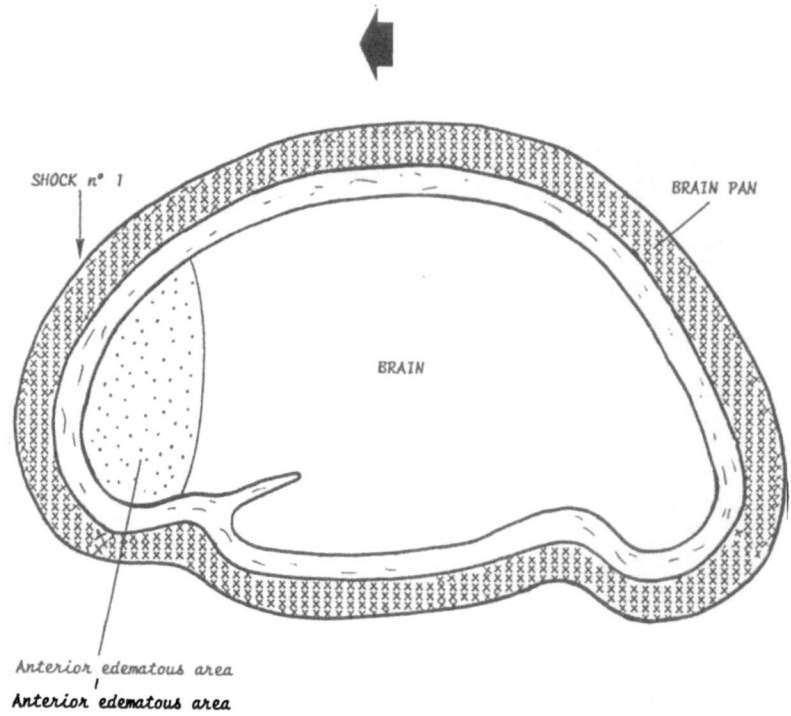

Fig. 5a. First edematous contusion area due to typical traffic accident.

5a). Then the brain is suddenly jerked back against the posterior wall, this movement provoking a second edematous contusion area (Figure 5b). Previous nervous lesions are responsible for vegetative storm, which occurs before brain death damages the cardiovascular system. Arterial pressure and vascular resistances increase, heart rate and output decrease, and endothelial lesions appear (Figure 6).

Cardiac failure has to be urgently treated, for example, when brain stem engagement occurs. The logistics of MultiOrgan Procurement (M.O.P.) have to begin at the scene of the accident by using mobile medical unit procedures. Winning time is the challenge of M.O.P. efficiency.

Brain death process and consequences

The edema spreads inexorably at the expense of the vascularization process and brain cells. Due to the fact that bony structures are not extendible, the edema can compress the entire central nervous system, including the brain stem. Thus, the process is irreversible (Figures 7 and 8).

When the brain stem is destroyed:

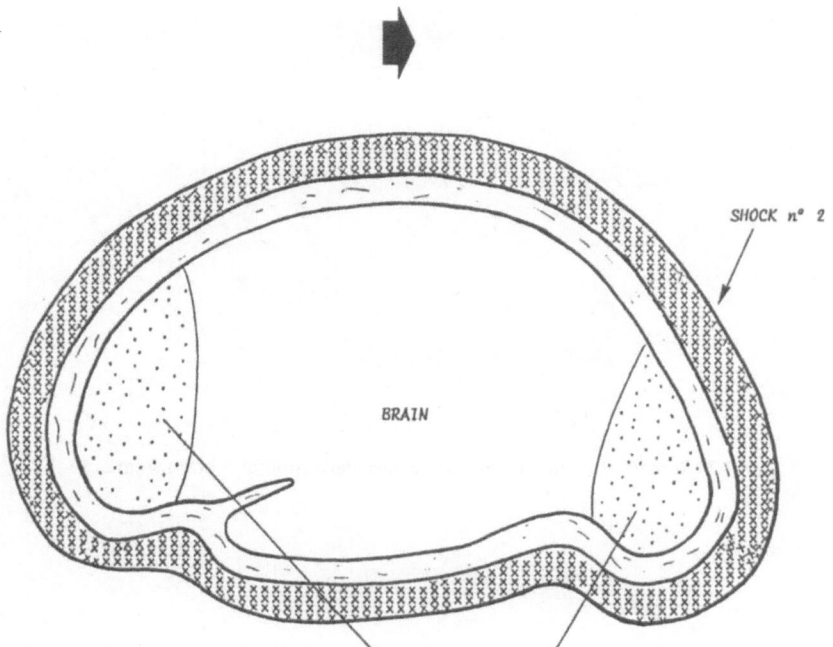

Fig. 5*b*. Second edematous contusion area due to typical traffic accident.

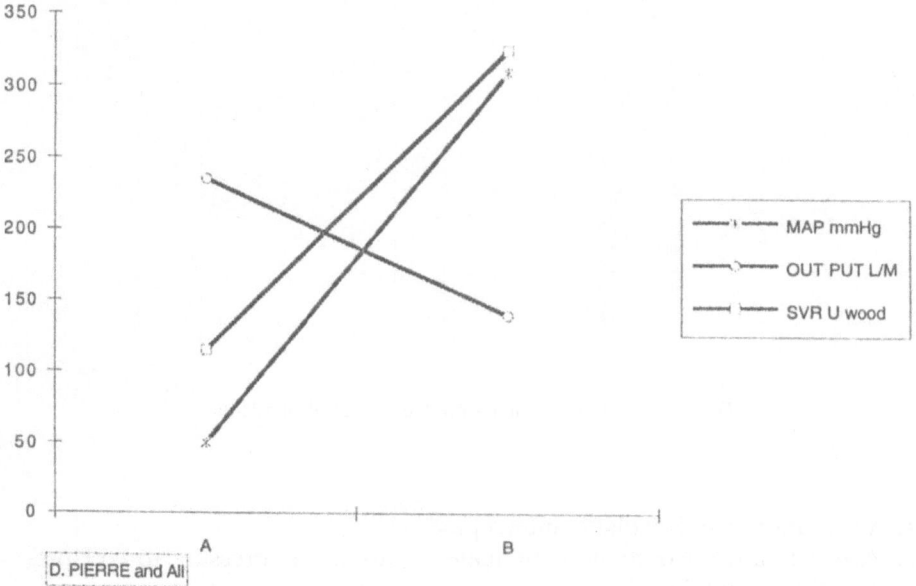

Fig. 6. General circulation vegetative storm.

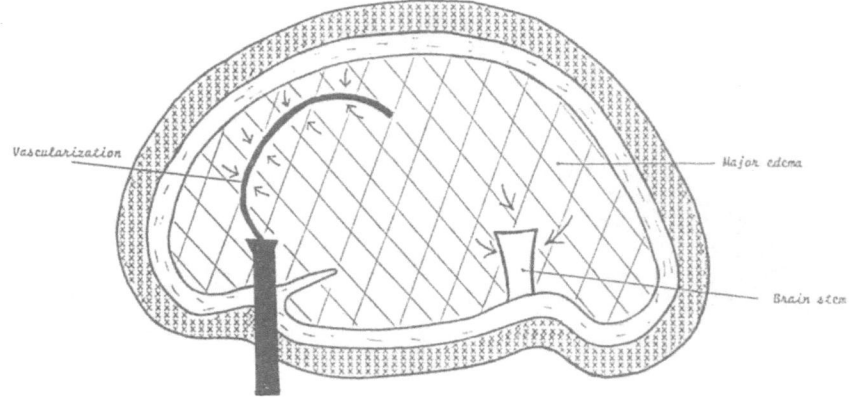

Fig. 7. Spread of edema compressing vascularization and brain stem.

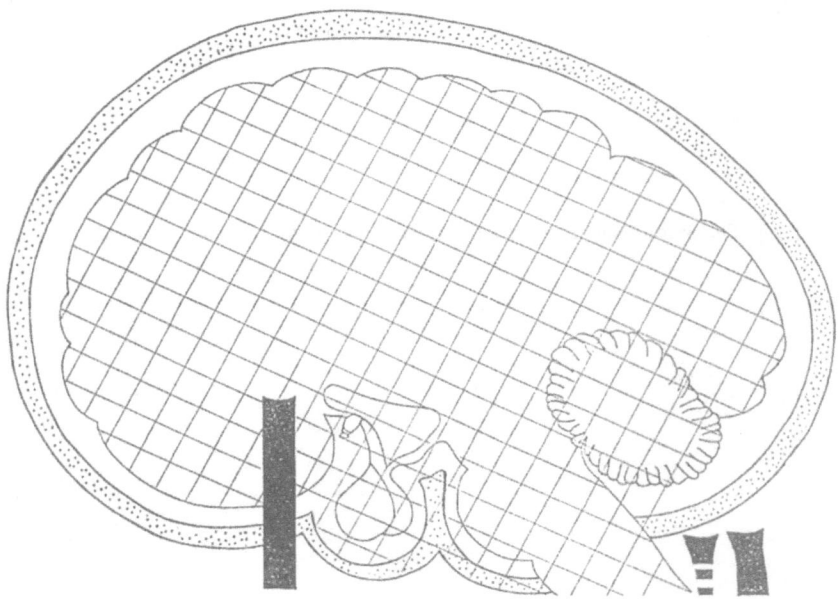

Fig. 8. Complete vascular stop due to spread of edema.

1. Ventilation is irremediably interrupted
2. Arterial vasoconstriction is eliminated, causing the pressure to collapse, resulting in paralysis
3. Cardiac activity weakens due to suppression of the sympathetic nervous

system stimuli, and, consequently depletion of peripheral catecholamines occurs.

In 50% of the brain dead population, a left ventricular function decrease is discovered. The hypophysis initially protected by the sella turcica is also damaged. On the vital plane, the anterior lobe plays a part in homeostatis of thyroid and corticosuprarenal hormones.

TSH reduction decreases emission of the cardiotropic hormone T3 as a study of a Lyon brain death unit shows:

A significantly low T3 hormone level is prevalent in the brain dead potential multiorgan donors population (80%) [4, 6, 11, 14, 16, 17].

Table 1.

Hormones	Number of donors	Results (mean)	Normal
TSH (mUI l^{-1})	76	0.84 ± 0.82	$2.18\ p < 0.001$
T3 (nmol l^{-1})	76	0.98 ± 0.54	$1.8\ p < 0.001$
T4 (pmol)	76	16.1 ± 4.7	$18\ p = 0.01$

The decrease of cardiotropic T3 hormone is due to TSH decrease and to a significant reverse T3 increase, which stops T4 T3 conversion. The mechanism of cardiac catecholamines depletion due to T3 failure is probably both a decrease in catecholamine receptors and a direct effect of metabolic drug action (Figures 9a, 9b, 10).

Suppression of ADH causes diabetes insipidus due to lack of renal tubular reabsorption.

Apart from hormonal depletions, a high number of ICU parameters are disturbed, as shown by the retrospective Lyon study. The statistics for 247 potential donors upon their arrival in the Lyon University Hospital brain death unit were:

Table 2.

Temperature	52% ↓	28% ↑
Blood pressure	36.1% ↓	8% ↑
Heart rate	1.6% ↓	46% ↑
Haemodynamic instability	35%	
Kaliemia	42% ↓	10% ↑
Central veinous pressure (ventilation pressure included)	62% < 5 m H_2O	20% < 0 m H_2O
Polyuria	80%	
Respiratory alcalosis	50%	
Hematocrit	71% ↓	
Prothrombin	87% ↓	
Fibrinogen	20.7% ↓	

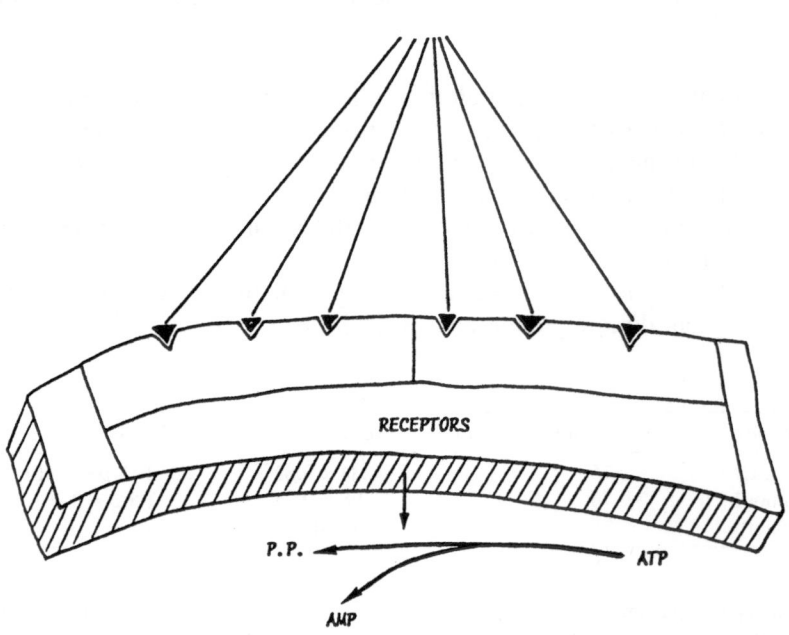

Fig. 9*a*. Mechanism of cardiac catecholamines depletion due to T3 failure. With T.H. (T3).

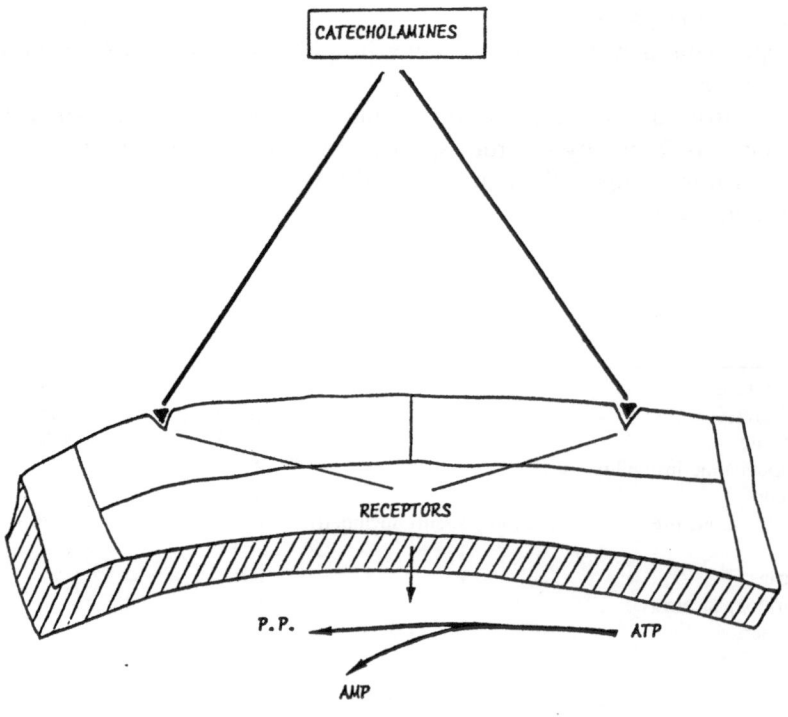

Fig. 9*b*. Without T.H. (T3).

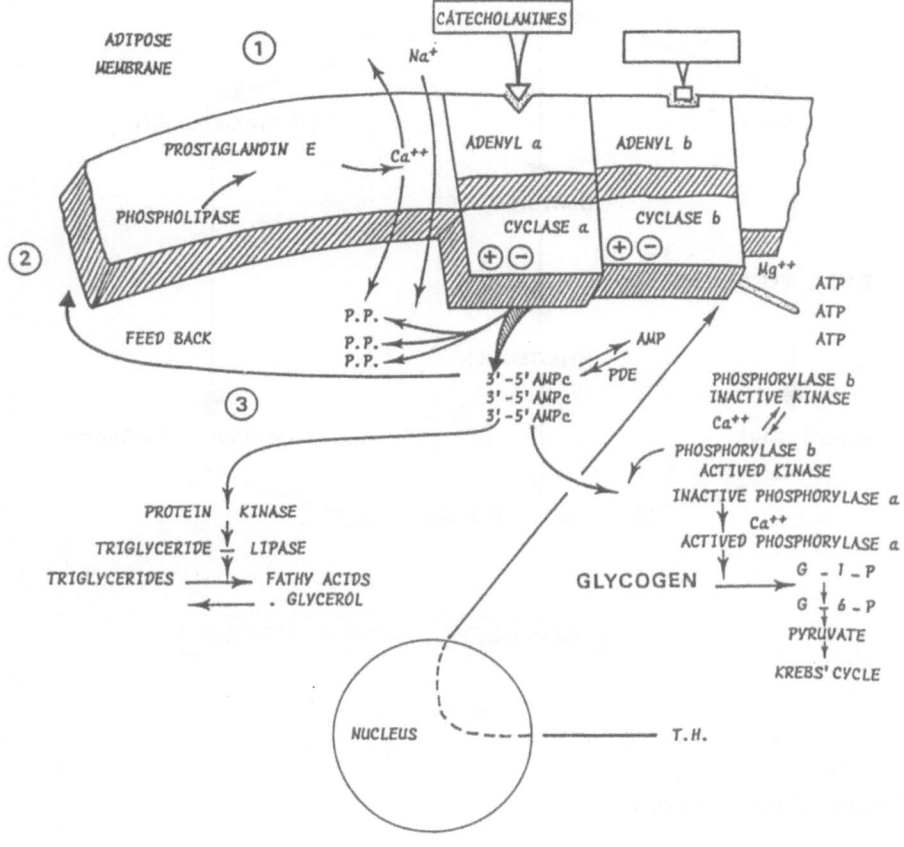

Fig. 10.

Physiologic functions controlled and equilibria maintained [7]

Main physiologic functions such as haemodynamic, ventilation, fluid and electrolyte balance, kidney output, temperature and coagulation all have to be controlled. Equilibria must be maintained as follows:

- arterial pressure >65 mmHg
- central veinous pressure >5–15 m H_2O
- urine output h^{-1} = 100–150 l
- temperature >36°C
- normoxia, normocapnia
- normokaliemia, normonatremia
- normophosphatemia [8]
- enough coagulation factors

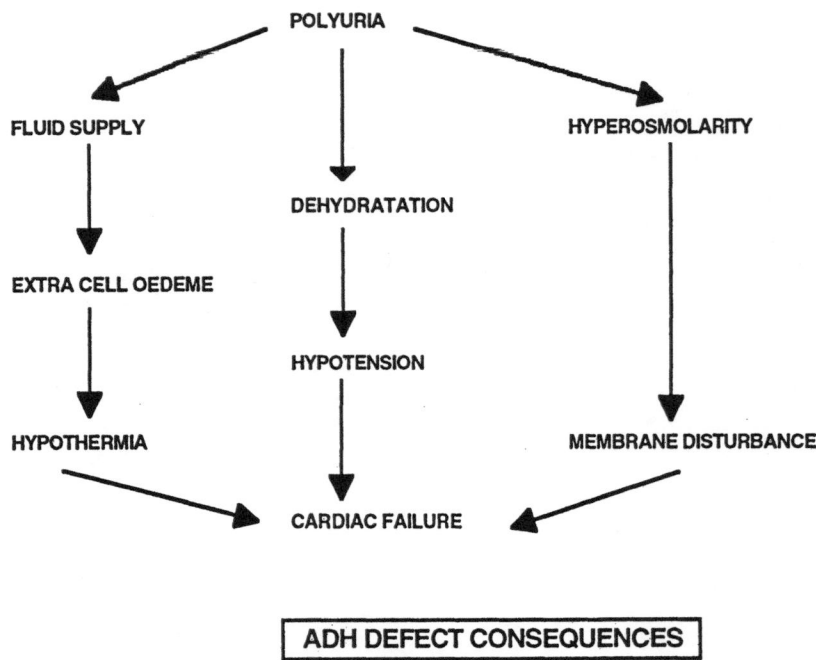

Fig. 11.

Combined examinations

Clinical exam is classical. This includes the circumstances of death, general clinical exam, weight, height, corporeal surface measures, patient background and therapies.

Combined general biological and specific examinations are completed. These include blood ionogramm, glycemia, calcemia, creatinemia, blood arterial gazes, blood cells formula with platelets, toxicological check-up, bacterial cultures, virus tests – such as HIV, HCV, HBs, CMV, EBV – chest X-rays, ECG, cardiac echography if possible, etc.

Immunology tests. These include blood group, antibodies, HLA-DR cross-matching.

Available I.C.U. monitoring equipment

For these procedures, an ECG, arterial pressure checker, cardioveter, automatic syringes, ventilator, electronic thermometer, heating blankets and other equipment is used.

Brain dead donor maintenance

Manipulations
Monitoring parameters are classical but the donor has to be maintained outside the ICU, especially during manipulations, transports, X-ray exams and operating room procedures.

Avoiding heart dysfunction or cardiac arrest has to be the major preoccupation. Manipulations of brain dead potential donors are always deleterious for heart function. In view of this, in Lyon University Hospital a special brain dead donor bed was designed. Its levels can be changed according to the height of operating or angiography tables and the heating mattress, which avoids temperature decrease, is always linked to that special bed.

Arterial pressure maintenance
Two aims of maintaining arterial pressure are:

1. Struggle against hypovolemia mainly due to neuro ICU procedures. Vascular liquid infusion can be used, for example, plasma expenders such as albumin or frozen plasma (which also gives coagulating factors), red cells, colloids, hydroxyethylamidon starch [13], Ringer liquid, ionic supplies, etc.
2. Fight cardiac failures, especially when there is high central veinous pressure, using Dopamine 5 Gmg kg^{-1} min^{-1} or Dobutamine 5 Gmg kg^{-1} min^{-1} [9, 18].

Temperature maintenance
Temperature is maintained to:

- Struggle against hyper- or hypothermia
- Struggle against anaerobic bacteria using, for example, penicillin or metronidazole

Ventilation
Ventilation of the brain dead is particularly important because of reduced brain oxygen consumption. Physiologically the brain needs 20% oxygen. However, hyperventilation has to be avoided; ventilator parameters have to be decreased against respiratory alcalosis. A ventilation heating system also fights against temperature decrease.

Hydroelectrolytic equilibrium
Hydroelectrolytic equilibrium depends on ionogramms, for example:

- hypernatremia implies dilution and hypokaliemia implies $1\,h^{-1}$ KCL supply
- plasma expenders are actually useful

Urine output maintenance

Oligoanuria can be treated with haemodynamic supports and with diuretics such as Furosemide 2–30 g kg^{-1} and Mannitol 20% – 2 l kg^{-1}. Polyuria can be treated with hypotonic solutions, plasma expenders or ADH supplies.

Brain death diagnosis

Diagnosis of brain death could depend on a logistical point of view and not only on legislation. Current ancillary diagnosis methods can be summarized as follows:

– EEG, for example, is often a cause of time lost for several reasons.
– Auditory evoked potentials are the reference exam of New York Hospital.
– Transcanial or carotidian doppler explorations can signal the time of brain death.
– Specific HMPAO isotopic scintigraphy, if available, is very useful [20–21].
– Digitalized or classic cerebral angiography explorations shorten the length of time in diagnosing circulatory arrest and confirming brain death.

General and medical public refusals: What can we do?

The European Donor Hospital Education Programme has the goal of sensitizing public hospitals for developing organ procurement. The French E.D.H.E.P. programme is not only involved in psychological information but, also, in general information about multiorgan and tissue procurement and transplant data because the problem is not only the number of donors but how to best use these donors. The limits of this programme are financial; for example, only 10 seminars will be organized in France in 1993 for approximatly 3,000 ICUs.

The European Transplant Coordinators Organization (ETCO), Euro Transplant, France Transplant, Organizacion Nationale de Trasplantes and UK transplant performed a great number of TC education meetings for many years, but it is very difficult to get full-time and enduring transplant coordinators. It is also very difficult to set up this position in each hospital. For example, in France only 24 TCs, including 7 regional TCs are full-time (14 of them are in 2 regions – Centre East and South East). Further, there are many problems for TCs, such as no professional recognition, personal careers and short basic levels in many countries.

General public information has to be spread everywhere but that information must give a positive view of transplant results, for example, via sports figures, normal, professional activities and so on.

Organization

France [3] and Spain [9] have similar organ procurement organizations, each with three levels of regional, local and national coordination, which probably have a positive effect on multiorgan procurement and multiorgan dispatching. But, in France, which has a national presumed consent law, there are significant differences in the number of donors and total organ procurements according to regional policies. General M.O.P. hospital policy was developed early in France Transplant Regions 3 and 6, which explains approximately 26% more organs (Figure 12). In France Transplant Region 3 (Auvergne, Bourgogne, Rhône Alpes, La Réunion), for example, 156 organs were obtained in 1993 as a result of general hospital procurement. The multiorgan procurement activity in the general hospitals explains the place of *FT* Region 3 in European statistics (Figure 13).

One point we have to mention is that refusals are less important in general hospitals (9.8%) than in university hospitals (26.2%) in France Transplant Region 3, despite good organization among university hospitals including, for example, local TCs and use of the brain death bed (Figure 14).

Transplant coordination for *FT* Region 3 comprises 1 intensive MD, 1 chief nurse, 4 nurses and 2 secretaries. The population is 8.1 million inhabitants and there are 5 university hospitals and 48 general hospitals (general

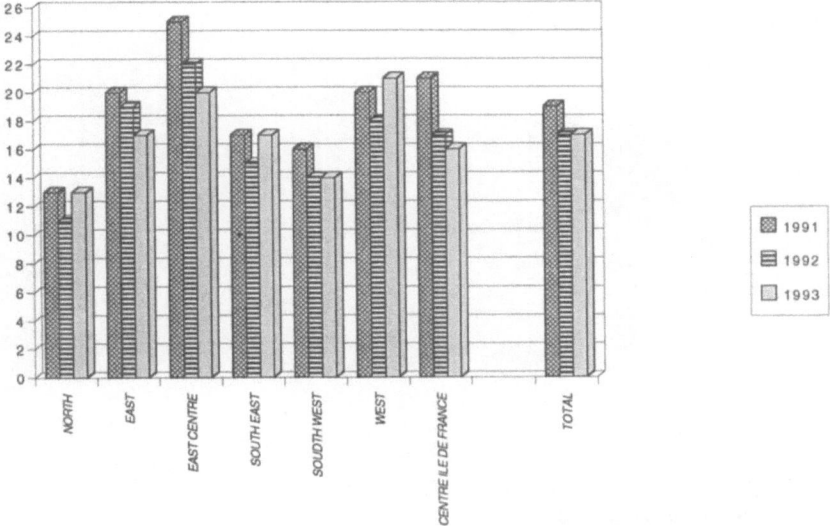

Fig. 12. Regional donors in France (pmp).

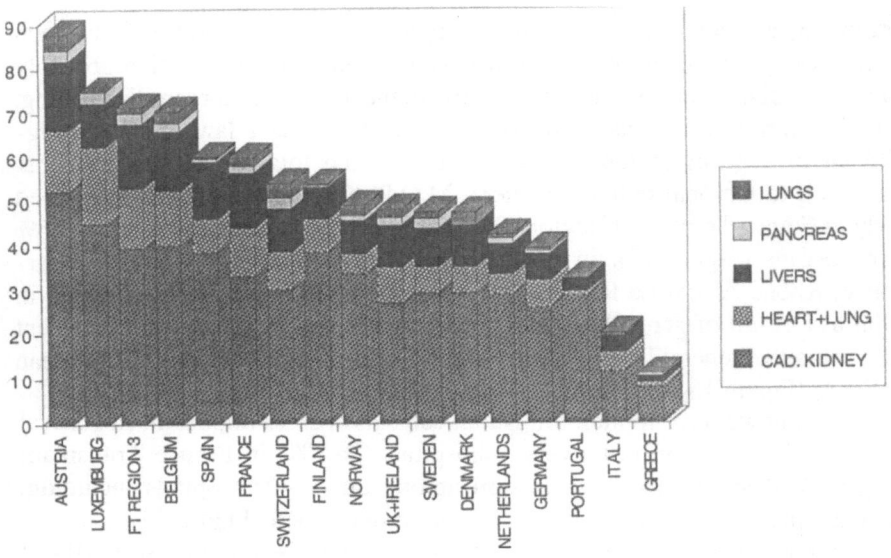

Fig. 13. Total organ procurement (pmp) in Europe 1993.

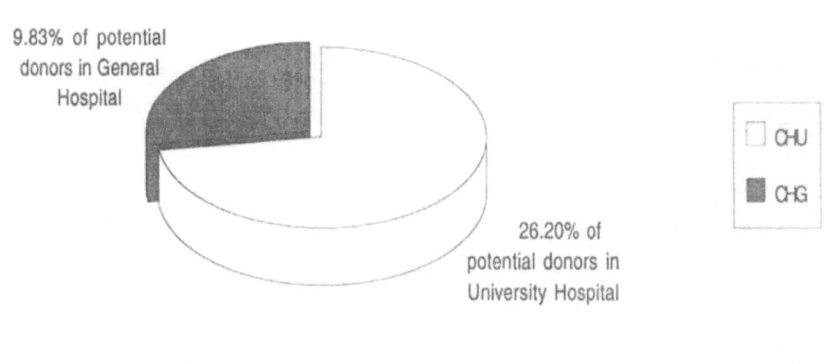

Fig. 14. Refusals in university hospitals versus general hospitals 1993.

hospitals are connected with regional transplant coordination). Regional transplant coordination has to:

1. organize general logistics such as road and air services and collecting biological exams, and the synchronized arrival of surgical teams; and
2. dispatch organs according to national and regional rules.

The particularity of France Transplant Region 3 is the mobile TC nurse, who helps each hospital in any way necessary for local coordination, intensive care or surgery procedures.

Conclusion

The population of western Europe is 376.8 million inhabitants. We could expect at least 2,000 additional cadaveric donors if we can increase the European mean from 14.7 to 20 donors pmp. If the multiorgan procurement mean could be moved from 64.7% pmp to 80% pmp we could expect 5,765 more organs. If the European mean of all organs procured could be increased from 44.6 pmp to 70 pmp, 9,570 additional organs could be available.

Are there organ shortage solutions?

Increasing the potential number of available organs involves many factors:

- The first is a supportive law in each country (the opting out philosophy is actually the best).
- The second is good organization including, if possible,

  - high-level, full-time medical transplant coordinators,
  - national organization with three levels of local, regional and national coordination (i.e. France and Spain),
  - available regional human means.

- The third factor is a new concept, which could be called European Transplant Procurement Management. This could eventually include eastern countries.

Acknowledgements

The authors would like to thank Mrs D. Minarro for excellent assistance in preparing this manuscript.

References

1. Cochat P, Lavocat MP, Floret D, Berthier JC, Teyssier G. Réanimation des enfants en état de mort cérébrale en vue d'un prélèvement d'organes à but thérapeutique. Arch Fr Pediatr 1988; 45: 703–8.
2. Colpart JJ, Moskovtchenko JF, Finaz de Villaine J, Mercatello A. La mort cérébrale: diagnostic, physiopathologie, conduite à tenir Cahiers d'Anesthésiologie. Tome 35, juillet 1987: 291–304.
3. Colpart JJ, Noury D, Cochat P, Kormann P, Moskovtchenko JF. Organisation de la transplantation d'organes en France Pédiatrie 1991; 46: 313–22.
4. Colpart JJ, Bret M, Coronel B, Mercatello A, Yatim A, Bouttin B, Moskovtchenko JF. Significant low TSH and T3 hormon level prevalent in brain dead multiorgan potential donors population. Transplant Clin Immunol 1991: 366.
5. Colpart JJ, Moskovtchenko JF, Mercatello A, Tognet E, Martin X, Faure JL, Gelet A, Lefrancois N, Touraine JL. One year creatinine data after post cardiac arrest in situ kidney cooling Transplant Clin Immunol 1990; XXI.
6. Colpart JJ, Bret M, Coronel B, Mercatello A, Bouttin B, Moskovtchenko JF. Significant low T3 hormone level prevalent in brain dead multiorgan potential donors population. Proceedings of the Seventh Congress ETCO; 1991 Oct; Maastricht, The Netherlands.
7. Colpart JJ, Guillot B, Bouttin B, Maillefaud B, Saury G, Touraine JL, Moskovtchenko JF. Potential multiorgan donors: a retrospective study of virus incidence. Proceedings of the Seventh Congress ETCO; 1991 Oct; Maastricht, The Netherlands.
8. Colpart JJ, Bret M, Coronel B, Mercatello A, Maillefaud B, Guillot B, Moskovtchenko JF. Are brain dead donors sudden cardiac arrests due to blood phophorus level decrease. Transplant Clin Immunol 1992: 365.
9. Colpart JJ, Bret M, Coronel B, Mercatello A, Laurent V, Bouttin B, Guillot B, Maillefaud B, Saury G, Moskovtchenko JF. Monitoring and management of multi-organ donor. Transplant Clin Immunol 1992; XIV: 277–84.
10. Duke PK, Ramsay MAE, Paulsen AW, Gunning TC, Roberts LC, Swygert TH, Valek TR. Intraoperative hemodynamic heterogenecity of brain dead organ donors. Transplant Proc 1991; 23(5): 2485–6.
11. Goarin JP, Jacquens Y, Cohen S, Guesde R, Le Bret F, Arengo A, Clerque F, Viars P. Effets de la triiodothyronine (T3) sur l'hémodynamique et la fraction d'éjection du ventricule gauche (FEVG) du donneur. Ann Franç Anesth Réa 1991; 10: R114.
12. Harms J, Isemer FE, Kolenda H. Hormonal alteration and pituitary function during course of brain stem death in potential organ donors. Transplant Proc 1991; 23(5): 2614–6.
13. Laurent V, Coronel B, Bret M, Mercatello A, Colpart JJ, Touraine JL, Moskovtchenko JF. Use of hydroxylethylamidon in organ donor resuscitation. Proceedings of the Transplantation Society Congress; 1992; Paris.
14. Mariot J, Jacob F, Voltz C, Perrier JF, Strub P. Evaluation of tri-iodthyronine and cortisol treatment in the brain-dead patient. Ann Fr Anesth Réanim 1991; 10: 321–8.
15. Masson F, Thicoipe M, Maurette M, Pinaquy C, Leger A, Erny P. Perturbations de l'hémodynamique, de la coagulation et de la glycorégulation induites par la mort cérébrale. Ann Franç Anesth Réa 1990; 9: 115–22.
15. Mercatello A, Roy P, Sing K Ng, Choux C, Baude C, Garnier JL, Colpart JJ, Finaz J, Petit P, Moskovtchenko JF, Touraine JL, Dubernard JM. Organ transplant from out of hospital cardiac arrest patients. Tansplant Proc 1988; XX(5): 749–50.
16. Orlowski JP, Spees EK. The use of thyroxine (T4) to promote hemodynamic stability in the vascular organ donor: a preliminary report on the colorado experience – Munksgaard 1991. J Transplant Coordination 1991; 1(1): 19–22.
17. Pennefather SH, Bullock RE. Triiodothyronine treatment in brain-dead multiorgan donors – a controlled study [letter to editor]. Transplantation 1993; 55 (6): 1443.
18. Quesada A, Teja JL, Rabanal JM, Cotorruelo JG, Espadas FL, Reganon GD. Inotropic

support in 50 brain-dead organ donors: repercussion on renal graft function. Transplant Proc 1991; 23: 2479–80.

19. Vedrinne JM, Coronel B, Vedrinne C, Dorez D, Colpart JJ, Mercatello A, Motin J, Estanove S, Moskovtchenko JF. L'évaluation échographique de la fonction ventriculaire gauche chez le patient en état de mort cérébrale permet-elle de prédire le bon fonctionnement du greffon chez le receveur? Ann Franç Anesth Réa 1993; 12: R177.

20. Yatim A, Colpart JJ, Tognet E, Bret M, Mercatello A, Moskovtchenko JF, Peyrin JO. Intérêt du 99 Tc HMPAO dans le diagnostic de la mort cérébrale. J Med Nucl Biophy 1992; 14(1): 58–63.

21. Yatim A, Mercatello A, Coronel B, Bret M, Colpart JJ, Moskovtchenko JF, Peyrin JO. 99 Tc-HMPAO cerebral scintigraphy in the diagnosis of brain death. Transplant Proc 1991; 23(5).

22. Optimal use of cadaver kidneys for transplantation

GERHARD OPELZ & THOMAS WUJCIAK

During the last two decades the success rate of renal transplantation has steadily improved. This has led to a widening of acceptance criteria for transplantation. Patients who, 10 years ago, would have been excluded for reasons such as advanced age or complicating secondary diseases, are nowadays readily accepted for the transplant waiting list. As a result, the pool of potential recipients has been increasing in all countries. For example, in the geographical area served by the Eurotransplant Organization (Germany, the Netherlands, Belgium, Austria and Luxemburg), the number of patients on the transplant waiting list has increased from approximately 4,000 in the year 1982 to more than 11,000 in 1992. Unfortunately, the number of available cadaver kidneys has not increased at a similar pace. In 1982, Eurotransplant reported approximately 1,500 cadaver kidney transplants and, by 1992, the number has increased to 3,100. As a result, the gap between the number of patients waiting for a transplant and the number of transplants realized has widened from year to year.

Although less restrictive acceptance criteria are the main reason for the longer waiting lists, the shortage of donor organs is further aggravated by the re-listing of patients who have rejected their graft. Transplant rejection thus carries a double penalty: the recipient loses his independence from the dialysis machine and again has to compete in the pool with other patients who are waiting for their first transplant, which decreases the chance of all patients for receiving a transplant soon. It is therefore obvious that all possible measures must be taken to ensure long-term graft survival in as many recipients as possible.

We and others have suggested that the outcome of transplants can be predicted based on a number of influential factors [1, 2]. Unfortunately, many of these factors are patient characteristics that cannot be altered, such as advanced age, metabolic diseases such as diabetes or oxalosis, highly reactive preformed lymphocytotoxic antibodies as an indicator of sensitization, or other complicating medical conditions. To selectively allocate donor kidneys to patients who are free of complicating conditions would predictably lead to a higher success rate. However, it would also discriminate against

J.L. Touraine et al. (eds.), *Organ Shortage: The Solutions*, 161–165.

Table 1. Influence of HLA matching on survival of first cadaver kidney transplants

Number of HLA-A + B + DR mismatches	Number of patients studied	Graft survival rate at 5 years (% + SE)		
		All transplants	Local kidneys	Shipped kidneys
0	2527	71 ± 1	71 ± 3	71 ± 2
1	5326	64 ± 1	64 ± 2	63 ± 1
2	11230	61 ± 1	64 ± 1	60 ± 1
3	14805	60 ± 1	61 ± 1	60 ± 1
4	11358	57 ± 1	60 ± 1	55 ± 1
5	6128	53 ± 1	53 ± 1	54 ± 2
6	1963	50 ± 1	53 ± 2	49 ± 4
Regression		$p < 0.0001$	$p < 0.0001$	$p < 0.0001$

All recipients and donors were typed for HLA-A and HLA-B antigen split specificities.

the less fortunate patients who are equally in need of transplants, albeit with a lesser chance of success. It would be unacceptable for ethical reasons to deprive these patients of their chance to receive transplantation treatment.

Considering these various aspects, it would seem desirable to allocate donor organs in such a way that all potential recipients, once they were accepted for the transplant waiting list, would have an equal and fair chance of receiving a donor kidney. This could be accomplished, for example, by a simple lottery system or by distributing the donor organs according to the potential recipients' waiting time in the pool. However, the drawback of such an approach is that established scientific facts relating to donor-recipient histocompatibility would be neglected. This would result in a relatively poor success rate. On the other hand, if histocompatibility (HLA matching) were used as the sole criterion for kidney allocation, patients with rare HLA phenotypes would be discriminated against because many of them would not be transplanted at all. We have therefore developed an allocation algorithm that takes into account the frequency of a patient's HLA phenotype and thereby allows the utilization of HLA matching without the undesirable effect of producing an unacceptably large fraction of "long waiters" in the recipient pool.

The basis for using HLA matching as an important criterion for organ allocation is shown in Table 1. The transplant success rate declines significantly as the number of mismatched HLA-A, -B, -DR antigens between recipient and donor increases ($p < 0.0001$). Importantly, HLA matching improves graft outcome both in patients who were reported to be poor candidates because of the presence of complicating conditions and in patients in whom complicating factors were absent (Table 2).

Table 1 shows in addition a comparison of HLA matching results for kidneys that were procured and transplanted in the same center with kidneys

Table 2. Influence of HLA matching on graft survival in patients with or without additional risk factors

Number of HLA-A + B + DR mismatches	Graft survival rate at 5 years (% ± SE)	
	Patients without risk factors	Patients with risk factors
0	72 ± 2	69 ± 3
1	66 ± 2	54 ± 2
2	64 ± 1	53 ± 1
3	63 ± 1	50 ± 1
4	60 ± 1	50 ± 1
5	54 ± 1	47 ± 2
6	54 ± 2	44 ± 3
Regression	$p < 0.0001$	$p < 0.0001$

that were shipped from one center to another. In both sets of transplants there was a highly statistically significant correlation of HLA matching with graft survival.

When HLA matching is used as the sole criterion for kidney allocation, several undesired side effects are produced. We performed computer simulations based on realistic background conditions in order to obtain information on changes in the recipient pool. Starting from the current patient distribution in the Eurotransplant waiting pool, we found that strict HLA-oriented kidney allocation would increase the number of patients who are waiting in the pool for longer than three years from currently 22% to 31% within a three-year period. Moreover, the likelihood of obtaining a kidney with zero or only 1 HLA-A, -B, -DR mismatch would decline, on average, from a current 64% to only 53% after three years. This unfavorable recipient pool evolution can be avoided by considering the likelihood of a given patient to obtain a good match (depending on the HLA phenotype) and the time period that a patient has already waited for a transplant. When the likelihood that a better match will be obtained in the future is very small, kidneys are allocated to patients with rare phenotypes even if the HLA match is less than perfect. Because transplant centers do not like to export kidneys to other centers unless they receive approximately an equal number of kidneys in return, the allocation method was refined to also consider each center's kidney exchange balance. Moreover, a bonus for local transplantation was built into the model in such a way that a kidney is assigned to a recipient of another center only if that recipient has at least two fewer HLA mismatches than the best-matched local patient. The computer algorithm on which this allocation model – called XCOMB – is based, was published in detail [3, 4].

Table 3 shows the results that can be obtained with the XCOMB allocation method, starting from a recipient pool corresponding to the current Eurotransplant waiting list and assuming that increases in the numbers of recipi-

Table 3. Comparison of kidney allocation methods

Allocation method	HLA-A + B + DR mismatches (% of patients)		
	0–1	2–3	4–6
Random	1	24	75
XCOMB	46	51	4
Reported to CTS study	21	54	25

Table 4. Influence of pool size on HLA matching (XCOMB method)

Pool size	HLA-A + B + DR mismatches (% of patients)		
	0–1	2–3	4–6
10,000	46	51	4
1,500	33	61	6

ents and donors would follow the pattern observed during the last three years. Compared to a random allocation of donor kidneys, without regard to the HLA match, the XCOMB method allows for a much higher rate of well-matched transplants. The rate of good matches is also considerably higher than that of actually performed transplants which were reported to the Collaborative Transplant Study from European centers during the last five years. Importantly, this favorable HLA match distribution can be obtained without increasing the rate of "long waiters" and without decreasing the chance of obtaining good HLA matches for those patients who remain in the pool.

Many countries or groups of cooperating transplant centers maintain recipient waiting lists that are much smaller than the 10,000 patients listed on the Eurotransplant waiting list. We therefore tested whether the XCOMB allocation method would also be suitable for a smaller recipient pool. The results of a computer simulation based on the current waiting lists of eight selected transplant centers in Germany, containing a total of approximately 1,500 patients, are shown in Table 4. Although the HLA match distribution of transplants is not as favorable as that for a pool of 10,000, the result is clearly superior to that obtained with random allocation and is considerably better than the results of transplants reported by European transplant centers to the Collaborative Transplant Study (Table 3).

Compared with a cadaver kidney allocation policy that does not take HLA matching into account, the XCOMB method results in an improved HLA match distribution. Compared with a kidney allocation policy that is based strictly on the HLA match, the XCOMB method has the advantage of avoiding the accumulation of "long waiters" and of maintaining a stable likelihood in the pool for obtaining good matches. To our knowledge, the XCOMB kidney allocation model is superior to other allocation methods currently in use because it intelligently combines the factors: HLA match, future match probability, preference for local use of donor organs, kidney exchange balance and waiting time.

References

1. Henninge M, Köhler CO, Opelz G. Multivariate prediction model for kidney transplant success rates. Transplantation 1986; 42: 491.
2. Thorogood J, van Houwelingen JC, Persijn GG *et al.* Prognostic indices to predict survival of first and second renal allografts. Transplantation 1991; 52: 831.
3. Wujciak T, Opelz G. Computer analysis of cadaver kidney allocation procedures. Transplantation 1993; 55: 516.
4. Wujciak T, Opelz G. A proposal for improved cadaver kidney allocation. Transplantation 1993; 56: 1513.

23. Organ procurement in Spain: The national organization of transplants

R. MATESANZ, B. MIRANDA, C. FELIPE & M.T. NAYA

Introduction

The growing shortage of cadaveric organ donors remains the major obstacle
to the full development of transplants. There is a growing discrepancy between organ supply and demand. Consent laws, although effective when fully
accepted, as in Austria, or partially accepted as in Belgium, have not been
introduced in most countries [1]. Organ shortage reflects not only a shortage
of donors, but also a failure to make use of existing donors. To overcome
this problem, a model of organization has been adopted in Spain, which is
based on a decentralized transplant coordinating network comprising 3 levels
– national, regional and local (i.e. hospital) – with organ procurement as a
specific goal. Since 1989, when the National Organization of Transplants
(ONT) was started, a 50% increase has been achieved in the number of
kidneys available for transplantation and an increase of more than 100% has
been realized for other solid organs.

Because of the potential relevance for other countries we briefly describe
this organization.

Description of environmental characteristics

Spain is a southern European country with 38.4 million inhabitants. It is
divided into 17 autonomous regions. The National Health System comprises
all facilities and public services devoted to health. Health counselors in the
17 Autonomous Communities, together with 17 members of the Central
Administration, constitute the Interterritorial Council for the National
Health System. The body is presided over by the Minister of Health and
Consumer Affairs and is specifically in charge of the coordination of health
policies. Today, public health assistance is available for 99% of the population.

The Spanish transplant law, approved by the Parliament in 1979, is technically quite similar to the laws of other western countries. Brain death is

J.L. Touraine et al. (eds.), *Organ Shortage: The Solutions*, 167–177.
© 1995 *Kluwer Academic Publishers*.

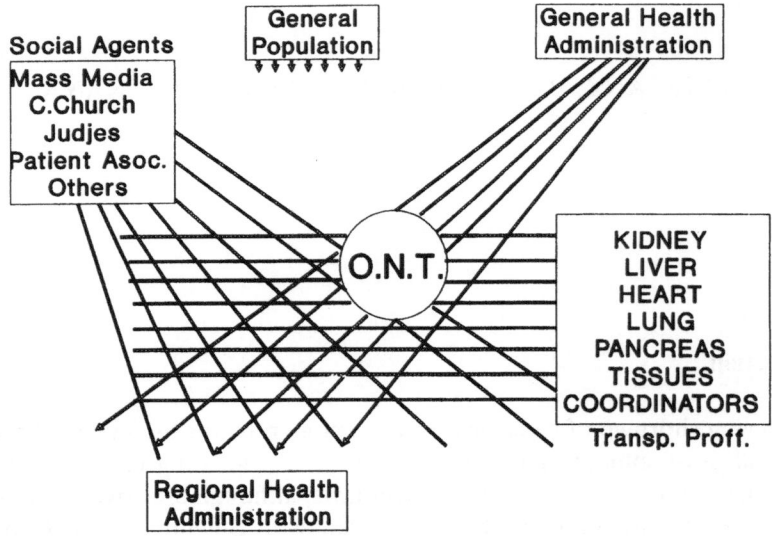

Fig. 1. Number and composition of Spanish transplant coordinating teams.

defined as the "total and irreversible loss of brain function" and must be certified by 3 doctors unrelated to the transplant team. Signs of brain death must be explored clinically and documented by silent EEG during a period of 30 minutes. Such explorations have to be repeated twice within an interval of no less than six hours. These signs are valid unless the patient is hypothermic or exposed to drugs with known brain-depressive action. Organs are obtained after informed consent of the family. The law also states that no compensation can be paid for donation, nor for grafted organs.

The first kidney grafts were performed in Spain in 1964 in Catalonia and Madrid. Thereafter, annual activity remained stable during the sixties and seventies. It increased progressively during the eighties after the law was approved by the Parliament in 1979. After a maximum number of renal grafts in 1986, the number decreased by 20% from 1986 to 1989.

Spanish coordinating teams and network: The ont

In September 1989, the ONT was started as an organisation attached to the Spanish Department of Health. Its central office is located in Madrid. From the beginning, it negotiated transplant policies. ONT emphasized the necessity that one person or group of persons must be responsible for the coordination of organ procurement and transplantation for each potential donor and each hospital. These teams were to interact with each other and with

Coordinating Teams
Spain 1993 (N=122)

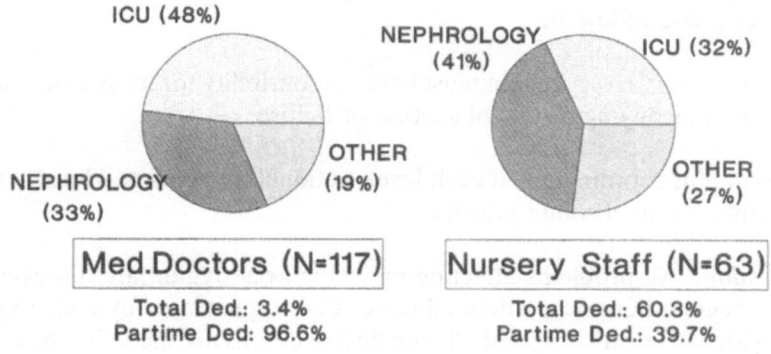

Med.Doctors (N=117)
Total Ded.: 3.4%
Partime Ded: 96.6%

Nursery Staff (N=63)
Total Ded.: 60.3%
Partime Ded.: 39.7%

Fig. 2. Coordinating role of ONT.

Table 1. Profile of the transplant coordinator in Spain

Qualification	Physicians	Nurses
Dedication	Part-time	
Dependence	Medical Director of the hospital	
Origin	Intensive Care Units	
Continuity	Temporary (2–4 years)	
Location	Within the hospital	
Main aim	Organ procurement	
Increasingly involved in	Management of resources	
	Educational Programes	
	Relations to Media	

the Regional and National Coordinators. The transplant coordinating net-work was then conceived at 3 levels: national, regional and local. The ONT advised that a medical doctor should be in charge in each hospital. Preferably, they should belong to intensive care or renal units and a staff nurse should also be attached to each transplant program. This implies that a medical doctor plus 3 nurses should be appointed in hospitals with renal, liver and cardiac transplant teams, and one person only in hospitals with no transplant team. If a hospital procures organs without having a transplant team, the coordinators are dedicated only part-time to coordinating tasks.

The profile of Spanish transplant coordinators is summarized in Table 1. As can be seen, they depend directly on the medical director of the hospital and not on the chief of a transplant unit, and they are increasingly involved in administrative tasks and relations to social groups other than sanitary ones. These networks have been developed over the past 4 years. In 1989, scarcely 25 coordinating teams were active in Spain, 122 are working today, one in each potential donor hospital. Figure 2 summarizes the origin and other characteristics of Spanish coordinators.

To adapt the coordinating network to Spanish needs, five basic principles were set up and followed:

Decentralization. Every region must have responsibility for its own decisions, and the accompanying results of success or failure.

Main aim. For coordinators at each level, national, regional and local, organ procurement is an absolute priority.

Cooperation. All problems affecting more than one region are discussed in the Interregional Council, where all regions are represented by their respective Regional Coordinator, and all technical decisions are made by consensus amongst National and Regional Coordinators.

Tasks of the central office. ONT acts as a service agency. It does not only arrange transport of organs or transplant teams. It elaborates and updates statistical data. It maintains the waiting lists and registries of transplant activity, and keeps interested social or professional groups informed. A telephone line has been established that works 24 hours a day, seven days a week, to answer any question or doubt concerning donors, organ procurement or organ transplantation. Finally, ONT promotes organ and tissue procurement and sharing, and guarantees the transparency of the entire process.

Relation to social agencies. All transplant coordinating teams are in close touch with social agencies that have potential influence on transplant activity and organ procurement (Figure 2). Especially media relations are carefully carried out. Specifically designed educational programs are being developed to offer transplant coordinators the best strategies to transmit messages to media professionals. Close contact and successful collaboration are also carried out with patient associations and judges and coroners.

Organ procurement figures

In 1989, 14.3 donors pmp were available in Spain; this rate increased to 17.8 in 1990, 20.2 in 1991, 21.7 in 1992 and 22.6 in 1993. This compares favourably with rates in other western countries, which have remained stable or have even decreased during the last 3 years (Figures 3 and 4). There are substantial differences among regions affecting the organ procurement rate, neverthe-

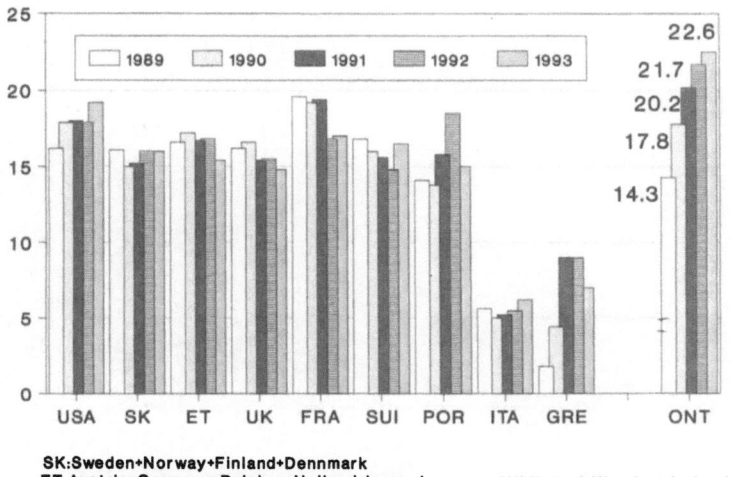

ORGAN DONORS
Annual Rate (p.m.p.)

SK:Sweden+Norway+Finland+Dennmark
ET:Austria+Germany+Belgium+Holland+Luxemburg   UK:United Kingdom+Ireland

Fig. 3. Annual rate of cadaveric organ donors in different countries and transplant organizations (pmp: per million population).

less, it must be emphasized that rates from some regions like Canarias or Euskadi (38.5 and 36 donors pmp, respectively) are probably near the maximum pool that can be achieved (Figure 5).

During 1993, multiorgan removal was performed in 70.5% of cases, i.e. solid organs other than kidneys were also removed; the respective figures for 1989, 1990, 1991 and 1992 were 30%, 50%, 64% and 69%. The number of organs removed each year increased from 1,409 in 1989 to 2,670 in 19932, i.e. + 89% (Figure 6).

In June 1992, a new road traffic law was approved. This law fortunately led to a significant decrease in the number of traffic road deaths: from 150 deaths pmp in 1991 to 121 in 1993 (i.e. 21.3% decrease). An 11.3% increase in the organ donor pool was seen during the same period (Figure 7). This was due to an improvement in donor detection, obviously with important changes in their characteristics. Figure 8 shows age variations and Figure 9 the differences in the cause of brain death, ACVA now being the most frequent.

Conclusions

In many countries a real decrease in the number of available organs for transplantation has been observed in recent years. The rate of potential donors has been reported to vary between 2.8 and 3.7/100 hospital deaths

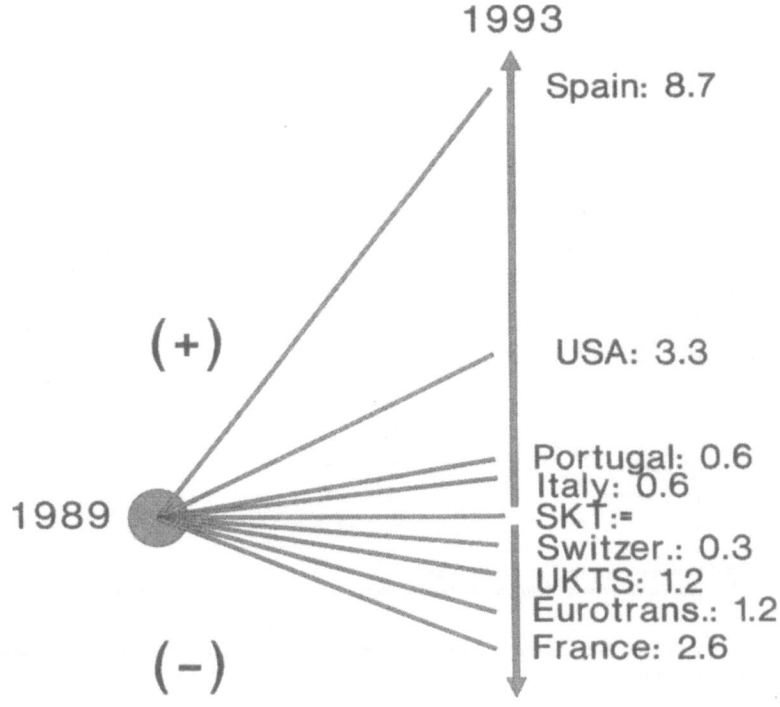

Fig. 4. Variations in the organ procurement rate during 1989–1993 in different countries.

[2] and between 40 and 100 donors pmp/year [3]. A large discrepancy exists between the number of potential donors and the actual number of organs procured. The Spanish experience shows that the problem is not a lack of suitable donors but, rather, a failure to use potential donors. Such failures may occur in any step of the following sequence: donor identification, consent of relatives, clinical management of the donor or procurement of the organ.

In 1991, the rate of patients accepted for renal replacement therapy rose to over 60 new patients pmp in most European countries [4, 5]. This was due in part to acceptance of elderly and high risk patients. Although not all are transplant candidates, the waiting lists grew in parallel. Consequently the transplantation capacity was exceeded, so that most patients now have to wait for more than 5 years to receive a renal graft.

The mortality of patients while awaiting other solid organ grafts is not negligible. In Spain, 6.4% of liver patients and 5% of cardiac patients died in 1992 while awaiting a transplant [6], and even higher figures have been reported in elsewhere [7]. These percentages may increase further in the future because of wider acceptance of therapeutic procedures due to increasing experience and improvement of results.

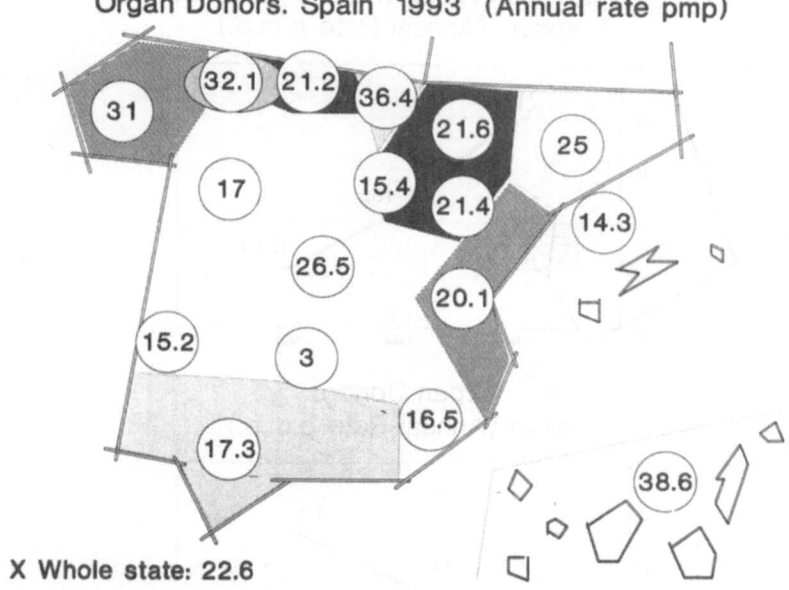

Fig. 5. Organ procurement rates in different regions during 1993.

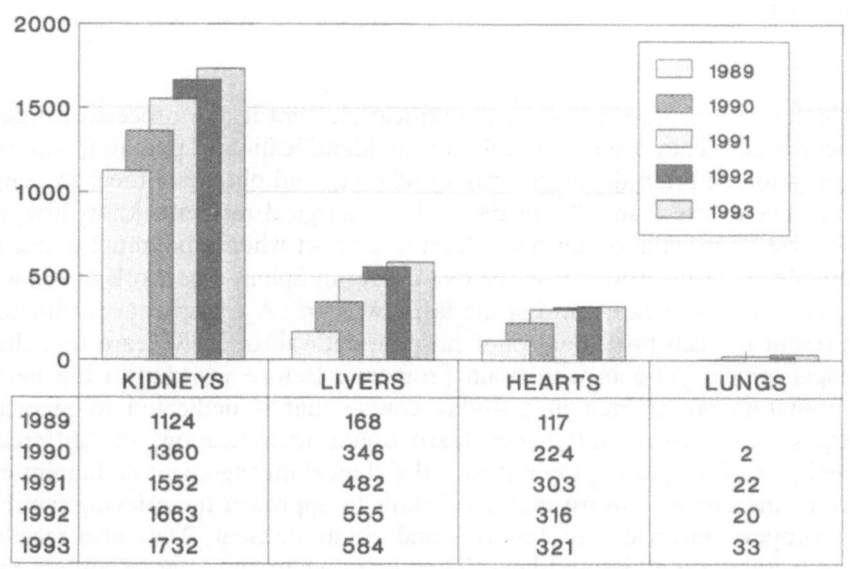

	KIDNEYS	LIVERS	HEARTS	LUNGS
1989	1124	168	117	
1990	1360	346	224	2
1991	1552	482	303	22
1992	1663	555	316	20
1993	1732	584	321	33

Fig. 6. Total organs removed with transplantation purposes during the last three years in Spain.

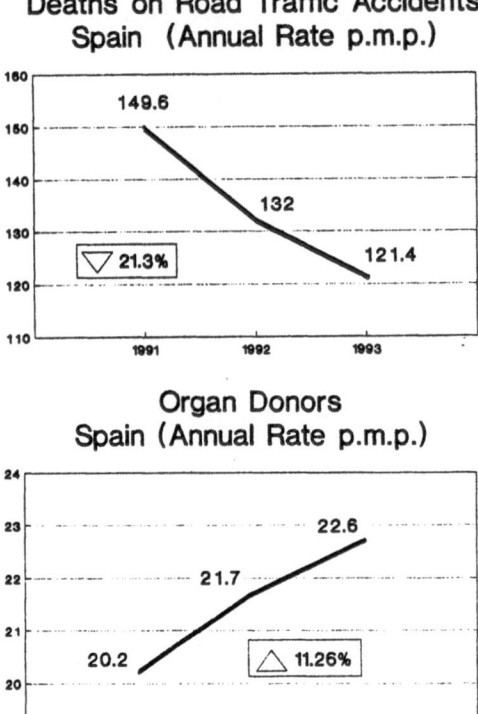

Fig. 7. Evolution of the rate of mortal traffic road accidents pmp and organ donors pmp in Spain: 1991–1993.

Health care professionals are the critical element in the process of organ procurement. They are responsible for the identification of potential donors, certification of brain death, informing relatives and obtaining their consent. In the USA, less than 50% of medical and surgical residents know how to recognize a potential donor and whom to contact when a potential donor is available [8]. This problem can be overcome. In Spain, a network of trained people has been created during the last few years. A transplant coordinator is present in each potential donor hospital with an intensive care unit that accepts critical patients with brain problems. Before working in the field, coordinators are trained in a 4–day course that is dedicated to medical doctors and nursery staff. They learn donor identification, the different techniques of diagnosing brain death, the clinical management and mainten-ance of the donor, and psychological skills to approach the grieving family, give support, interview the relatives and obtain consent. They also receive some lectures on ethics and laws. They learn when and how to contact the coordinating office. Also, basic information concerning solid organ and tissue transplants is given.

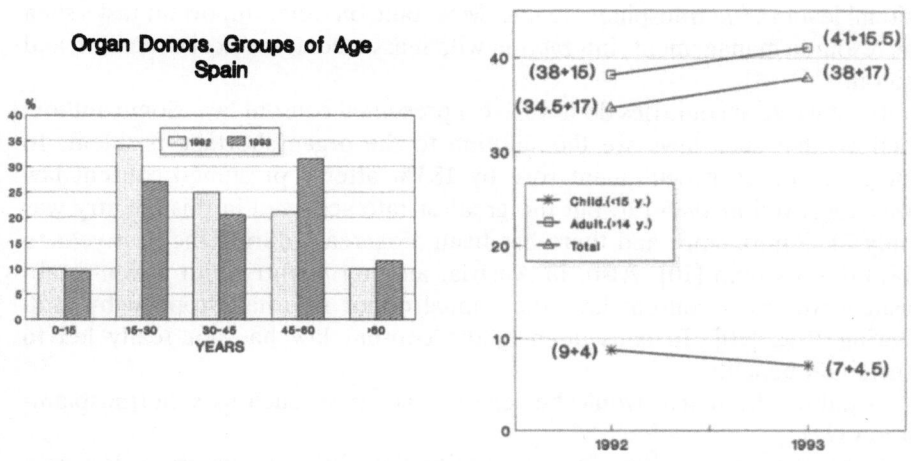

Fig. 8. Organ donors' characteristics in Spain: age.

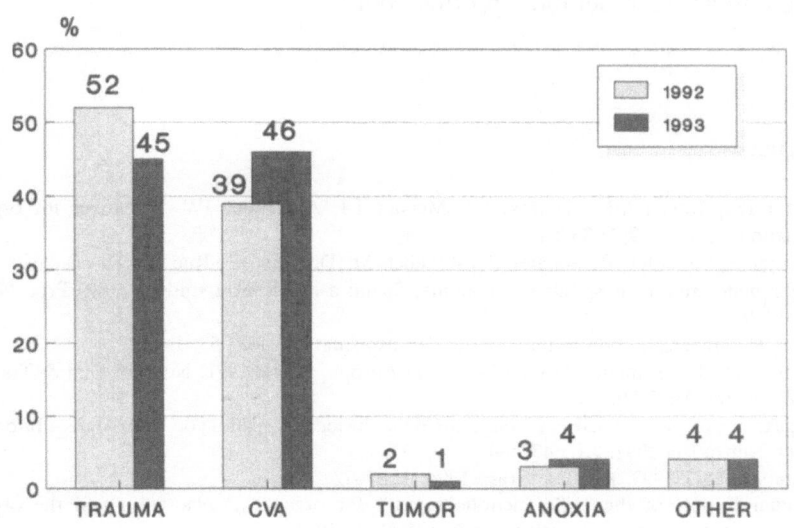

Fig. 9. Organ donors' characteristics in Spain: cause of brain death.

This program started two years ago and today 80 coordinators have been trained in such courses. The Spanish transplant coordinators are directly accountable to the hospital medical director and work at a similar professional level as the transplant teams. Most take on other important tasks such as resource management, interaction with mass media, medical education and so on.

Most western countries do not have a presumed consent law. Some authors believe that such laws are the solution to the organ shortage problem. In Belgium, organ procurement rose by 183% after a presumed consent law was approved in 1986 [9], but the greatest rate achieved in this country was only 21 donors pmp, and there has been a decrease during the past year to 18.3 donors pmp [10]. Also, in Austria, another country with a well-established presumed consent law, the annual donor rate has dropped by 12% during 1992 [10]. In consequence, the consent law has not really led to sustained benefits.

Another alternative would be scientific advances such as xenotransplantation [11].

However, while waiting for future scientific advances, one must do something now to improve organ procurement. We feel that our approach indicates that organ procurement can be improved by organisational efforts on the national, regional and local levels [12, 13]. In Spain, this has led to a rise in organ procurement even though no change in law has been made.

We do not really know whether the particular approach used in Spain to organize organ procurement and transplantation can be directly applied to other countries with different health systems. Nevertheless, we hope the information on the Spanish system can be useful when organizational structures are under consideration in other countries.

References

1. Kittur DS, Hogan MM, Thukral KJ, McGaw LJ, Alexander JW. Incentives for organ donation? Lancet 1991; 338: 1441–3.
2. Espinel E, Deulofeu R, Sabater R, Mañalich M, Domingo P, Rué M. The capacity for organ generation of hospitals in Catalonia, Spain: a multicentre study. Transp Proc 1989; 21: 1419–21.
3. First R. Transplantation in the nineties. Transplantation 1992; 53: 1–11.
4. Report on Management of Renal Failure in Europe, XXII, 1991. Nephrol Dial & Transp 1992; 7(supp 2): 7–29.
5. Registro Nacional de Dialisis y Trasplante de la Sociedad Española de Nefrologia – Informe 1990. Nefrologia 1992; XII: 471–84.
6. Memoria ONT 1993. Rev Esp Trasp 1994; 3: 67–72.
7. Annual Report of the U.S. scientific registry for organ transplantation and the organ procurement and transplantation network. UNOS, 1991.
8. Spital A, Kittur DS. Barriers to organ donation among housestaff physicians. Transp Proc 1990; 22: 2414.

9. Roels L, Varenterghem Y, Waer M, Gruwez J, Michelsen P. Effect of a presumed consent law on organ retrieval in Belgium. Transplant Proc 1990; 22: 2078–9.
10. Eurotransplant newsletter, 1993; number 107 (Sept.).
11. Najarian SJ. Overview in Xenotransplantation studies: Prospects to the future. Transp Proc 1992; 24: 733–8.
12. Mijares J, Perdigo L, Neyro MT, Arrieta J, Montenegro J, Aranzabal J. Donor detection and organ procurement in the Basque Autonomous Community: general data. Transp Proc 1991; 23: 2543.
13. Mañalich M, Cabrer C, Garcia Fages LC, Valero R. Method of organ procurement: transplant coordination team. Transp Proc 1991; 23: 2546.

24. Integrated ways to improve cadaveric organ donation

B. MIRANDA, R. MATESANZ, C. FELIPE & M.T. NAYA

Background

The growing shortage of cadaveric organ donors remains the major obstacle to the full development of transplants. Organ and tissue transplants are probably the only sanitary field that cannot be supported solely by research and financial resources. We need the participation of the entire society to cover the most important part of the process: the donors. Without them the transplants cannot proceed. Given the enormous benefits of transplants, there exists an overriding commitment to continue the drive to increase organ donation rates. Although transplants save thousands of lives and transform the quality of life of thousands more, many people die or remain on renal replacement therapy because the organ supply falls drastically short of actual demand.

The binomial *donation/transplantation* is indivisible. Nevertheless, historically the second part has received much more attention from the point of view of research and resources: only 2% of abstracts received at the Congress of the International Society of Organ Transplantation, held in Paris in 1992, referred to the topic: "Organ procurement and preservation" [1]. The same could be observed a year later at the congress of the European Society of Organ Transplantation in Rhodos [2]. Fortunately this concept is now changing. All transplant professionals are concerned about organ shortage and ways to improve it. This can be seen in some editorials of specialized magazines, but there are still very few papers representing research work in this field. Health departments are also starting to demonstrate their concern, supporting some initiatives such as national and international working groups and expert meetings. Pharmaceutical companies, also, are now more prone to dedicating financial resources to support the development of educational and research programmes on this topic. A clear example of this progressive change is the fact that this prestigious international meeting is dedicated to the intention of finding solutions to the dilemma.

Donaton/transplantation is a complex process involving different steps, starting and ending in the *society*, this being its main feature (Figure 1). As

J.L. Touraine et al. (eds.), *Organ Shortage: The Solutions*, 179–190.
© 1995 *Kluwer Academic Publishers*.

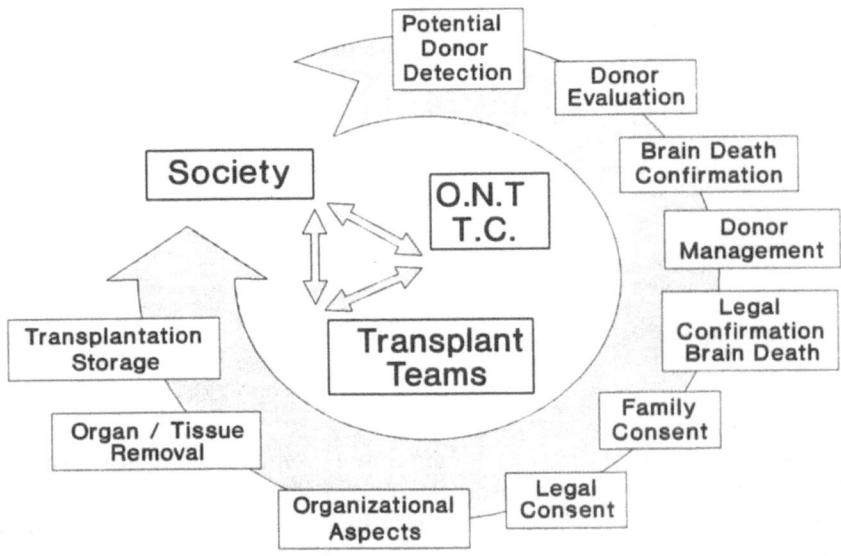

Fig. 1. The donation/transplantation process.

A. Caplan testified before the US Congress in 1990, ". . . Transplants are not specially related to costs or techniques but with Ethics. Transplants are the only field of health that could not have existed without the participation of the society. It is the citizen who, during his life or after deceased, makes possible the graft of his organs or tissues. Without these donations transplants would have not been developed . . . " [3]. We should always keep this in mind: the donation/transplantation process starts and ends in the society; the citizens are its motor and its main beneficiaries. Health professionals are obviously necessary since donors and recipients cannot keep in contact by themselves, but do not forget, we are there only to help and be useful; we will never be the protagonists. Our overall aim must be the optimization of the donation/transplantation process in order to alleviate the organ shortage.

Process overview

Following the proposed schema, the process would start with the potential donor detection, considering potential donors all people that can be diagnosed as having brain death. All these potential donors must be evaluated, looking carefully for any pathologic contraindication representing a potential risk for the recipient. After that comes the necessary clinical and legal confirmation of brain death. During the time spent for all these requirements it is necessary to mantain the haemodynamic stability of the donor within a

Table 1. Organ Donor Pool in different areas

	Kentucky 1988	Madrid 1992	Euskadi 1993
Inhabitants	3.4 M.I.	4.8 M.I.	2.1 M.I.
Deaths	35009	35039	
Deaths pmp	10297	73009	
Brain death	173	269	120
Brain death pmp	50.8	56	57
Denied consent	92 (53%)	50 (18.6%	9 (7.5%)
Medical contraindications	43 (25%)	79 (29.4%)	35 (29%)
Effective donors	38 (22%)	140 (52%)	76 (63.5%)
Effective donors pmp	11.2	29	36.2

See [5] for the Kentucky data. Reproduced with permission of A. Navarro (Madrid) & J. Aranzábal (Euskedi).

very narrow range to preserve the viability of the organs. In the case of a legal or social requirement of family consent, (the case of most countries [4]) we have to approach the family and interview them to request consent. Independent of this requirement, complete family support is mandatory. We also have to prepare the hospital for a multiorgan procurement procedure. The coordinating office should always be contacted to offer the donor; the organs will then be shared following the previously accorded criteria and all logistic support for organs or teams travelling will be prepared. Once the removal of organs and tissues is finished, these will be grafted or stored. This large and complex process, involving more than 100 health professionals and consuming sometimes more than 2 days, cannot be left to a free evolution. Every step must be previously protocolized to avoid any improvisation. Nevertheless sometimes difficulties arise and the donor is lost. It is very important to identify those problems and promote solutions, making the process increasingly easy and smooth.

Potential donor detection

This constitutes the starting point and is probably the most difficult step to make routine.

Knowledge of the environmental characteristics in our area of work is mandatory: infrastructure of the hospitals, mortality of the area, incidence of traffic accidents, cerebrovascular accidents and cerebral tumors, health resources, etc. We must be able to point to where the neurosurgery teams are located, to which hospitals accident victims are transferred, etc. Moreover, we need an approach to the potential organ donor pool in our scope of influence. This can be acheived in two different but complementary ways: with prospective or retrospective methods.

We need a potential donor registry, where data can be collected in prospective or retrospective ways. Table 1 shows summaries of three examples of potential donor registries. The Kentucky registry was built using a retrospective method, a revision of all medical records of dead people in the area studied [5]. The two Spanish registries used prospective methods. Hospital transplant coordinators filled in forms for all brain deaths detected in their hospitals and sent them to the regional coordinator. Studies of the entire region were then carried out [6, 7]. In all cases, a conclusive number of potential donors per million population (pmp) fell into a very narrow range and were very similar to other reported figures [8]. This is of particular importance since we are talking about different countries and different working methods.

Following the calculation of potential donors pmp, it is necesssary to analyze the causes of loss of donors, which is why the study must be exhaustive. Table 1 shows the different rates and causes of loss of donors in the Spanish and American studies. In this way, the prospective registries can be compared with a retrospective one, to acquire more reliable information about donor detection in our area. This also avoids errors such as over- or underestimation of the potential donor pool.

Once the problems are diagnosed, it becomes easier to make potential solutions available. If, for example, a lack of donor detection is demonstrated by a particular hospital, it is mandatory to start a detection programme there. This would be carried out by the transplant coordinator and would include:

- Educational programs for health staff about the donation/transplantation process
- Daily revisions of the list of patients accepted in the hospital
- Follow-up of patients accepted with a Glasgow score <7
- Daily visits to all hospital units that have potential donors

In a study carried out in Barcelona over a period of 5 years, it was reported that approximately 30% of potential donors are detected by the transplant coordinator during these daily visits and controls [9].

Donor evaluation

Once the potential donor is detected, he/she must be evaluated to determine the viability of the organs. Standard protocols for donor evaluation must be developed and followed carefully to ensure that there is no potential risk for the recipient. These procedures will also be useful in analyzing the donor's characteristics and its outcome. These characteristics are constantly changing, since both organ shortage and the growing experience of transplant teams broaden the criteria for acceptance of organs [10]. Moreover, this evaluation procedure also contributes to the detection of concrete problems in specific areas (i.e. if a hospital only has young donors dying because of traumatic brain damage).

Brain death diagnosis and certification

Clinical criteria necessary for the diagnosis of brain death are clear and well explained in specialized publications. They are standard worldwide and widely accepted. Nevertheless, we found differences in the necessary legal criteria to be met in each country. Transplant coordinators are responsible for meeting these legal requirements. The coordinator is also responsible for the custody of all certifications and tests required by the law.

In our country, judges and coroners must be called in when the cause of death is traumatic; this represents less than a half of all donations. It is important to keep these professionals informed about the donation/transplantation process. The topic must be included in their educational programmes and close contact between health and law professionals working in this field needs to be maintained. There is no agreement on the cases for which judges can deny their consent for donation. For some lawyers, there is no reason for a legal denial when all requirements are observed; for others, organ donation can interfere with the development of an indictment in some cases of presumed murder. In the region of Madrid, up to 4% of potential donors are lost every year due to judicial denials [6]. This is an area that needs urgent attention.

Donor management

During all the time necessary to evaluate the donor, to achieve family consent as well as legal requirements, and to organize the logistics of the harvesting procedure, it is necessary to maintain the viability of the organs. This phase, called "donor maintenance and management", is not a punctual phase, but prolonged work during all the other processes. Depending on the other requirements, this can be prolonged up to 24 hours or more, during which time it is necessary to maintain the haemodynamic stability of the donor to ensure a good perfusion to organs and tissues. It is a direct responsibility of the doctor in charge of the intensive care unit, but we cannot forget that it also depends on the rest of the process. As a consequence, the responsible of the whole becomes also responsible of this part. Moreover, detection of possible problems affecting the positive development of the procedure is important to avoid losing time. Looking again at the Barcelona study [9], it was reported that, of 399 cases, 55 (14%) presented haemodynamic impairment or uncontrollable sepsis, contraindicating harvesting. In the multicenter study of Madrid [11], this problem was present in 29 of 269 potential donors (11%). The promotion of educational and research programs in this field should be mandatory to minimize such problems. New techniques or therapeutics that could be helpful must be widely spread. As has been stated

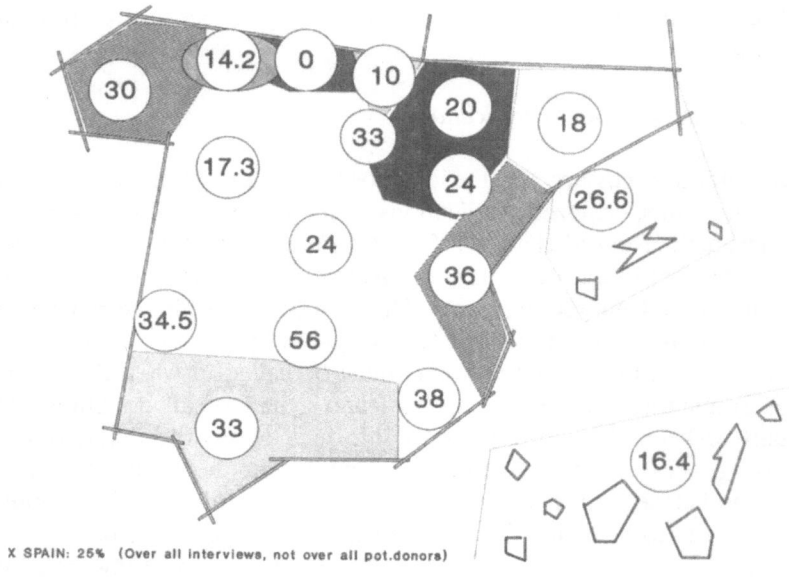

Fig. 2. Family refusal rate (%) in Spain during 1993.

previously, extra time loss must be avoided since time runs against us in the entire process.

Family approach

Approaching the family represents a key point of the process and the most sensitive, since it is based on the relation with human drama that death represents. In most countries family consent for donation is mandatory [4]. This has led to a great debate between authors sustaining the absolute necessity of strict presumed consent laws, and authors supporting the consultation of relatives.

In a recent Spanish survey it was stated that most citizens are against a change in the current practice and that only 5.7% believe that harvesting should be performed without requesting the family's wishes [12, 13]. Reasons provided by the general population in support of this attitude include that presumed consent represents an abuse of authority or an insult to the relative. It seems clear that such a change would find signficant social rejection, at least in Spain. The family refusal rate in our country has remained stable during recent years: 26.7% in 1992 and 25% in 1993, with a great variability among different areas (Figure 2) [14]. This led to the loss of more than 300 potential donors and, subsequently, more than 600 kidneys to be grafted in Spain during 1993. Some factors influencing the family decision within these circumstances must be taken into account.

Table 2. Study on family refusals and outcomes

Cause	No.	Change in attitude		Absolute negative	
		No.	%	No.	%
Lack of/inaccurate information provided to family					
Brain death	50	43	86	7	14
Corpse integrity	25	25	100	0	
Family opposed	22	14	64	8	36
Lack of information about donor's wishes	27	21	78	6	22
Social claims	16	12	75	4	25
Previous negative of the donor	14	4	29	10	71
Religious causes	13	12	92	1	8
Family wants the grief at home	10	9	90	1	10
Problems with hospital staff	5	3	60	2	40
Assertive negative	2	1	1		
	184	144	78	40	22

Reproduced with permission of P. Gomez et al., Alicante, Spain.

Public attitudes towards organ donation. As stated in a recent survey, in Spain more than 90% of the general population has a favourable opinion about donor's families and transplant procedures [13]. The problem arises when there is a lack of information about the wishes of the deceased. In this situation, only 54% of US citizens and 50% of the Spanish population would donate the organs of their relatives [13, 15]. The immediate conclusion is that people should be encouraged to speak about donation and transplantation and to transmit their wishes to their relatives, in order to facilitate their decision at a particular and difficult moment. According to the same survey [13, 15], in this case, 93% and 94% of Spanish and North American people, respectively, would give a positive answer to the request.

This message can be transmitted to the general population directly through conferences or meetings with different social groups, through campaigns, or in the schools. The development of audio-visual materials can be promoted. A 24–hour-day telephone line, working 7 days a week, is very useful to answer the doubts or questions of the general public. Of course, the most important carrier to transmit the message is the media. Media relations are of capital importance to achieve our aim.

Family attitude. We have commented on the percentage of refusals among potential donor's families. At this particularly sensitive moment, the family's answer will depend not only on their own attitudes but, also, on the way the option is presented. The causes of denied consent do not vary very much between countries. Available data from the USA [5, 15] have shown that most denials are related to:

- Doubts about brain death: 60% of US citizens believe that brain death equals death, but 30% believe that it is a comatose state and 10% don't know.
- Conflicts of interest: 34% of Americans think that there is a black market for organs and 58% are sure that poor people do not have the same opportunities as the rich.
- The family has a negative attitude.
- The person(s) requesting organ donation was not comfortable presenting the option.
- Timing and place were not appropriate: the requesting interview must be decoupled from communication of the death, in this way allowing the family the necessary time to accept the drama. This point has also been stated in a French study [16].

Causes of denied consent in Spain have been studied in different regions and hospitals, but we would like to comment on a particular study carried out in Alicante during 5 consecutive years [17]. A summary of the results is presented in Table 2. Among 184 negative responses upon first contact, 144 (78%) were reversed and consent could be achieved. As can be seen, most doubts refer to brain death assumption and corpse integrity, but there are also cases in which the response can be easily changed using the appropriate arguments and approach. When denied consent is due to the previous negative response of the potential donor, the negative attitude of the family or problems with the hospital staff, then consent is not so easy.

There are some points that need special attention regarding family approach:

- The approach should be made by specially trained staff.
- It is necessary to make a complete approach and offer of help, not only a requesting interview.
- The first approach should be carefully prepared, gathering all available information about the family members and deciding the timing and place.
- We can never transmit that we are in a hurry.
- All interviews need to be evaluated in a follow-up by the coordinating team, and all previous errors should be avoided. Most frequent errors are: to get angry, not to follow the rhythm of assimilation of the relatives, to interrupt the family, etc.
- Never forget we are there to help and be useful and never to disturb anyone.

Health professionals' attitudes. Data from the Partnership for Organ Donation reports that sometimes the family is not approached (20% of all potential donors) [5]. The reasons given are:

- Donation is viewed as compounding the family's grief.

- Staff is concerned about a perceived conflict of interest.
- Staff is uncomfortable with the idea of donation or presenting the option.
- There is a lack of awareness of the process or criteria.

Nevertheless, families should always be approached. Further data provided by the Partnership for Organ Donation [15], and data from a Spanish study carried out in Malaga [16], have demonstrated that families could also benefit from donation. The two groups studied the consent of families when requested one year after death or more. Among donor families, 86% believe that donation provides a positive outcome of death, 89–100% would donate again and 79% think that donation helps the grieving families. Among families that have denied consent, 30% would have changed their minds.

It is clear that responsibility for consent rests not only with the family, but also with the requesting staff, who should be correctly trained to deal with this step of the process with the help of psychologists and communication experts.

Organizational aspects

The coordinating office must always be alerted when a donor is available in a hospital. Donor data should be provided to assure correct sharing of the organs, depending on criteria for allocation previously accepted by all involved groups. Organs and/or team transport arrangements are then made (Figure 3). At the donor hospital, the transplant coordinating team is responsible for preparing for a multiorgan harvesting procedure. During the entire process, the coordinating team at the hospital and the staff of the coordinating office remain in close contact, providing continuous support to all people involved, health professionals and other social groups. More than 100 people participate in each process and, therefore, it is necessary for someone to be coordinating their efforts.

Organ allocation rules constitute a very important part of the organizational aspects. In Spain, organ sharing criteria are discussed every year. Medical criteria are accorded by ONT and transplant team representatives, and geographical criteria by ONT and local health administration representatives. These criteria are reviewed at the beginning of the year according to the results and transplant figures from the previous year.

ONT in Spain remains the organization responsible for guaranteeing the transparency of this particular step of the process.

After the harvesting of organs and tissues, and the grafting or storage of them, we finally return to society, where recipients are waiting for these organs and tissues. We then become the vehicle that transforms the organ donors into available organs to be grafted on recipients, allowing life to continue.

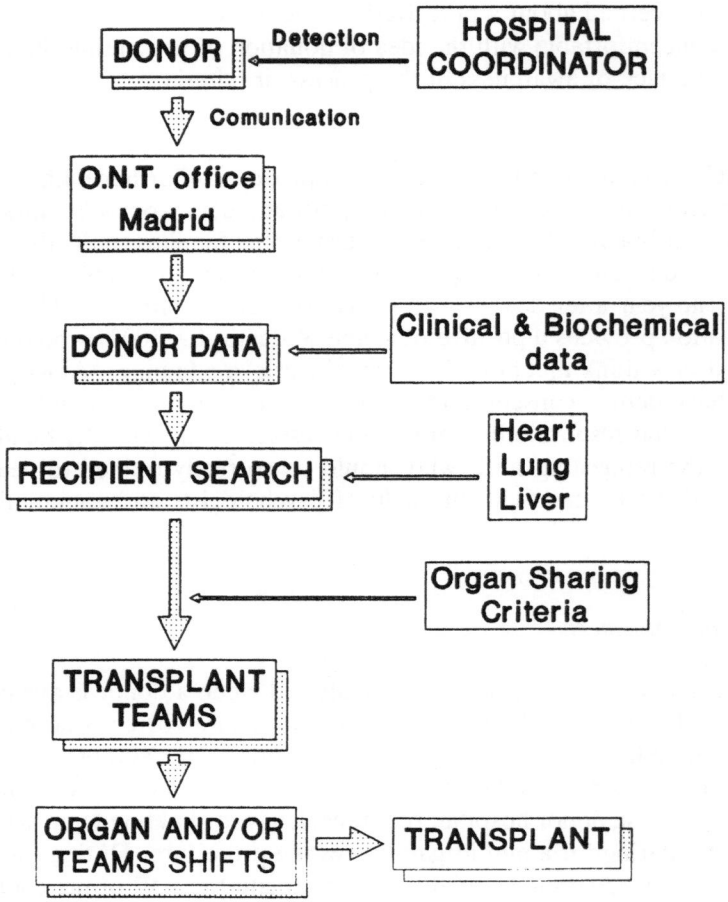

Fig. 3. Transplant coordination from the Central Office of the ONT.

Final remarks

Donation/transplantation is a complex process in which all steps must be carefully executed. The participation of the whole organ procurement organization is of capital importance, and there must be someone with a complete overview of the process, being responsible for the whole. A profile of transplant coordinators and the functions of the central office functions have been stated elsewhere in this congress (Dr. Matesanz contribution) and we will not reiterate.

The secret of organ procurement, if it exists, is the assumption of the concept that all of us (transplant teams, organ procurement professionals and society as a whole) benefit from transplants; we are all traveling in the same boat, so we must all work in the same direction, with the same objectives. If we are able to keep society informed about our work and its results, if we have a health system able to support such programmes and well-trained professionals to deal with them, and if we maintain a good organization, we will probably achieve good results. We cannot forget that our main aim is to obtain valuable organs to offer to recipients and that our work must be based on a clear list of key points:

- Diagnosing problems and providing solutions
- Analysis of available data and information to all professionals involved
- Promoting the development of educational and research programmes
- Participating in the transplant policy of the health department
- guaranteeing the transparency and equity of the process

Transplant and organ procurement professionals must be trained, so that together they can represent the necessary bridge that keeps donors and recipients in contact, since these individuals cannot achieve this contact themselves.

References

1. The Jean Hamburger Memorial Congress. Proceedings of the Fourteenth International Congress of the Transplantation Society; 1992 Aug 16–21; Paris.
2. Proceedings of the Sixth Congress of the European Society for Organ Transplantation; 1993 Oct 25–28; Rodos, Greece.
3. Caplan AL. Testimony to the Subcommittee on Health and Environment of the United States Congress. In: Matesanz R, Miranda B, editors. Etica y trasplante de organos. Rev Esp de Trasp 1993; 2(supp 1): 8.
4. Miranda B. Legislación y trasplante de organos y tejidos. In: Matesanz R, Miranda B, editors. Trasplante renal – algunos aspectos prácticos. Madrid, Spain: Grupo Aula Médica, 1994: 26–51.
5. Garrison NR, Bentley FR, Raque GH, Polk HC, Sladeck LC, Evanisko MJ. There is an answer to the shortage of organs. Surg Gyn Obstet 1991; 173: 391–6.
6. Navarro A, Escalante JL, Andres A, et al. Donor detection and organ procurement in the Madrid Region. Transp Proceed 1993; 25: 3130–1.
7. Aranzábal J, et al. Organ procurement evolution in the Bask Country. Proceedings of the Sixth Congress of the ETCO; 1993 Oct 22–25; Rodos, Greece.
8. First R. Transplantation in the nineties. Transplantation 1992; 53: 1–11.
9. Cabrer C. Aplicación del diagrama ASME al proceso de obtención de órganos para trasplante [tesis doctoral]. Barcelona, Spain: Facultad de Medicina, Universidad de Barcelona, 1994.
10. Organización Nacional de Trasplantes. Memoria 1993. Rev Esp de Trasp 1994; 3: 71.
11. Oficina Regional de Coordinación de Trasplantes. Memoria de Trasplantes 1992. Consejeria de salud de la CA de Madrid, Dirección General de Planificación, 1992: 49.
12. Martin A, et al. Donación de organos para trasplante: aspectos psicosociales. Nefrologia 1991; XI(supp 1): 62–8.
13. Martin A, Martinez JM, Lopez JS. La Donación en España: un estudio sobre los aspectos psicosociales. In: Matesanz R, Miranda B, editors. Coordinación y Trasplantes. Madrid: CEA, 1994 (in press).

14. Organización Nacional de Trasplantes. Memoria 1993. Rev Esp de Trasp 1994; 3: 72.
15. Gallup Poll. The USA public's attitudes toward organ transplantation – organ donation (G087073). Princeton, New Jersey: Gallup Organization, 1987.
16. Frutos MA, Blanca MJ, Rando B, Ruiz P, Rosell J. Actitudes de las familias de donantes y no donantes de organos. Rev Esp de Trasp 1994 (in press).
17. Gómez P, Santiago C, Moñino A. La entrevista de donación y la relación de ayuda. In: Matesanz R, Miranda B, editors. Coordinación y Trasplantes. Madrid: CEA, 1994 (in press).

25. Training the transplant procurement management (TPM) coordinator

M. MANYALICH, C. A. CABRER, L. C. GARCIA-FAGES, R. VALERO, L. SALVADOR & J. SANCHEZ

The application of a new technology needs knowledge of the technology, training and the necessary economic resources (material and human). However, in the field of transplantation the major impediment and limiting factor at present is the lack of sufficient organs and tissues.

This obvious truth has been disregarded in many national and institutional transplant programmes which have spent a large part of their budgets on acquiring knowledge from other more developed counties or on programmes of experimental training.

To some degree, transplant teams foresaw this problem and took the first steps toward solving it by creating the post of Transplant Coordinator. In Europe, coordinators were usually created through the support of transplanting teams who needed someone to organize the path from donation in the intensive care unit to the extraction of organs in the operating theatre. This organizational assistance was gradually assistance was gradually extended to the follow-up of patients transplanted, according to the case, including the problems, great or small, that might arise.

In the U.S.A., where Transplant Coordinators have developed more or less the same functions as in Europe, instead of establishing themselves within the transplant teams, they have been organized independently in O.P.O.s (Organ Procurement Organizations) or O.P.A.s (Organ Procurement Agencies), and work in parallel with the transplant teams. Both in Europe and America, functions are usually divided between the Procurement Coordinator and the Clinical Coordinator, depending on the phase of transplant to which they are dedicated. Their professional background is usually social work, administration, nursing or medical technician.

In our country Transplant Coordination was born in Catalunya, and was officially regulated in 1985 with the holding of the first course on Transplant Coordination. and the administrative order that to be acredited as such, each Transplanting Hospital or generating centre would need a Transplant Coordinator. The first coordinators were nephrologists who organized renal extractions. Progressively other specialities were introduced into coordination, parallel with the development of other transplant programmes –

J.L. Touraine et al. (eds.), Organ Shortage: The Solutions, 191–195.

cardiac, pancreatic, hepatic, etc. Surgeons, I.C.U. doctors, anaesthetists also became coordinators, creating teams of doctors and/or nurses with progressively more clinical and organizational responsibilities, who had to negotiate solutions and make decisions – all of which signified a much greater role than that carried out by the first coordinators.

The Transplant Procurement Management (TPM) Coordinator is a professional who facilitates the technology of transplantation, trying to cover the needs of the greatest possible number of patients (recipients). The function of the TPM is the procurement and distribution of organs and tissues for transplantation.

What is the TPM profile?

Coinciding with the actual situation in Spain, the basic profile is: a medical specialist with hospital experience, full time, having transplantation as his principal objective, and always available, which, given the obvious needs for doctors to be off duty at times, means that working in teams is necessary. TPM Coordination is a profession and needs training and time for learning. Knowledge which, once absorbed, should not be abandoned in favour of another specialization or occupation.

Coordination should be embarked upon as a profession and not as a job on the way to other goals. The greatest qualities necessary are skill in human relations and lack of any aversion to treating and talking about death, as this is the frontier continually crossed in their field of work – death of the donor, life for the recipient.

The knowledge required may be acquired without problems, independent of the original specialization, although specialists in anaesthesiology, reanimination and intensive care will have greater experience in donor maintenance, the diagnosis of brain death and the correct way of approaching the families of critical patients. It is also necessary to be familiar with the general scheme of transplantation, the existing laws and regulations, systems of preservation and the form of transporting organs and tissues. Fundamentally they must know: Who can be an organ donor? Where are donors to be found? And, also, they must be motivated to detect donors with the aim of fulfilling their mission: to increase the number of cadaveric extractions.

To fulfill this objective, the coordinator should be familiar with all the means of obtaining organs and tissues – living related donor, cadaveric donor through brain death, heart attack or exitus – not forgetting the possibility of xenotransplantation in the future. However, the focus of attention and principal work area must be entirely related to the critical patient, that is, the intensive care and emergency units.

I believe it is possible to see in our country a clear chronological difference between the first coordinators of the eighties and the TPM Coordinator of the nineties, which is reflected in the improvement in the generation of organs in Spain. The TPM Coordinator has four functions: Clinical, Research, Educational and Managerial.

Clinical

This function focuses on the procurement of organs and tissues, and is dividable into 4 categories:

Detection. Active, through visiting intensive care units, notification by I.C.U. doctors or by administration, or by daily checking of the admissions list. We also carry out quality control of detection through the weekly list of hospital deaths, looking for undetected potential donors.

Follow-Up. By applying the American Society of Mechanical Engineers (A.S.M.E.) Diagram we follow all possible organ donors – patients with a Glasgow coma score <7, without absolute contraindications for donation. This diagram allows us to analyze the distinct phases of the organ generation process, time employed, possible delays, the causes of abandoning the process (non-evolution to brain death, family refusal or clinical contraindication), and the complete evolution until the extraction of organs and tissues.

Support. For the process to be carried out satisfactorily, all the necessary resources must be available – laboratories, transport, specialists, nurses, anaesthesia, machines, material, etc. – to allow the process to take place anywhere and at any time.

Quality Control. The TPM Coordinator must assume responsibility for the viability of the donor, with all the clinical explorations, analyses and complementary tests that this entails, and by these means facilitate the evaluation of the viability of organs and tissues by the coresponding transplant teams, while at all times assuring the correct distribution of organs and tissues.

Research

This function looks into possible new ways of generating more organ donors, the viability of organs and, with other specialists, into donor maintenance, brain death, social evaluations of families, etc.

Educational

Transmission of the transplant culture and the donation of organs both to health professionals and the general public in another responsibility of the TPM Coordinator. This includes participation in the training and education of future TPM Coordinators.

Management

To achieve the desired goals, the TPM Coordinator must be prepared to accept responsibility for and make decisions about the use of resources (material and human). Study and analysis permits differentiation of the different processes involved, allowing the cost for each process; organ generation, transplant of the different organs and tissue banks to be calculated. By relating these costs to transplant results (survival rates), cost-effectiveness and cost benefit figures may be obtained. This enables the evaluation of relevant technology by the TPM coordinator who can then facilitate decision-making on the adequacy of therapies and activities.

Organizational Position

The sum of responsibilities and relations entailed by the different parts of the job make the efficient and comfortable performance of the necessary clinical and management tasks difficult when situated in an existing hospital service (nephrology, surgery, intensive care, etc.). For this reason, ubication in a unit independent of other services, although closely linked functionally with transplant teams is ideal. Hierarchically, the unit should answer to the Medical Director in medical matters and the hospital management in administrative ones. Perhaps the best formula would be to create a medical adviser to oversee transplants (TPM Coordinator), analogous to the situation in the industrial world where the Product Manager is responsible for a product from the purchase of raw materials to the point of sale, answers to the senior management and is independent of purchasing, production, sales, etc.

Why transplant procurement management?

Simply because in English, the name corresponds well to the functions described for the TPM Coordinator, functions which outside Spain are not performed by Transplant Coordinators. We believe it will be easier to convince the rest of the world that there are TPM coordinators in Spain who achieve excellent results in the generation of organs, than to spend years explaining how "the Spanish Transplant Coordinator is different".

What *is* different are the results obtained in the generation of organs (donors/pmp) in Spain, which leads the world ranking since 1991, and has resulted in a recommendation from the Transplant Committee of the Council of Europe, supporting the Spanish oganizational structure and the holding of training courses for TPM Coordinators such as the course of Barcelona.

What is the training for TPM Coordinators? What is the educational method?

As the Catalan author Josep Maria de Segarra said, a person is formed by learning, accepting what is learned, and practising what is accepted. Educational methods for children (pedagogy) are well developed, but not so those for adults (andragogy). Adults only learn what is interesting and useful to them. The process of learning and acquisition of knowledge should be base on an integrated system which uses the three areas of knowledge: Cognitive, Attitudinal and Sensory-Motor, with their respective functions of memory, integration and automatism.

The quality of learning also depends on which senses are employed in the transmission of skills and attitudes. Thus in oral learning, 70% of knowledge acquired is remembered after 3 hours, but only 10% after 3 days; likewise, with visual learning, 72% is remembered after 3 hours, but only 20% after 3 days. However, in interactive learning, the high degree of participation and student–teacher interaction means that these figures increase considerably: 85% is remembered after 3 hours and 65% after 3 days. In other words "Listen and forget, see and remember, do and learn".

We use an interactive method based on the learning by experience model of David A. Kolb. Each student begins with a concrete experience and, by adding more information through learning, is able to make reflexive observations. For this reason, before the course we send a pedagogic dossier containing the basic theoretical information the student needs, thereby facilitating reflexive observation which, together with the accumulation of data imparted during the course, leads to improved abstract conceptualization of knowledge acquired. Through guided and relevant simulations we aid the development of active exprimentation which, with repetition, instruction and practice results in learning to add to the initial concrete experience.

26. Surgical optimization of multi-organ procurement

M. DAWAHRA, X. MARTIN, P. CLOIX, L. TAJRA
& J.M. DUBERNARD

Introduction

The sometimes strange behaviour of individual surgeons and the uncoordin-
ated and delayed arrival of procurement teams have created a need for a
rapid, effective technique that reduces potential errors during procurement
and might allow for the removal of organs from unstable donors. The aim
is that a single surgeon should take charge of the donation and coordinate
the efforts of the respective teams [1].

A technique of multiple organ procurement was first described by Starzl
et al. in 1984 [2]. Since that time, many modifications have been reported,
the most recent being the total abdominal evisceration of Nakazato et al.
[3]. Controversies still remain concerning the surgical strategies between
initial organ perfusion and initial dissection. The excellent preservation properties of the UW solution permits more of the dissection to be performed
ex vivo. In our institution, we use the technique of organ perfusion before
dissection of organs as it is easy to perform by less-experienced surgeons.

Incision

The complete midline incision from the suprasternal notch to the symphisis
pubis (Figure 1) is the most currently performed, even in the case of procurement of abdominal organs only. This incision allows excellent exposure and
convenient proximal control of the great vessels.

Preparation for in situ cooling of abdominal organs

Immediately after incision, one must be ready to harvest the maximal number
of organs in case of cardiac arrest. It is therefore necessary to be ready for
immediate perfusion and cooling of the abdominal and thoracic organs.

Access to the distal aorta, vena cava and ureters is obtained by medial

J.L. Touraine et al. (eds.), *Organ Shortage: The Solutions*, 197–205.
© 1995 *Kluwer Academic Publishers.*

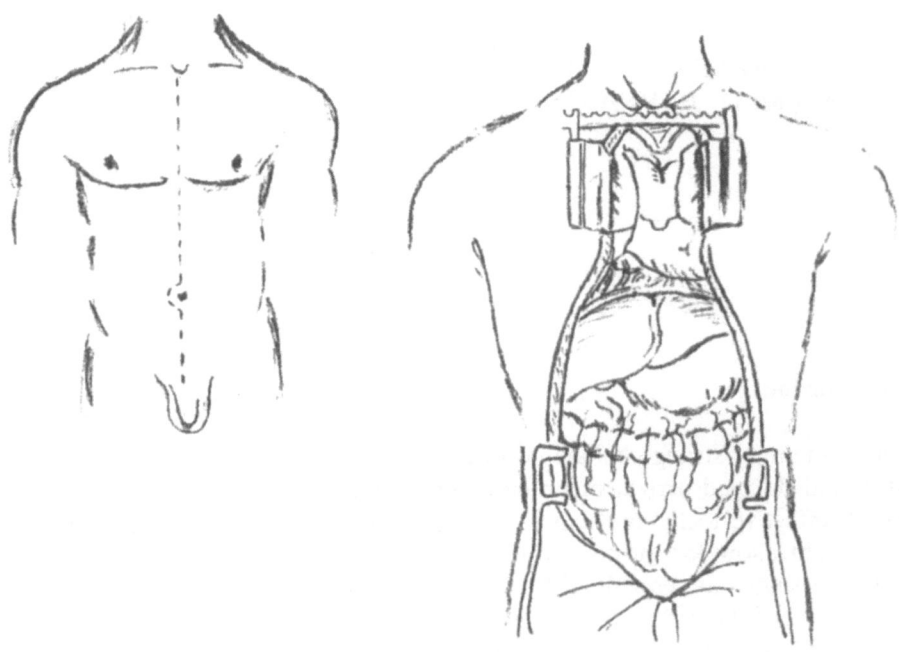

Fig. 1. Xyphopubic and sternotomy incision for multiorgan donation.

mobilization of the right and left colon and the distal part of the small bowel
after incision of the white line of Toldt. A Kocher maneuver is outlined to
free the duodenum and with blunt dissection the head of the pancreas is
mobilized. On the left side, a defect is created in the sigmoid mesocolon by
ligation and division of the inferior mesenteric vessels. The left ureter can
then be identified as well as the right one. The distal part of the aorta and
IVC are dissected free and encircled (Figure 2). Upward dissection of the
anterior surface of the aorta is continued until the left renal vein is encountered crossing the aorta from left to right. The aorta is looped at the level
of the inferior mesenteric artery, as well as vena cava, below the entry of the
renal veins. At this time, aortic cannulation is performed allowing emergency
cooling in case of donor cardiovascular instability.

Sometimes, arteries to the lower renal pole originate from the iliac artery
and aortic cannulation through the opposite iliac artery becomes necessary
in order to provide perfusion of such anomalous arteries.

Isolation of the celiac axis and proximal aorta

After the lateral portion of the left triangular ligament of the liver is taken
down, the aorta is mobilized as it passes through the crura of the diaphragm

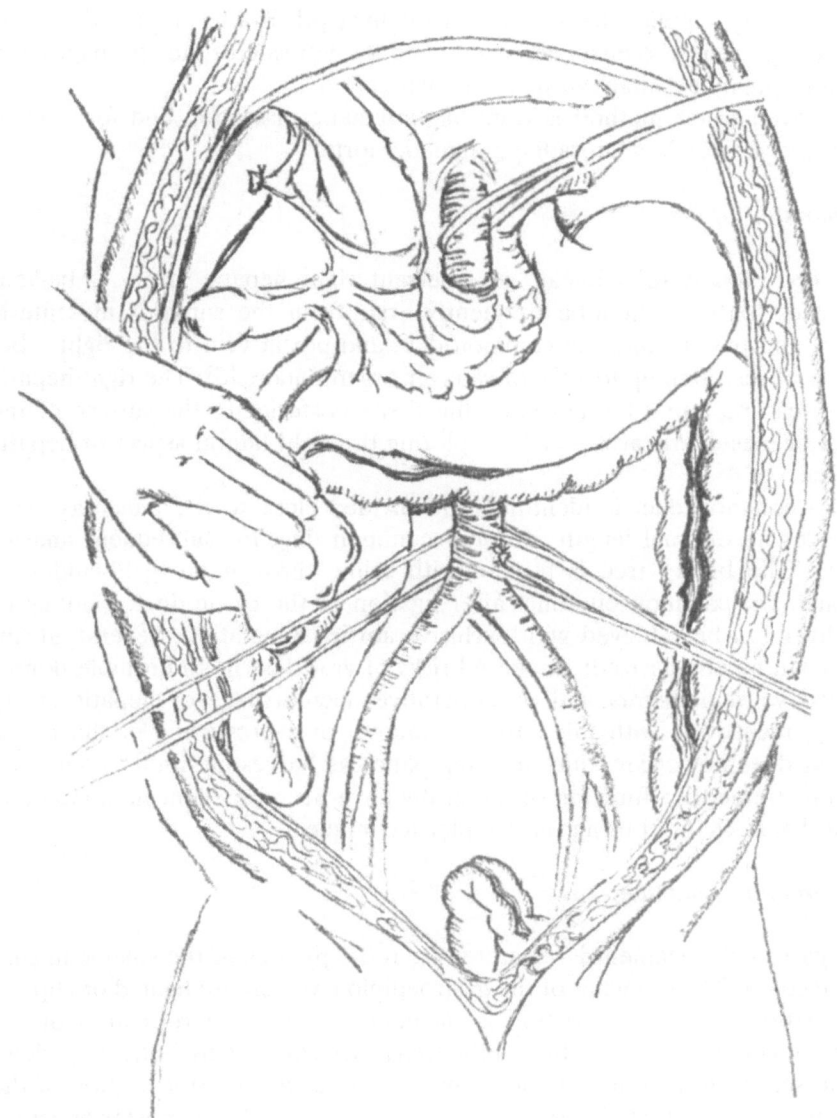

Fig. 2. Preparation of the aorta and inferior vena cava for cannulation and isolation of the proximal aorta and celiac axis.

and celiac lymphatic structures, which are divided, usually with electro-cautery. The aorta superior to the celiac axis must be individualized to be clamped (Figure 2). Its dissection begins on his right side in the avascular space. In approximately 20% of donors, an aberrant branch from the left gastric artery supplies the left lobe of the liver [4]. If a left replaced hepatic artery is present, the dissection is done on the left side of the esophagus and aorta to prevent damage of liver vascularization.

An even faster method is transdiaphragmatic dissection and location of the distal descending supradiaphragmatic aorta.

Preparation of the liver

The first step is to delineate an aberrant right hepatic artery. Aberrant branches to the right lobe frequently arise from the superior mesenteric artery and pass behind the common duct and portal vein to the right lobe. This is observed in up to 13% of cadaver organ donors [5]. The right hepatic artery can be found by dissecting the tissue posterior to the surface of the superior mesenteric artery or by exploring the right lateral aspect of hepatic pedicle.

The common duct is identified and divided close to the pancreas. This provides an optimal length of donor common duct for subsequent anastomosis. The biliary tree is flushed with saline through the gallbladder or through the common bile duct after ligation of the cystic duct. Cooling of the liver can be achieved with exclusive aortic cannulation. Several advantages can be emphasized: decreased risks of graft loss in an unstable donor, limited warm ischemia and intraoperative haemorrhage or hepatic artery injury, moreover, with this latter technique, over-pressuring of the portal system does not occur, thus allowing pancreas harvesting under good conditions. Immediate function of the grafts have been excellent in animal and clinical studies [6, 7] using this simpler technique.

Preparation of the pancreas

The gastrocolic ligament is separated from the pylorus to the splenic flexure of the colon. The branches of the gastroepiploic vessels are ligated or clipped before division. The dissection is facilitated by upward retraction of the stomach and inferior retraction of the transverse colon. This maneuver allows the lesser sac to be entered and allows access to the anterior portion of the spleen. The short gastric vessels are ligated and divided. The posterior aspect of the spleen is dissected. The spleen is used as a handle to expose the lienophrenic ligament, which is divided. After the spleen is freed, the small vessels between the mesocolon and the retroperitoneum are divided. Dissection can then be conducted fom the left to the right and separation of the tail of the pancreas from the retroperitoneum is performed. At this point, identification of the splenic vein that runs the posterior aspect of the tail of the pancreas will help to lead the dissection on the right. Dissection is then conducted to the neck of the pancreas.

When a whole pancreas is harvested, the surgical procedure is the same concerning dissection of the spleen and distal pancreas. The superior mesenteric vessels are identified at the inferior margin of the pancreas. A loop is placed on the duodenum at the pyloro duodenal junction and at the duodenojejunal angle.

Cooling procedure

When preparation of the organs is complete, cooling and perfusion can take place and organ harvesting can be performed.

The preferred sequence of removal is heart or heart/lung first, liver and/or pancreas second, and kidneys last. The separation of the abdominal organs is often done in vivo. However, an en bloc specimen of abdominal organs can be harvested after preservation fluid flush and the separation of the organs can be performed on the back table.

The thoracic and abdominal teams then coordinate cardiopulmonary arrest. The distal abdominal aorta previously cannulated is connected to a gravity flush system with preservation solution. The abdominal team ligates the isolated distal abdominal IVC and perfusion of the abdominal organs via the aortic canula is performed (Figure 3). Slushed iced saline is also poured in the peritoneal cavity and the pericardial sac to complete the cooling process. For adult patients, a total amont of 5.0 liters of preservation fluid is flushed through each of the aorta. This allows the abdominal organs to be generously cooled and flushed, while assisting the thoracic team in removing the heart and lungs. The amount of infusate is variable and guided by decoloration of the organs and cooling, which is judged by touch and sight. Frequently, the intestines and pancreas become chilled and bloodless while the liver remains discolored and still feels warm. Many institutions have reported graft pancreatitis caused by excessive in situ flushing of the donor pancreas and have suggested restricting the flushing volume to 2–3 l [8]. Depending on the speed of the thoracic team's cardioplegia and removal of the heart and lungs, this cooling process should take about 5 to 15 minutes. The suprahepatic IVC is also opened as soon as possible as an extra precaution against over-distension of the liver. With the evolution of multiorgan harvesting, at present, cooling is usually performed via cannulae placed in the lower abdominal aorta; this technique permits simultaneous en bloc perfusion of kidneys, pancreas and liver. The meticulous and time-consuming procedures necessitating ligation and/or coagulation of numerous small vessels are thereby avoided.

Liver retrieval

The hepatic artery is identified within the gastrohepatic ligament deep in the lymph node at the superior margin of the pancreatic head. The main trunk is followed to the left, to the origin of the celiac axis. In case of isolated liver retrieval, the celiac axis is kept with an aortic patch. In donors weighing

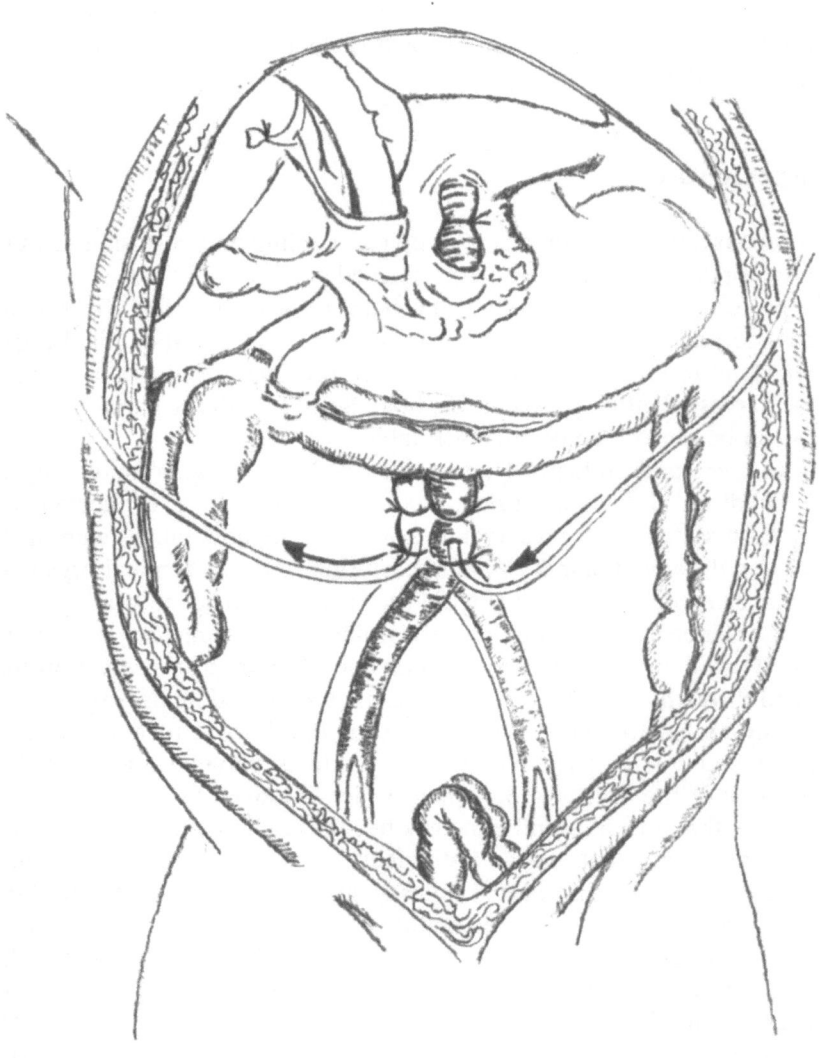

Fig. 3. Cooling of abdominal organs.

more than 30 kg, procurement of the aortic patch is not always necessary; further, this technique cannot be used in small children or in retransplants where the aortic patch is used as an arterial conduit [8]. The gastroduodenal vessel and the right gastric branch of the hepatic artery are divided close to their origin to maintain the vascularization of the head of the pancreas through the superior pancreaticoduodenal arcade if a whole pancreas is

simultaneously harvested. The splenic artery is identified at the origin during
the dissection of the hepatic artery.

The liver is mobilized by incision of its ligamentous attachments to the
diaphragm. Initially the liver is retracted to the patient's left and the right
triangular ligament is divided. The liver is then retracted to the right and
the left ligament is totally divided. Finally the ligamentum teres is divided
and, in cases in which reduced-sized liver transplantation is planned, the
entire ligamentum teres is preserved because it can be used to partially cover
the cut surface of the liver. These ligaments can be left long for subsequent
attachment to the diaphgram of the recipient. The superior aspect of the
liver is dissected free by incising the anterior diaphragm back to the suprahepatic IVC. A rim of diaphragm is left attached to the suprahepatic vena
cava. It is convenient to insert a finger in the suprahepatic vena cava lumen
avoiding cutting wounds. The IVC is divided proximal to the entrance of the
renal veins.

Pancreas retrieval

A Kocher maneuver is performed to mobilize the duodenum and the head
of the pancreas. The supraduodenal portal vein is divided just below to the
coronary vein. If the portal vein is too short, subsequent lengthening, using
a tubular venous graft, is possible. The remnant of tissue is trimmed along
the superior border of the pancreas and common hepatic artery and near the
stumps of the superior mesenteric artery and splenic artery. The segment of
duodenum corresponding to the head of the pancreas is transected using
a GIA automatic stapling device. In order to reduce the risks of fungal
contamination, antifungic solutions can be injected in the duodenal segments.

In the case of simultaneous harvesting of liver and total pancreas three
situations may occur:

– Vascularisation of the liver is normal, the arterial supply of the pancreatic
  graft is represented by the celiac axis via the splenic artery and superior
  mesenteric artery on the same aortic patch. Liver transplant is taken with
  the common hepatic artery.
– In the case of a left hepatic artery, the celiac axis is left in continuity with
  the common hepatic artery and the left gastric artery. Pancreatic graft will
  be vascularized by superior mesenteric artery and splenic artery. Both
  vessels can be prolonged using the iliac bifurcation as a Y plasty (Figure
  4).
– When an aberrant right hepatic artery originating from the origin of the
  superior mesenteric artery is present, the initial portion of the superior
  mesenteric artery is reserved to the hepatic team. The distal portion of
  the superior mesenteric artery can be revascularised retrogradely by an
  arterial graft, or the right hepatic artery can be divided close to the head
  of the pancreas and re-implanted to the gastro-duodenal stamp.

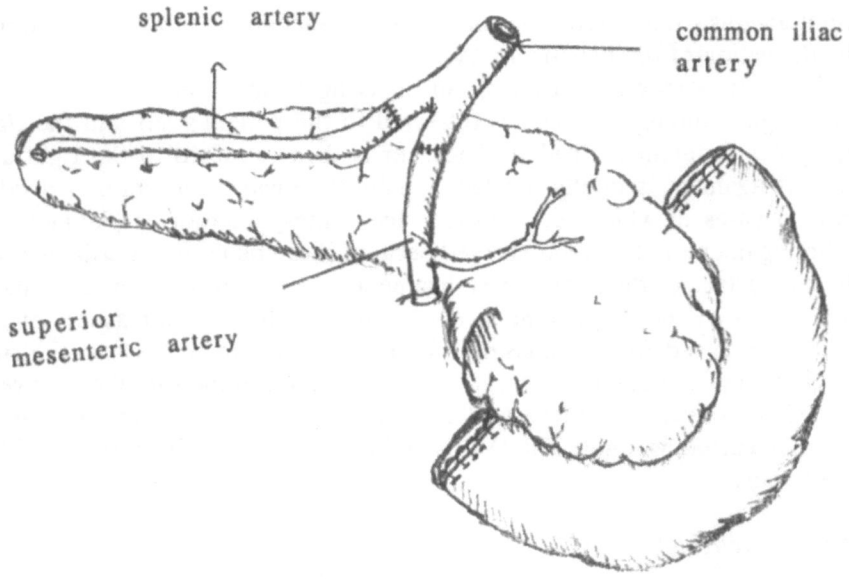

splenic   artery

common iliac
artery

superior
mesenteric   artery

Fig. 4. Arterial reconstruction of the pancreas graft.

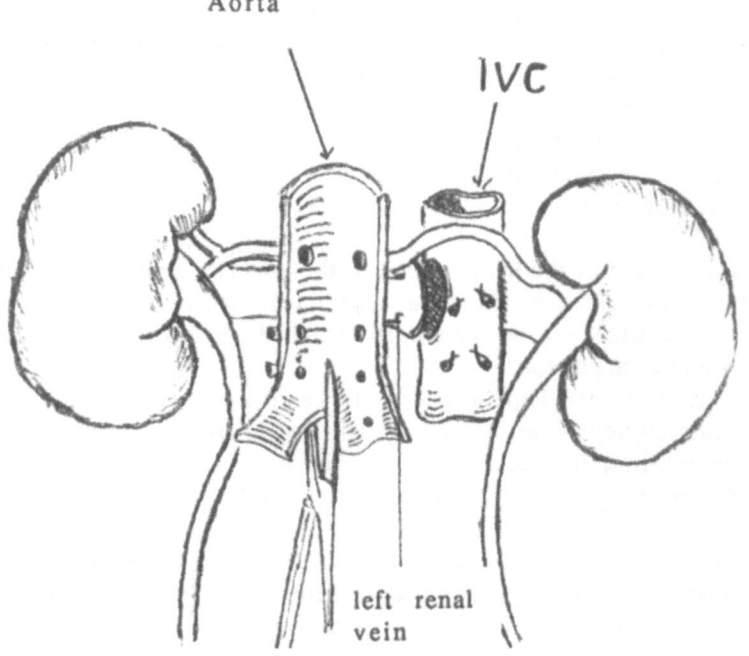

Aorta

IVC

left renal
vein

Fig. 5. The left renal vein is divided close to IVC.

Removal of the kidneys

The cannulae in the IVC and aorta as well as the ureters marked with loops are gently retracted anteriorly, keeping track of these four structures while dissecting the kidneys. Posterior attachments of the kidneys are cut, staying close to the posterior ligaments and muscles covering the vertebral bodies, and continuing until the proximal aorta and IVC are reached.

Once the posterior dissection is completed, the residual attachments between the gastrointestinal tract and the anterior surface of the specimen are divided. The kidneys are taken out en bloc. When separating the kidneys, it is most convenient to turn the specimen over. The posterior wall of the aorta is incised, allowing a perfect view of renal arterial branches from inside the lumen. The left renal vein is transected close to the IVC (Figure 5).

Conclusion

Multiple abdominal organ procurement should enable the kidneys, the liver and the whole pancreas to be removed. Simultaneous procurement of the liver and pancreas is always possible, and the keys to a successful technique are flexibility and adaptibility, allowing rapid access and in-situ flushing to avoid warm ischemia, without compromising the viability of any organs.

References

1. Margreiter R, Königsrainer A, Schmid Th, Takahashi N, Pernthaler H, Ofner D. Multiple organ procurement – a simple and safe procedure. Transplant Proc 1991; 23(5): 2307–8.
2. Starzl TE, Hakala TR, Shaw BW Jr, Hardesty RL, Rosenthal TJ, Griffith BP, Iwatsuki S, Bahnson HT. A flexible procedure for multiple cadaveric organ procurement. Surg Gyn Obstet 1984; 158: 223–31.
3. Nakazato PZ, Concepcion W, Bry W, Limm W, Tokunaga Y, Itasaka H, Feduska N, Esquivel CO, Collins GM. Total abdominal evisceration: an en bloc technique for abdominal organ harvesting. Surgery 1992; 111(1): 37–47.
4. Dubernard JM, Sutherland DER. International handbook of pancreas transplantation. Dordrecht, The Netherlands: Kluwer Academic Publishers, 1989: 71–130.
5. Shaffer D, Lewis WD, Jenkins RL, Monaco AP. Combined liver and whole pancreas procurement in donors with a replaced right hepatic artery. Surg Gyn Obst 1992; 175: 204–7.
6. Bittard H, Chiche L, Mouzarkel M, Douguet D, Benoit G. Study of kidney and liver viability in the rat after exclusive aortic perfusion using intracellular ATP measurement. Urol Res 1992; 20: 415.
7. Boillot O, Benchetrit S, Dawahra M, Porcheron J, Martin X. Early graft function in liver transplantation: comparaison of two techniques of graft procurement. Transplant Proc 1993; 25: 2642.
8. Nghiem DD. Simultaneous recovery of whole pancreas without arterial reconstruction in the multiple organ liver donor. Transplant Proc 1990; 22(2): 614–5.

27. The place of anatomy in liver transplantation: Multiplicity of possibilities and optimization of the utilization of cadaveric and living donors' organs

TRINH VAN MINH

Referring to the problem addressed by this conference, "Organ Shortage: The Solution?", anatomy has its small place in liver transplantation because it is the basis of all creations and modifications of surgical techniques to increase and optimize the utilization of available donor sources:

- reductive resection for paediatric transplantation [1, 2, 6, 10, 14, 15, 23];
- splitting into two, three, even (doubtfully) four grafts [3, 4, 9, 11–13, 16, 17];
- partial procurement from a living donor [5, 7].

In this paper I would like to focus on the last two points and discuss the following three: multiplicity of anatomic possibilities and surgical limitations; right half–left half liver splitting in cadaveric donors; and right lobe–left lobe liver splitting in living donors.

Multiplicity of anatomic possibilities and surgical limitations

Until now, surgical practice seems to have been limited to a few habitual liver splitting methods: right half–left half, right lobe–left lobe and right half–left lobe. That is using only two main fissures: the sagittal and umbilical. However, there are many other methods that have not yet been exploited: the right, the left lateral and the inter-subsegmentar splits (between VI and VII, and particularly between VIII lateral and VIII medial of our liver segmentation, an intermediary portal fissure which corresponds approximately to the limit between the right and the middle hepatic venous territories) [21, 24, 25].*

I say "not yet exploited" because all these divisions are not readily applicable as they were anatomically demonstrated, but have to be considered and studied to be adaptable to relevant surgical splitting techniques.

In this field there are two main difficulties. The first is that there are only three great hepatic veins interposed between five main portal territories:

J.L. Touraine et al. (eds.), *Organ Shortage: The Solutions*, 207–212.
© 1995 *Kluwer Academic Publishers.*

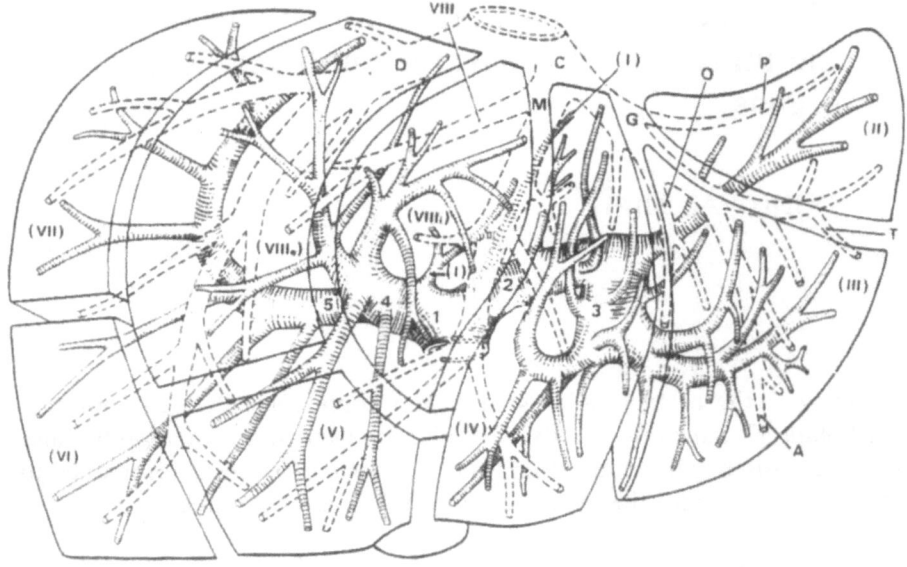

Fig. 1. Typical disposition of the two main intrahepatic structures and segmentaiton of the liver.

posterior (VI + VII), anterior (V + VIII), medial (IV), antero lateral (III), and postero lateral (II) (Figure 1), and each graft must have its own triad portal pedicle and suitable hepatic vein drainage.*

The second difficulty consists of multiple anatomic variations of different intrahepatic structures: portal veins, hepatic veins, hepatic arteries and biliary ducts [8, 9, 18–27]. Hence, the role of anatomy is to study and clearly demonstrate to surgeons those anatomic inconveniences that can interfere with their surgical techniques; not to disappoint and discourage them but to help them and suggest ways to discover other eventual possibilities or modifications.

On the right half–left half liver splitting (in a cadaveric donor)

We have an important landmark: the sagittal (or principal) fissure with the middle hepatic vein just inside.* The question is whether to make the section on the right or on the left of the vein.

The common tendency seems to agree with Bismuth et al. [3], to take a splitting planus on the left.

However, according to our statistical study [22, 26], the sagittal fissure is found passing over the portal bifurcation in 43.33% of cases, on its left in 30% of cases, and on its right in only 26.66% of cases. The middle hepatic vein is found here as well. The right disposition of the middle hepatic vein corresponds more often to cases with a long right portal branch, rarely to cases with a mean or short right portal branch, and never to cases with a duplication of the right portal branch (where it is always above the left portal branch).*

Therefore, I think that in most cases it is simpler to make the split on the right of the middle hepatic vein, leaving this vein to the left half of the liver, and covering any eventual variation of sliding of tributaries of the left hepatic vein on the middle hepatic vein. (The section of the left portal branch just at its origin remains possible in these cases for preserving the portal trunk in continuity with the right portal branch) [27, 28].*

In only the few cases where the middle hepatic vein is found on the right of the portal bifurcation, over a long right portal branch, and especially when this vein is hyperdeveloped and deviated to the right half of the liver [21], is it more practical and prudent to take the splitting planus on its left. Fortunately in these cases, there is always a compensative development to the right of tributaries of the left hepatic vein for the drainage of the medial segment (IV).* (That was probably the case of the split liver grafting realized by Bismuth et al. in 1989, where "an accessory middle hepatic vein for the quadrate lobe" was noticed.)

On the right lobe–left lobe liver splitting (in a living donor)

In a normal anatomic view* the limit of the umbilical fissure on the upper surface of the liver often overlaps a little to the left of the insertion of the falciform ligament, and the fundus of it is just occupied by the postero-anterior portion of the left portal branch (the umbilical recess of Rex 1888, or the porto-umbilical sinus of Ton That Tung 1937).

Left lobectomy was conceived to be done on the left of the umbical recessus. Transplant surgeons, however, seem to prefer a split on its right because it is easier to get a unique portal pedicle for the graft, that is, the transversal portion of the left portal branch [5].

In this manner, portal branches to the medial segment (IV) are sectioned; and the portally devascularized segment is no longer useful to the right lobe or the left, to the living donor or the infantile recipient. So, what may happen then?

No necrosis is however observed (as confirmed by one of the authors, Dr. Boillot, pers. comm.). I think that this may be due to possible termino-terminal portal and/or arterial anastomosis between the two halves of the liver at some levels, particularly at the gallbladder bed.

Thanks to those anastomosis, in some of our corrosion casts (but not in all), the coloured plastic injected in the anterior segment portal vein (or right paramedian vein of Couinaud) passed largely into some inferior portal branches of the medial segment [21].* Minute arterial anastomosis between both halves of the liver and between superficial extrahepatic and profound intrahepatic arteriolar networks were also observed at different levels – at the gallbladder bed, at the subcapsular space of the liver surface and at ligament insertion zones (in our other specimens with a fine injection of coloured plastic or gelatine solutions).

Moreover, surgeons tried to get further assurance by a possible preservation of an arterial branch to the medial segment. The real results of this procedure have to be proved by experimental surgery.

All the same, the portally devascularized segment (IV) remains functionally excluded, therefore wasted. And for a living donor, the operation corresponds to a left hemihepatectomy and not a left lobectomy.

New propositions for partial liver procurement from a living donor

According to the need of the recipient, I think that it is always better to minimize the split of the living donor, for best preserving him from risk. Furthermore, it is easier to persuade a donor to give a minimal part of his liver to save the life of his relative, with maximal safety for his own life.

Thus, besides *left half liver splitting*, which is more serious for the living donor but more profitable for a bigger child or even an adult recipient, I would like to propose other solutions more limited in parenchyme withdrawal, therefore more acceptable for the donor while adaptable to smaller recipients.

A true *left lobe splitting* must be done on the left of the umbilical recessus, sectioning the two portal pedicles, II and III, at their origin, and leaving all the remaining for the right lobe of the living donor. The grafting will be more complicated for the surgeon, who has to deal with two portal anastomosis. But the operation is feasible, with the previous preparation of two suitable portal branches while realizing the hepatectomy on the recipient. Such a left lobe split is also applicable to a left lobectomized recipient as an auxiliary graft (in fulminant hepatitis, for example).

The *subsegment II splitting and the subsegment III splitting* will simplify the number of portal pedicles and are more conservative for the living donor, but the relevance for the recipients must be taken into consideration because of their variable small size and form (they seem to be smaller in Vietnamese patients, but big enough in French patients to be adaptable to small child recipients).

Between the two, I prefer subsegment III, because there is no great problem with its vasculo biliary pedicles and because it is more constant and more often well developed in size. There are more anatomic problems with subsegment II, due to its incompatible hepatic venous drainage and its limits and variability in size (which is sometimes very atrophied in our specimens).*

Conclusion

In summary, there are many anatomic possibilities for split liver procurement, therefore many alternatives from which to choose, according to the need of the recipients, the adaptability of anatomic variations and the safety of cadaveric or living donor organs.

The problem is to make the best choice for different circumstances. Preoperative anatomic considerations and explorations are necessary for each case. In regard to some problems and some new propositions concerning the living donor, I think that further surgico-anatomical and surgico-experimental studies are necessary for giving better answers.

This is also one of our proposed projects, which we hope to discuss with some surgeons at this conference, for a possible future collaboration.

Acknowledgements

I would very much like to thank the Foundation Marcel Merieux and the Organizing Committee of the C.I.T.I.C. for having organized this meeting and engaging specialists of different disciplines in profitable discussions and possible cooperations for a major common objective: contribution to the solution of organ shortage in transplantation.

Notes

*Double slides projections were shown that cannot be reproduced in this paper.

References

1. Bismuth H, Houssin D. Reduced sized liver graft for hepatic transplantation in children. Surgery 1984; 95: 367–70.
2. Bismuth H, Houssin D. Partial resection of liver graft for orthotopic or heterotopic liver transplantation. Transplant Proc 1985; 17: 279–83.
3. Bismuth H, Morino M, Castaing D, et al. Emergency orthotopic liver transplantation in 2 patients using 1 donor liver. Br J Surg 1989; 76: 722–4.
4. Boillot O, Miranda F, Cloix P, et al. Transplantation hépatique après bipartition réglée du greffon chez deux receveurs. Lyon Chir 1992; 88: 5.
5. Boillot O, Dawahra M, Porcheron J, et al. Transplantation hépatique pediatrique et donneur vivant apparenté. Ann Chir 1993; 47(7): 577–85.
6. Broelsch CE, Edmond JC, Thistlethwaite JR, et al. Liver transplantation including the concept of reduced size liver transplantation in children. Ann Surg 1988; 208: 410–20.
7. Broelsch CE, Edmond JC, Whitington PF, et al. Application of reduced size liver transplants as split graft, auxilliary orthotopic grafts, and living related segmental transplants. Ann Surg 1990; 212: 368–77.
8. Couinaud C. Le foie: Etudes anatomiques et chirurgicales. Paris: Masson Edit., 1957.

9. Couinaud C, Houssin D. Controlled partition of the liver for transplantation. Anatomical limitations. Paris: Couinaud Edit., 1991.
10. Edmond JC, Whitington PF, Thistlethwaite JR, et al. Reduced size orthotopic liver transplantation: use in the management of children with chronic liver disease. Hepatology 1989; 10: 867–72.
11. Edmond JC, Whitington PF, Thistlethwaite JR, et al. Transplantation of two patients with one liver. Analysis of a preliminary experience with "split liver" grafting. Ann Surg 1990; 212: 14–22.
12. Houssin D, Couinaud C, Boillot O, et al. Controlled hepatic bipartition for transplantation in children. Br J Surg 1991; 78: 802–4.
13. Houssin D, Boillot O, Soubrane O, et al. Controlled hepatic bipartition for transplantation in two recipients: surgical technique, results and perspectives. Br J Surg 1993; 80: 75–80.
14. Otte JB, Salizzoni M, De Hemptinne B, Kestens PJ. Il trapianto di fegato. Archivo ed atti della Società Italiana di Chirurgia. Masson-Milano, 1987: 143–51.
15. Otte JB, De Hemptinne B, Salizzoni M. Reductive hepatic resections and liver transplantation. Proceedings of the XXVI World Congress of the International Surgeons; 1988 July 3–9; Milan.
16. Otte JB, De Ville de Goyet J, Alberti D, et al. The concept and technique of the split liver in clinical transplantation. Surg 1990; 107: 605–12.
17. Pichlmayr R, Ringe A, Bubernatis G, et al. Transplantation einer spenderleber auf zwei empfanger (splitting transplantation): eine neue methode in der weiterenwicklung der leber-segment transplantation. Langenbecks Arch Chir 1988; 373: 127–30.
18. Van Minh T. Multiplicité des variations bilaires des voies biliaires principales. Essai de classifications. Revue Medicale Hanoi 1973: 169–88.
19. Van Minh T. Les variations des voies biliaires intrahépatiques. Correlations et rapports avec la veine porte. Trav Sc de la Fac de Med de Hanoi 1975: 217–29.
20. Van Minh T. Reconsiderations sur les variations biliaires et les dispositions hypoportales des voies biliaires intrahepatiques. Trav de la Clin Chir de l'Hop HN Viet Duc Hanoi 1975: 217–29.
21. Van Minh T, editor. Le varianti anatomiche del sistema portale intrahepatico. In "Le resezioni epatiche per via transparenchimale. Ton That Tung". Torino: Minerva Medica, 1985: 1–67.
22. Van Minh T. À Propos de l'anatomie chirurgicale du foie. Quelques aspects nouveaux. Revue Medicale Hanoi 1988; 82–8.
23. Van Minh T. Subdivision of the anterior segment and hepatic veinous segmentation of the liver. Surgical signification in reductive resections for liver transplantation. Proceedings of the XXVI World Congress of the International College of Surgeons; 1988 July 3–9; Milan.
24. Van Minh T, Paletto AE, Salizzoni M. Surgical anatomy of intraparenchimal structures of the liver. Proceedings of the XXVI World Congress of the International College of Surgeons; 1988 July 3–9; Milan.
25. Van Minh T. La segmentation du foie et les variations anatomiques du système porte. Ann Chir 1990; 44(7): 561–9.
26. Van Minh T, Galizia G. L'importanza de la scissura principale nella chirurgia del fegato. Chirurgia 1991; 4(9): 425–31.
27. Van Minh T. Sur la possibilité de division d'un foie en deux transplants. Hanoi 1989 (Communication to Pr Cassia G, Brescia, and to Dr Galizia G, Napoli, Italy); In Vietnamese: Hình Thái Học (Morphology) Hanoi 1991; 1: 1–5.
28. Van Minh T. Considerations anatomiques à propos d'une possibilité de division d'un foie en deux transplants. Abstract (poster) of the 26th CITIC 1994 June 13–15, Lyon.

28. Detection of anti-HLA class I IgG antibodies by ELISA

I. MERCIER, L. GLANVILLE, L. ELLINGSON, L. IGOUDIN,
N. VANPOUILLE, A. SEGERS, P. POULETTY & R. BUELOW

Introduction and results

An ELISA for the detection of anti-HLA class I IgG antibodies (PRA-STAT™) was developed and compared to microlymphocytotoxicity (Figure 1). ELISA plates were coated with a panel of soluble HLA (sHLA) antigens isolated from the culture supernatants of 46 different EBV transformed phenotyped B cell lines (Table 1). A schematic drawing of the assay format is shown in Figure 2. After the incubation of the ELISA plates with test serum, bound antibodies were detected using a peroxidase-conjugated anti-human IgG antibody. To evaluate if a serum specimen contained specific anti-HLA class I antibodies, each serum was tested, in parallel, in sHLA antigen containing wells and one well containing no sHLA antigen. The OD in the antigen-containing well minus the OD in the no antigen well allowed differentiation between positive and negative reactions to the particular antigens contained within each well. Serum samples containing no anti-HLA class I IgG antibodies (n = 80) gave negative results when tested by PRA-STAT. 102 specimens from patients on a kidney transplant waiting list were tested by PRA-STAT in five different laboratories and %PRA values were calculated (Figure 3). The correlation coefficients (r) of test results ranged from 0.89 to 0.96 (Table 2), indicating a high reproducibility of %PRA values determined by PRA-STAT. The same set of 102 serum samples was also tested by lymphocytotoxicity six times in five different HLA laboratories (Figure 4). The correlation coefficient (r) of lymphocytotoxicity test results ranged from 0.57 to 0.94 (Table 3), indicating that the reproducibility of PRA-STAT assay results is higher than the reproducibility of lymphocytotoxicity assay results. 61 of the 102 samples gave identical test results in all six lymphocytotoxicity assays. The lymphocytotoxicity test results of these specimens were compared to those obtained by PRA-STAT (Table 4). The agreement between PRA-STAT and lymphocytotoxicity results was 93%, the specificity 94% and the sensitivity 93%.

Endpoint titration of several patient specimens demonstrated equivalent sensitivity of PRA-STAT and lymphocytotoxicity (Table 5).

J.L. Touraine et al. (eds.), *Organ Shortage: The Solutions*, 213–220.
© 1995 *Kluwer Academic Publishers*.

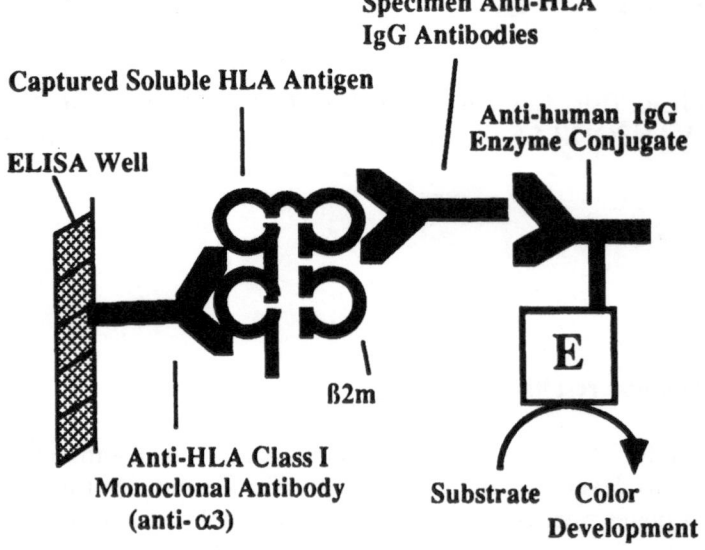

Figure 1. Principal of the PRA-STAT assay.

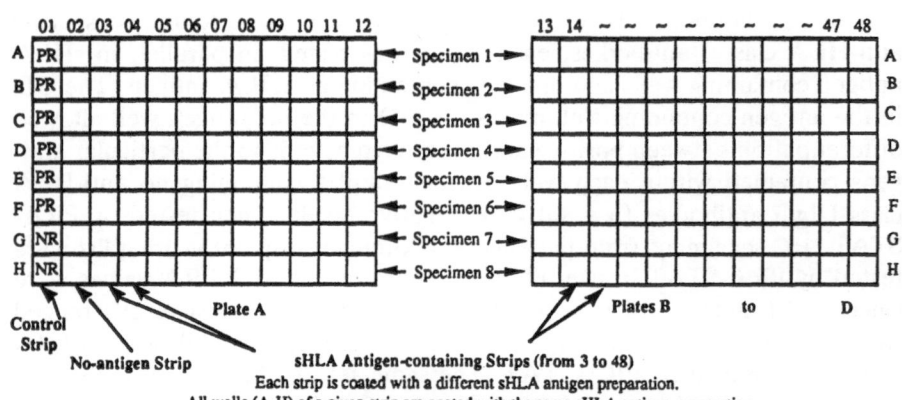

Figure 2. ELISA plate format.

Conclusion

Detection of anti-HLA class 1 IgG antibodies by PRA-STAT is a reliable alternative to lymphocytotoxicity testing. The agreement between lymphocytotoxicity and PRA-STAT test results was 93%. ELISA technology offers several advantages over lymphocytotoxicity: (i) standardization of HLA antigen panel and reagents, (ii) specificity for anti-HLA class I IgG antibodies, (iii) objective read-out of test results, (iv) higher reproducibility.

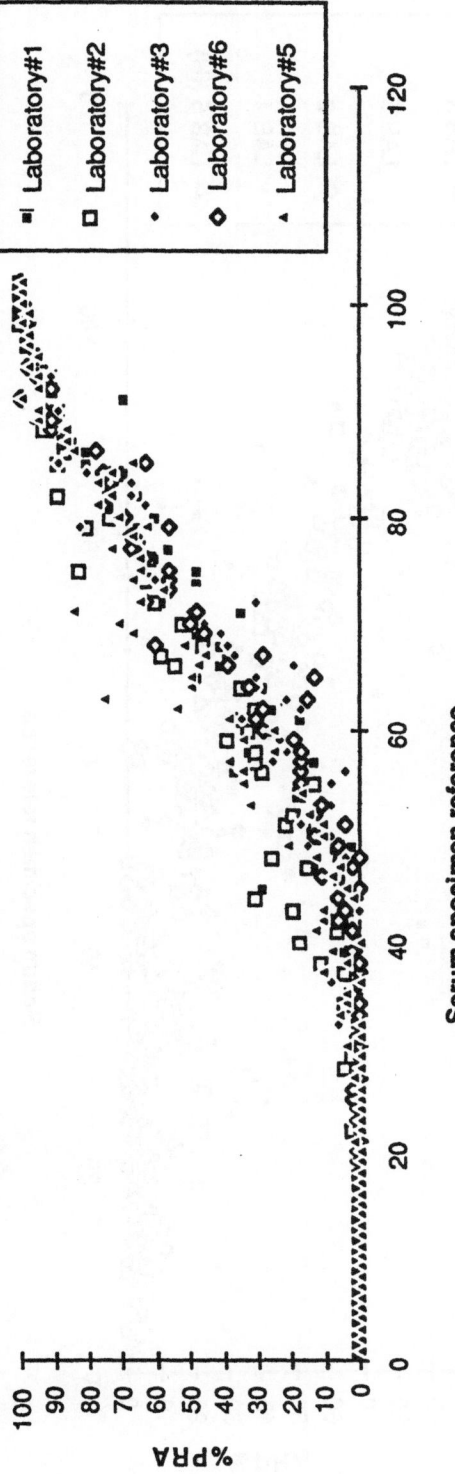

Figure 3. Interlaboratory (n = 5) reproducibility of %PRA values by ELISA (PRA-STAT™).

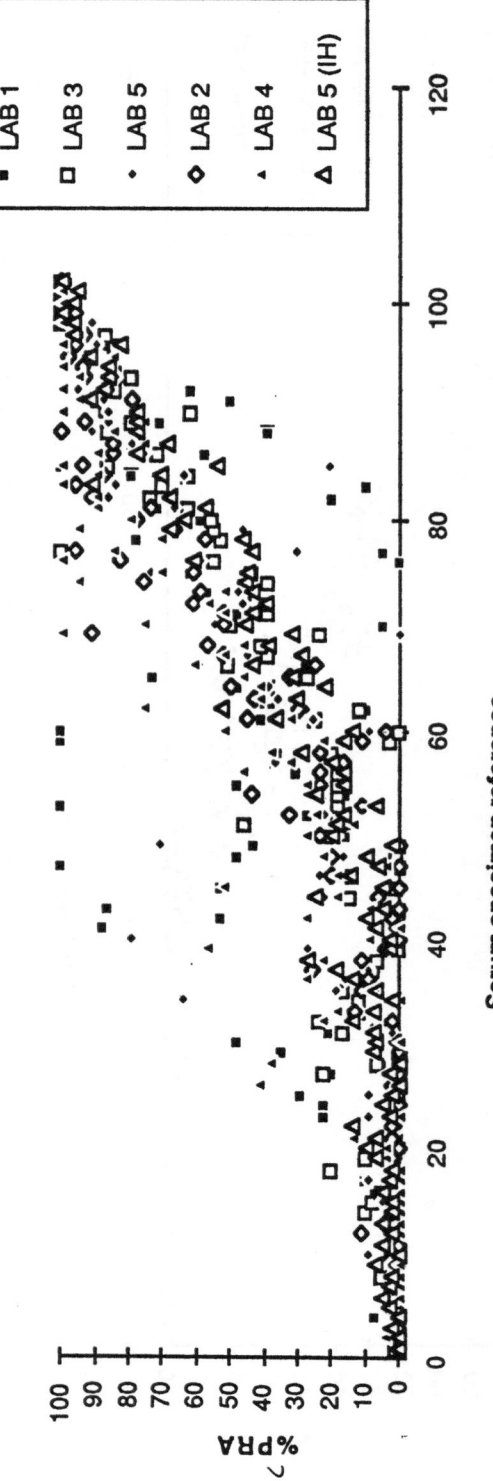

Figure 4. Interlaboratory (n = 6) reproducibility of %PRA values by lymphocytotoxicity.

Table 1. sHLA antigen preparations were derived from cells with the following phenotypes

Strip #	Plate	Cell phenotype
01	A	Control Strip: B7, for reference testing only
02	A	No-antigen strip (sHLA-antigen negative)
03	A	A1, B52
04	A	A30, B18
05	A	A24, B55, B61
06	A	A23, B14
07	A	A32, B38
08	A	A29, B61
09	A	A1, B41
10	A	A24, B60
11	A	A31, B60
12	A	A31, B62
13	B	A1, B57
14	B	A24, B14
15	B	A1, B61
16	B	A24, A26, B51, B61
17	B	A28, A33, B38, B58
18	B	A11, A32, B39, B62
19	B	A3, A23, B50, B55
20	B	A11, A33, B51, B54
21	B	A3, B27, B35
22	B	A2, A29, B41
23	B	A2, B54, B62
24	B	A2, A33, B7, B14
25	C	A2, A28, B8, B50
26	C	A3, A29, B7, B44
27	C	A26, B39, B44
28	C	A33, B45, B58
29	C	A31, A32, B13, B51
30	C	A3, A11, B18, B52
31	C	A1, A23, B35, B49
32	C	A2, A34, B8, B41
33	C	A1, A30, B8, B63
34	C	A2, B52, B63
35	C	A2, A26, B49, B57
36	C	A24, B27, B44
37	D	A2, A25, B18, B45
38	D	A2, A24, B27
39	D	A11, A25, B7, B37
40	D	A1, A2, B39, B58
41	D	A25, A30, B13, B55
42	D	A2, B13, B60
43	D	A29, A32, B35, B45
44	D	A2, A3, B18, B50
45	D	A24, A28, B44, B49
46	D	A1, A2, B8, B27
47	D	A2, A23, B49, B55
48	D	A24, B57

Table 1. Continued

Allele specificities and number of times represented in panel of sHLA antigen preparations

Allele specificity	# Times in panel
A1	8
A2	14
A3	5
A11	4
A23	4
A24	8
A25	3
A26	3
A28	3
A29	4
A30	3
A31	3
A32	4
A33	4
A34	1
B7	3
B8	4
B13	3
B14	3
B18	4
B27	4
B35	3
B37	1
B38	2
B39	3
B41	3
B44	4
B45	3
B49	4
B50	3
B51	3
B52	3
B54	2
B55	4
B57	3
B58	3
B60	3
B61	4
B62	3
B63	2

Table 2. Laboratory to laboratory correlation of %PRA values determined by PRA-STAT

	PRA-STAT Laboratory #1	PRA-STAT Laboratory #2	PRA-STAT Laboratory #3	PRA-STAT Laboratory #6
Laboratory #1 PRA-STAT	1			
Laboratory #2 PRA-STAT	0.93	1		
Laboratory #3 PRA-STAT	0.95	0.89	1	
Laboratory #6 PRA-STAT	0.96	0.91	0.94	1
Laboratory #5 PRA-STAT	0.95	0.91	0.93	0.96

Table 3. Laboratory to laboratory correlation of %PRA values determined by lymphocytotoxicity

	Commercial Tray			In-House Tray	
	Laboratory #1	Laboratory #3	Laboratory #5	Laboratory #2	Laboratory #4
Commercial Tray					
Lab 1	1				
Lab 3	0.58	1			
Lab 5	0.57	0.86	1		
In-house tray					
Lab 2	0.58	0.94	0.84	1	
Lab 4	0.57	0.88	0.81	0.93	1
Lab 5	0.61	0.94	0.89	0.94	0.89

Table 4. Comparison of PRA-STAT and cytotoxicity test results

	PRA-STAT Positive	PRA-STAT Negative
Microlymphocytotoxicity Positive	42	3
Microlymphocytotoxicity Negative	1	15

Table 5. Endpoint titration of serum specimens by PRA-STAT and lymphocytotoxicity

Sample #	Dilution	Cytotoxicity %PRA	Cytotoxicity test result	PRA-STAT %PRA	PRA-STAT test result
654	neat	23	pos	25	pos
654	1:04	13	pos	4	pos/neg
654	1:16	3	neg	0	neg
654	1:64	0	neg	nt	–
2351	neat	48	pos	15	pos
2351	1:04	10	pos	70	pos
2351	1:16	2	neg	37	pos
2351	1:64	0	neg	nt	–
853	neat	47	pos	37	pos
853	1:04	10	pos	11	pos
853	1:16	2	neg	4	pos/neg
853	1:64	2	neg	nt	–
P3068	neat	26	pos	2	pos/neg
P3068	1:04	0	neg	0	neg
P3068	1:16	0	neg	0	neg
P3069	neat	32	pos	13	pos
P3069	1:04	0	neg	0	neg
P3069	1:16	9	neg	0	neg
P3070	neat	30	pos	20	pos
P3070	1:04	0	neg	2	pos/neg
P3070	1:16	0	neg	0	neg
P3071	neat	23	pos	43	pos
P3071	1:04	0	neg	9	pos
P3071	1:16	0	neg	0	neg
P3072	neat	58	pos	26	pos
P3072	1:04	0	neg	2	pos/neg
P3072	1:16	0	neg	2	pos/neg

PART FOUR

Ethics and recipient selection

29. The foundations of the right to be grafted

ANNE MARIE MOULIN

Each century has been commonly characterized by a specific focus. In the same way that the Era of Enlightenment discovered happiness, and liberty haunted the Romantics, health seems to be the concern of our times. In fact, health might be considered a fundamental condition for both happiness and liberty. The French Revolution already acknowledged that "through public welfare, the (poor) patient is entitled to prompt, free, appropriate and *complete* medical care."[1] The right to health has been historically determined by the development of preventive and curative medical techniques, and still further amplified by recent medical discoveries.

With transplantation, medicine is engaged in an active process of immortalizing human nature. On the one hand, the right to transplantation clearly emerges as a product of the revolutionary right to health and the scientist' conception of the Enlightenment; on the other, it stands in a twilight zone, the transgression of borders, "between body and machine, between gift and commodity, individual and collective ownership, moral duty and abomination, death and life."[2] To examine the foundations of a right to transplantation, we have to compare the logic of unlimited scientific and technological progress to anthropological order, which is governed by different laws and, in short, places limits on progress.

The analysis of organ shortage, the object of our present conference, leads us to abandon the optimism and self-confidence that characterized the early days of graft surgery and to explore the rich contradictory trends underlying the putative right to transplantation.

Unlimited progress – the right to health and the right to transplantation

Let us first address the history of the right to health,[3] since the right to transplantation appears to be a recent offspring of this antiquated right. The right to health was already discernible in the French Constitution of 1848. In the Constituents' own words, the state must "raise all citizens to an ever higher degree of morality, enlightenment and well-being."[4] Health was a

J.L. Touraine et al. (eds.), Organ Shortage: The Solutions, 223–233.
© 1995 *Kluwer Academic Publishers*.

kind of moving target, clearly pointed to as one of the main objectives of the state and, significantly, was expected to progress along with scientific developments. This new type of right, instead of being placed alongside the "natural rights," back at the Origin of Man, was always pushed further ahead in the course of history, as something to reach for and not as something to restore to its original purity.[5]

Such new claims as the right to work and the right to health, emerging on the fringe, were received by political thinkers as a major threat to the established order. Tocqueville saw in them the eruption of the mob on the political scene. Since then, it has become common practice to oppose formal and eternal rights, "les droits-libertés," such as liberty of thought or word, transcending the limits of space and time, with the concrete historical claims, "les droits-créance," which take place in time and space and vary according to the context.[6]

The right to health is in fact a highly medicalized collection of rights linked to the availability of new medical goods, which reflects the rapid transformation of medical knowledge. Among them emerges the right to transplantation. Such a right was vindicated, as often happens, not in reference to an ideal right to establish by law, but in the context of a struggle between private interests. In France, some French citizens, discontented with the management of transplantation lists, vindicated their rights and their priorities over their foreign competitors.[7]

For the time being, the right to transplantation does not literally figure in the law. But, in the wake of other "third-generation rights,"[8] it is an obvious candidate for the status of subjective rights. A subjective right is a "right to," which those legislators, doctors and judges who hold the power of enforcing the right can apply with legal force. Its application in turn implies the existence of a large-scale technical system of transplantation with an allocation of services, and national and international regulatory measures.

Today's dilemma is between the impossibility of recognizing health as a purely individual privilege, a "natural one" (this was the position of the 18th century English philosopher Locke) and the immorality of admitting that this right is necessarily restricted and unequally distributed. If the right to transplantation belongs among historical claims – the rights that occur in time and space, to be imposed upon a third party – then we have to understand how the management of these rights is operated not only by the state, but by the members of the social body.

This means that we must investigate the philosophical foundations for the social construction of the right to transplantation. Along our philosophical voyage (which may seem to be a detour but is fundamentally relevant to the issue), we will have to understand how the physical body partakes in the definition of the individual. We will also reactivate the original sense of a current metaphor, the "social body". In so doing, we will face the contradiction between the addiction to unlimited technological progress and the limits set by our historically shaped sensitivity. The sensitivity to the integrity of the body beyond death, and to the exchange of bodily fluids or organs,[9] not unlike the body itself,[10] has a long history, which itself reflects the ambiguous or even corrupted aspects of medical progress.

The history of the western world follows two contradictory trends. The integrity of the dead body has always received attention, while torture and mutilation have been considered as punishments. On the other hand, fragmentation of the individual body has been praised as highly suggestive of collective entities transcending individuality and sheltering a redistribution of merits, virtues and . . . matter.[11]

The philosophical debate: The limits of the individual/collective body and soul

Descartes's mechanistic philosophy, to which we referred above, clearly made organ transfer an acceptable medical issue. In Cartesian philosophy, the soul/body dualism is represented by the duality between spirit and space. The basis for individuality has to be found in thought, and existence is a manifestation of thinking before it is an event of life.

While each individual soul is a substance, only global matter (or geometrical yspace) receives the full dignity of a substance: matter transfer is a mere accident of the substance, in scholastic words. It follows that the flux of shapes in space and time does not alter individuality. The body, not unlike a watch, can be repaired an infinity of times, with a supply of appropriate spare parts.[12] Iatromechanism favoured the implementation of grafting, as witnessed by the attempts of nose transplantation which took place in Italy at the end of the XVIth century.[13] Theologians discarded the localization of the soul in a specific organ[14] and left the way open for the surgeon's knife. Along Cartesian guidelines, human matter is likely to be reconstructed by man, pretty much in the same way that God will raise and reunite all bodies at the End of time.[15]

Descartes stands somewhere between the two main traditions of Western philosophy, Plato and Aristotle.

In Platonician philosophy,[16] the body is the host, or rather, the grave of the soul. Death is properly a delivery and the mortal spoil is readily disposable. On the other hand, according to Aristotle, who shaped the official Christian doctrine on the body/soul problem, matter has to be conjoined to spirit in order to give birth to an individual. Which means that corporality is an intimate part of the individual, and raises the question of the status of the body after death, keeping in mind the resurrection to come.

In the Middle Ages, much of the debate about the resurrection of the body and the relation between body and soul revolved around the issue of bodily continuity. Theologians worried not about whether the body was crucial to human nature, but about how the parts related to the whole, that is to say, how bits could and would be reintegrated after scattering and decay[17] on Judgement Day. The crucial question was: what accounts for the identity of the earthly and risen body? Questions of risen embryos, foreskins and fingernails, of the subtlety of glorified flesh, of how and whether God makes whole the amputee, the eunuch or the fat man were frantically discussed on many occasions among theologians.

Two main questions were addressed that seem to me pertinent to the present discussion:

- what belongs to the individual that needs to be preserved, at least temporarily, in the dead body?
- under what conditions can we invoke the existence of a collective human body which permits part transfer and coexists with autonomous individuals?

The debate on relics illustrates nicely the case in point.

Fragmentation in ancient times: The age of relics

Aquinas, although a supporter of Aristotelianism, denied continuity of form between body and cadaver. He said, for example, that the dead body of a saint is not identical to that saint during life. He was considered heretical by some, since he thus seemed to suggest that the relic was *not* the saint.

During the XIIth century, and parallel to the fashion of preserving relics for miracles, the habit spread among the aristocracy of dividing bodies and burying the noble organs[18] such as the head and the heart in different places, in order to extend the sphere of mystic or mundane influence attached to the dead. Relics are also suggestive of a donor pool. Augustine defines bodies as dearly loved garments, aids to memory and tools for the working of miracles.[19]

Relics[20] clearly illustrate the necessity of a material substrate for the implementation of a cure. They act as a mediation between this world and the other. They do not belong to the cadaveric order; they authorize the gift of life because they retain some spiritual virtue from their living possessor. We are today familiar with these transition forms between the living and the dead and the dissociations between the failure of some vital organs and the maintenance of some others, source of theological difficulties in accepting the medical criteria of death.[21]

During the Age of Relics, however, a strong concern for the integrity of the dead body balanced the mystic desire to dissolve identity for the sake of the community. In 1299, Pope Boniface VIII legislated against the practice of dividing bodies for burial and also included a prohibition of boiling bodies in order to recover and dispatch the holy men's bones throughout Christendom.[22] In Cosmas and Damian's miracle, very popular in XVth century paintings, the holy surgeons graft the black leg of a Moor slave, who is dead, onto their white patient. Curiously, they also attach the white leg onto the mutilated body in the grave. This gesture is not a baroque and absurd staging but reflects a strong commitment to bodily integrity. This issue is at the heart of the Moslem *ulema*'s present controversies over transplantation,[23] even if reluctance to accept grafting procedures may be tempered by the acknowledgement of an omnipotent god's ability to restore maimed or tortured bodies to their initial states.

On the other hand, the ignominious quartering of the body in the Middle Ages, and decapitation, the privilege of nobility in many European countries, remind us that fragmentation of the body could also be viewed as a kind of additional punishment in the civil rule. After the XVIth century, anatomical science made its way to Europe, thanks to royal patronage. The king generously donated four or five bodies from the destitute sent to the gallows. As the medical schools developed, academics demanded more bodies in order to acquire surgical competence. Among the lay public, the dissection of the poor, trapped in the hospitals, figured as an additional burden to the hardness of the times. In England, gangs of bodysnatchers ironically called "resurrectionnists" violated tombs and provided material for the medical schools, much to the anger and hatred of their contemporaries.[24] Dissection,[25] an initiation ritual in a medical corporation exempted from the current taboos on the body, has only recently disappeared from the student curriculum.

Today, it is clear that the intact condition of the body retains deep significance for our society. The rituals that surround death and allow neighbours and kin to view and touch the body, testify to the perception of a mysterious physical continuity in the person who still feels the warmth of homages after death.[26]

Eager to eclipse the healing power of the clerics, physicians, during their successful struggle against the Church at the end of the XIXth century, were unaware of the complexity of the functions they so light-heartedly assumed in lay garments. They were fascinated by the extension of their social power and by technological progress. They paid little attention to the symbolic mediations which lay on them, as witnessed by the present debate on the right to die and the recent emphasis on care for the dying. Doctors have become the true *passeurs* from this world to the other.[27]

Doctors "switch on" the cycle of transplantation themselves, and they may even do so according to the patient's degree of morality during life,[28] like the judges in the tribunal of the dead in Greek antiquity, according to Book X of Plato's *Republic*.

The transplantation crisis

Transplantation science has focused during these last few years on the rejection phenomenon, considered essential. Immunology has provided the general framework for biological research,[29] by putting the emphasis on rejection, or the impossibility of organ transfer from one individual to the other. The immunological agenda has included the investigation of similarities and differences in the human reservoir. The impossibilty of transfer has been circumvented by an "ingenious device of reason" in Hegel's words, here the quest for *minimal biological compatibility*, ascertained according to immunological criteria.

The crisis[30] of transplantation[31] peaked in France and other European countries along with the structural crisis in our political and economic system. A major symptom of the crisis receives due attention in this colloquium, namely, organ shortage.

This crisis is primarily scientific, insofar as the scientific criteria which guided the established networks in the 1960s have been reconsidered. Considering that the selection of donors was subject first to histocompatibility selection, we lived with the optimistic conviction that the best possible choice was being made.[32] The crisis has arrived with the awareness of multiple choice criteria and the idea that there might be some other rational decision. Secondly, these doubts appeared as the medical profession was being progressively questioned and demoted from its traditional position in terms of morality and prestige.[33] Thirdly, the multiplication of transplantable organs has offered the image of a carved body with empty eye sockets and brought back the nightmare of dissection, once considered as belonging to a vanished past.[34]

Transplantation brings together two contrasting sets of images: the merely mechanistic view of grafting, suggestive of an active process of repair and adjustment of "body parts",[35] and the perspective of strong continuity in the social body, between its living members and, also, between the living and the dead. In the latter perspective, the meaning of transplantation extends far beyond the surgical techniques currently being perfected to point to complex exchanges between individuals, exemplified in many ways throughout history.

The ethical question we pose today is of a transplantation system both socially and morally acceptable that lies at the junction of our conflicting views of science and culture, and indicates the necessity of "stitching up the paradigms."[36] Since transplantation has reached a degree hitherto unknown, the question is raised of the *global meaning* of the enterprise. The use of new potent immunosuppressive drugs and the alleviation of the HLA identity "straitjacket",[37] open a previously unexplored space, where prosecution (for not being transplanted) becomes thinkable, precisely as medical decisions become more perplexing. Hence, the necessity of assessing a new dimension of compatibility, *cultural compatibility*.[38] In a very specific way, popular assumptions and academic discourse about transplantation touch each other most closely here. Biological and cultural compatibility are two faces of the same coin.

In France, the 1976 Caillavet Law on organ transplantation was initially conceived to fully exploit the availability of cadaver organs in hospitals. The law was inspired by a spirit of confidence in the powers of reason and technical progress and, also, by the implicit assumption of social consensus.[39] Today doctors are worried. On the one hand, they loathe the idea of becoming the passive instruments of an all-powerful state and, on the other, they have lost the certainty of society's implicit consent, an obvious exception to our contractual, Roman-derived law.[40] The uneasy management of *implicit consent*, and the debate on the legitimacy of the family viewpoint suggest that the population is divided on the subject, profoundly attached to the implementation of a transcending right to health but equally prone to shrink from its consequences. People are more attached to the integrity of the dead body and related rituals than we might have expected. Their understanding of the division between body and corpse, life and death, does not follow the simplistic Cartesian scheme.

How can we improve the failing coherence between our beliefs and our practice? How can we save time for reflection, without imposing a moratorium, which would be damaging for the patients eager to wrench resurrection from doctors and society?

We have already mentioned the difference between "droits-liberté" and "droits-créance," in other words, between natural and "artificial" rights. In any case, the right to an organ transplant is unstably positioned between the two kinds of rights, since transplants are intended to prolong life but, also, to give life. Patients who have received transplants will easily speak of resurrection. Is the right to transplantation a mere extension of the right to health or is it something more flamboyant, the right to life,[41] which brings it into the vicinity of the "right to have a child," making transplantation an immediate challenge to the natural order? Transplantation seems, in fact, to be a rebirth more than a resurrection. Birth is the most socialized of all biological events; no wonder that transplantation must be registered and legitimized by the whole social body.

Besides, if the remedy is to be found in the body of the Other, to acknowledge such a right would amount to bringing back ancient slavery. When the impossibility of claiming a right on the body of another individual is blatant, then the mediation of the collective body is unavoidable. Our legal system, founded on the tradition of Roman law, deals only with abstract persons[42] and does not give word to a material body. How can we introduce the fiction of a material collective body with recirculating organs?

Here again we return to past and present anthropological intuitions, glimpses at cultures where such a material body exists and is treated as a reservoir of energy and healing cures. The body of the king, in some African cultures, highlighted by Frazer's famous book,[43] is a source of collective spiritual solace and material well-being and, as such, is periodicaly sacrificed in due time. The recycling of organs among the living in our modern societies is an equivalent example of sacrificial violence. The analogy may seem far-fetched to the modern reader who uneasily associates glittering modern technical skill with physical assault on the sacred body of the king[44] in so-called primitive cultures. However, the cannibal order[45] is here clearly an appropriate term for the culture of transplantation.[46] Put in milder terms, the very idea of socially useful and legitimate sacrifice seems to be essential to the development of modern transplantation, primarily because it blurs the otherwise important distinction between living donors and cadavers.

In contrast with the majestic epic of unlimited progress in the science of grafting, the anthropological dimension conflates different epochs and places as summarily illustrated above. In transplantation, the biological by itself does not found the cultural. To the contrary, cultural determinants have to be integrated into biological thinking. Transplantation finds its main inspiration in the natural paradigm of pregnancy, early assimilated to an alien graft from the male genitor, but it cannot be reduced to the mere imitation of nature. Its innovative character is indicative of its bold cultural status and the implicit transgression contained in it.

Identifying cultural compatibility

My thesis is that individual and societal consent must be strong, not only to respect the continuity of our law and its tradition in terms of the jurisprudence of the body, but also because transplantation, in order to work, must go through a revival of the individual's commitment towards social entities that transcend him.

Transplantation reveals unescapable dependencies of the living on the dead.[47] The process of immortalizing the human species reintroduces the dead into the social space, and vehicles the sense of guilt, sharpened by the suspicion of commercial transactions. What transplanter would deny that while their transplanted patients survive with the organs of others, they are themselves inhabited by the remembrance of their deceased patients? The modern alienation from the dead leads to some monstrous exclusions[48] and partly explains our present difficulties. Let us acknowledge that all cultures have dealt with this segregation process. In Ancient Greece, a coin was put into the mouth of the dead, so that he could pay his obol to Charo to be taken over, and would not wander like a ghost on this bank of the river Styx. In Bali, the coffin carriers shake the dead violently to make him lose his sense of orientation and prevent him from finding his way back home.[49] The anonymous character of donation no longer appears to be sufficient protection against nightmares and anxieties.

Transplants are subject not only to biological compatibility, but to a more general compatibility, which is harmonization with our society's cultural system. We must re-root science and techniques in their cultural environment if we are to avoid a fracture. This attempt to reestablish the continuity of the social debate is rendered essential by the current crisis.[50] This crisis opposes an idealistic ethic of transplantation that views the body as a person to a juridical and commercial realism that views the body as a thing, or even as an item whose market needs to be regulated.[51] Science thought it had conquered an autonomous space; instead it has to take into account a whole range of symbolic representations and elaborate what I have called cultural compatibility.

I would like to conclude with the concrete suggestion that together we need to elaborate a transplantation culture. Could we not relieve the general state of anxiety surrounding organ transplantation by officially admitting an established current of exchange between the living and the dead, and by considering the appearance of a new collective body, a social body that would be endowed with materiality? We need to think about a new sanitary order, no longer based exclusively on fear of diseases and swapping germs, but rather on the recognition that there is a positive value in biological exchanges. Only in this way will transplantation be able to reconcile certain archaic notions about the body, with its undeniable vocation as a representation of modernity.

References

1. DB Weiner, C Bloch and A Tuetey, editors, Procès-verbaux et rapports du Comité de mendicité de la Constituante, 1790–1791, Paris, Imprimerie nationale, p 391, quoted by DB Weiner, Le droit de l'homme à la santé, Une belle idée devant la Constituante: 1790–1791, Clio Medica, 1970, 5, p 210.
2. I. Braun and B Joerges, How to recombine large technical systems, the case of European Organ Transplantation, Wissenschaftszentrum Berlin für Sozialforschung, 1993, p 2.
3. Article Droit à la santé, Les mots de la bioéthique, G Hottois and MH Parizeau editors, Bruxelles, De Boeck, 1993, p 140–144; M Foucault, Un système fini face à une demande infinie, Sécurité sociale, L'enjeu, Entretien avec S Bono, Paris, 1983, p 39–63.
4. Constitution du 4 Novembre 1848, in P Ardant, Les textes sur les Droits de l'homme, Paris, Presses universitaires de France, 1993, p 58.
5. AM Moulin, AIDS and the history of the right to health, AIDS, health and human rights, Fondation Marcel Mérieux, 1993, p 67–73.
6. J Rivero, Les libertés publiques, Paris, Presses universitaires de France, 1981; Luc Ferry, Des droits de l'homme à l'idée républicaine, Paris, Presses universitaires de France, 1985.
7. N Herpin and F Paterson, Centralisation et pouvoir discrétionnaire, La transplantation rénale en France, Ethique des choix médicaux, J Elster and N Herpin, editors, Arles, Actes-Sud, 1992, p 37–62.
8. Let us just briefly mention the right to housing, to private life, not to speak of the right of being different. See Consécration et usage de droits nouveaux, Centre de recherches critiques sur le droit, Université de Saint Etienne, 1992.
9. F Héritier-Augé, Le sperme et le sang, Nouvelle revue de Psychanalyse, 1985, 32, p 111–122; P Oliviéro, La communication sociale des matériaux biologiques: sang, sperme, organes et cadavres, Cahiers internationaux de sociologie, 1993, 18.
10. J Léonard, Archives du Corps, La santé au XIXe siècle, Rennes, Ouest-France, 1986.
11. J-P Baud, L'affaire de la main coupée, Histoire juridique du corps, Paris, Le Seuil, 1993.
12. AM Moulin, Body parts, Transplantation Proceedings, 1993, 25, p 33–35.
13. G Tagliacozzi, De curtorum chirurgia per insitionem, Venise, 1597.
14. See for example Father Malebranche, a convinced Cartesian, in P Costabel, Les notions de corps et de soi à la fin du 17e siècle, Soi et Non-soi, M Bessis and coll., Paris, Le Seuil, 1990, p 251–265.

232   *A.M. Moulin*

15. "Everyman is summoned to resuscitate and thus invited to recover his personal integrity, transfigured and definitely in his possession in Christ our Lord", Solidarité et respect des personnes dans les greffes de tissus et d'organes, Conference of The French Bishops on Organ Donation, Documents épiscopaux, 15 October 1993.
16. See the dialogues such as *Phaedrus, Phaedo* . . . .
17. P Walker Bynum, Material continuity: personal survival and the resurrection of the body: a discussion in medieval and modern contexts, Fragmentation and redemption, essays on gender and the human body in medieval religion, New York, Zone Books, 1991, p 239–262.
18. J Le Goff, The head or the heart? The political uses of bodily metaphors in the Middle Ages, Fragments for a history of the body, M Feher, R Naddaff and N Tazi, New York, Zone Books, 1989, p 13–27.
19. Fragmentation and Redemption. . ., P Walker Bynum ed.
20. G Fichtner, Das verpflanzt Mohrerbein, zur Interpretation der Kosmas und Damian Legende, Med. Hist. J., 1968, 3, p 87–100; J Gelis et O Redon, Les miracles miroirs des corps, Université de Paris VIII ed., Paris 1983, p 23–50; P Browne, Reliques et statut social au temps de Grégoire de Tours, La société et le sacré dans l'antiquité tardive, Seuil, Paris 1985, p 171–178; The Cult of the Saints, Chicago University Press, Chicago 1981.
21. For Judaism and Islam see G Bernheim, Ethique juive et transplantation, D Boubakeur, Ethique islamique et transplantation, Ethique et Transplantation, Cilag, Club de la Transplantation ed., Bagneux 1994, p 39–45.
22. In the decree Detestenda feritatis in 1299.
23. V Risler-Chaim, Islamic Medical Ethics in the XXth century, Brill, Leiden 1993, p 28–43.
24. R Richardson, Dissection, death and the destitute, London, Routledge and Kegan Paul, 1988.
25. JL Valabrega, La relation thérapeutique, Paris 1965.
26. TA Kselman, Death and the afterlife in modern France, Princeton, NJ, Princeton University Press, 1993.
27. S Novaes's fine title for her forthcoming book on doctors and sperm donation, *Les passeurs de gamètes*.
28. On the selection of receivers of liver transplants, AL Spital, Unrelated donors: should they be used? Transplantation Proceedings, 1992, 24, p 2215–2217; PR Jeyarag et al., Liver splits, the answer to a low donor pool, Transplantation Proceedings, 1992, 24, p 1956–1957.
29. AM Moulin, Le dernier langage de la médecine, Histoire de l'immunologie de Pasteur au SIDA, Paris, PUF, 1991
30. NJ Delorme, La réforme de la transplantation d'organes, Concours médical, 1992, 114, p 3491–3493.
31. From past to present, J Hamburger, Transplantation d'organes: nouveaux problèmes éthiques, Actes Biologie et devenir de l'homme, Paris, Université de Paris (MUR), Paris, McGraw Hill, 1976.
32. L Degos, Le don reçu, Paris, Plon, 1990; see also, J Elster, Ethique des choix médicaux . . .
33. AM Moulin, Reversible history: blood transfusion and the spread of AIDS in France, AIDS and the public debate: historical and contemporary perspectives, C Hannaway, V Harden and J Paranscandola, editors, Amsterdam, IOS Press (in press).
34. On the phantasms of those who "donate their bodies to Science", A Hernandez, N Léry, Le don du corps et la mort, Ethique, 1993, 7, p 38–42.
35. AM Moulin, Body parts, the modern dilemma, Transplantation Proceedings, 1993, 25, p 33–35.
36. B Saint-Sernin, Suturer les paradigmes, Médecine et humanisme, Melun, Association Economie et Santé, 1992, p 121–124.
37. AM Moulin, Le dernier langage de la Médecine, 1991, PVF publisher, p 221.
38. AM Moulin, Droit à la santé et droit à la transplantation. La compatibilité culturelle, Ethique et Transplantation, Cilag ed., p 16–30.

39. The French philosopher François Dagognet went so far as to suggest that donating his own body was an implicit part of the contract between the individual and society, Corps réfléchis, Paris, Odile Jacob, 1990, p 84–85.
40. Cf. Marie-Angèle Hermitte, Consentement et prélèvement d'organe sur cadavre, Ethique et transplantation, Cilag, p 81–90.
41. A Comte-Sponville, A propos de la vie, du droit et de la morale, Ethique et droits de l'homme, Arles, Actes-Sud, 1988, p 275.
42. J-P Baud, L'affaire de la main coupée.
43. JG Frazer, The dying god, 1890.
44. Luc de Heersch, The sacrficial body of the king, Fragments for a history of the body . . . , p 387–394.
45. The title of a popular best-seller by the political thinker Jacques Attali on medicalization.
46. AM Moulin, Droit à la santé et droit à la transplantation. See also the notion of "culture d'accompagnement" in MA Hermitte, Consentement et prélèvement, Ethique et transplantation, p 81–90.
47. N Elias, La solitude des mourants, Détroits, 1987, p 50.
48. TA Kselman, Death and the afterlife in modern France . . .
49. D Napier, Foreign bodies. Performances, art and symbolic anthropology, Berkeley, University of California Press, 1992.
50. RD Guttmann, The meaning of "the economy of ethics of alternative cadaver organ procurement policies", Yale Journal of Regulation, 1991, 8, p 453–462; RD and A Guttmann, Organ transplantation: duty reconsidered, Transplantation Proceedings, 1992, 24, p 2179–2180.
51. G David: Entretien. Il est pervers de développer un marché du corps humain, Ethique, 1992, 22, p 125–128.

30. The graft survival curve: Ideology and rhetoric – Part II

RONALD D. GUTTMANN

Introduction

In a previous paper entitled "The Graft Survival Curve: Ideology & Rhetoric" [1], I attempted to understand and interpret the significance of the common language and concepts used by members of the transplantation community, with respect to the graft survival statistic and its visual representation, the graft survival curve. In the course of this analysis, it became clear that there were many scientific dimensions as well as possible political agendas in the presentation and promotion of survival statistics and survival curves. First, proper clinical studies and clinical trials use this type of primary or secondary endpoint associated with testing a hypothesis either with retrospective analysis or prospective methodology. Second, the same type of endpoint outcome measure is derived from the voluntary submission of data sent to various local, national and international registries. What became very clear in analyzing the nature of and the statements about graft survival statistics was that they obscurely reflected the continuation of a long-standing confrontation that has been known in the field of clinical transplantation: the battle over control of the rules of organ rationing between the cadres of immunologists and clinicians.

One of the earliest examples of graft survival curve representations is found in the 1946 paper by Medawar on skin grafts in rabbits [2]. The belief that the extrapolation of the data presentation of animal allograft studies, whereby graft survival analysis could be related to various genetically derived cellular markers, especially the major histocompatibility complex (MHC), has led to the strong belief by many that similar type-matching of organs between human donors and recipients is still the major and most clinically significant factor in graft survival. Since the debate is old, controversial, well known and stale, there is little that needs to be said about the morass of the conflicting literature that has led the debate, however, it is good to consider how such conflicts and tensions can cause the redefinition of concepts which changes neither the genetics nor the biological nor the clinical realities of

J.L. Touraine et al. (eds.), Organ Shortage: The Solutions, 235–241.
© 1995 *Kluwer Academic Publishers.*

transplantation. Löwy has given us an insightful analysis of this tension which led to the definition of clinical histocompatibility [3].

Patients

There is serious reason to be very critical about the graft survival statistic as the major outcome measurement for patients, since it focusses on the graft as an object, often to the exclusion or non-consideration of other factors of the patient's medical condition. It neglects to consider the real subject matter of clinical transplantation, the reversal of end-stage disease and rehabilitation of patients. What has also been surprising is the glib language about graft survival, the incessant referral to one- or two-year graft survival or, more recently, the "half-life" of grafts, a seemingly obvious attempt to humanize the vital organ, when there is really the need to reference a heterogenous population of patients, each of whom has an individual outcome and who collectively are much more complex than the graft survival statistic can ever represent.

Two of the major criticisms of the common approach to the survival statistic and graphic presentation are the need for dichotomization of complex data and the reduction of data to hardly meaningful clinical entities. If the nature of clinical transplantation was the function of the graft or a particular drug used, "yes or no", this approach might be acceptable, but a series of surrogates can never accurately reflect the complex clinical situation nor be used as any more than a superficial hypothesis suggestor for appropriately detailed prospective clinical studies. The therapies we use have significant side effects, patients may have other co-morbid illnesses, and outcomes can also be measured in terms of quality of life, social and physical rehabilitation, the reversal of medical problems and the occurrence of new medical complications.

The fact that certain centres can consistently achieve excellent outcomes, including graft survival, and the fact that certain early graft loss problems can be overcome by improved donor technical factors and good perioperative care should focus our attention on these centers for a more detailed medical analysis. Indeed center variation [4] and perioperative considerations [5, 6] are still considered important in a very recent literature. This is relevant to the early allograft loss issue which largely determines graft survival rates long term.

HLA

Without going into detail about the debate over the clinical significance of HLA-matching for organ transplantation, it needs to be said that given the good results that certain centers can obtain with adherence to effective therapy, obtaining good quality organs and providing high quality ongoing treatment and care, the debate over "the match" becomes trivial. However, "the match" as well as the "graft survival" statistic have become the jargon of the transplant community, the easy way to talk comfortably and authoritatively, especially when "average" rather than "excellent" becomes the standard. The effect of this type of discourse, I believe, is to subvert high quality discussion of the critical clinical studies needed, and the high quality education of a younger generation of physicians, nurses, and other interested parties, including patients. This endless debate misleads referring physicians and manipulates those sitting around the table making the rules of rationing organs to feel self-assured about the moral authority of their political activity.

As an experienced clinical transplanter, knowledgeable about the HLA-typing system and laboratory practice, there is little doubt that the selective processes that we already have in place, such as ABO compatibility and an accurate negative crossmatch, are the essentials in the laboratory contribution. It is acknowledged that the PRA percentage can be useful in some instances as can the anti-HLA specificities detected. While the "6–antigen match" may be relevant, provided it negates any proliferative tissue interaction between donor and recipient, the tissue typers hierarchical claim that 5 antigens matched or mismatched is better prognostically than 4, than 3, etc., has been dealt with in a superficial manner and is biologically unfounded given the complexities of clinical transplantation [7, 8]. The claims are rhetorical and the evidence is not critical. What the preoccupation with HLA does is similar to that of other current debates in diagnostic medicine, it creates the "geneticization" of an issue. Further, given the large degree of polymorphism of the HLA system, the bias of the match has already fueled the fires of claims of unfairness by ethnic minorities [9] and other explanations of the differences in graft survival are being offered [10, 11]. Therefore, not only are many of the genetic claims questionable, but their strength has given voice to those who wish to see one aspect of unfairness in the rationing system.

Registries

What has been of particular concern to me in recent years has been the rhetoric about graft survival statistics emanating from the registry organizations. The registries which have been traditionally *descriptive* in their output after collecting reduced data have become *prescriptive*, often with the agenda to advocate the use of one therapeutic regimen instead of another, rather than continue the traditional registry role of generating findings which could be the basis for a serious scientific prospective study [12–15]. Prescribing by the proprietors of the organization should be regarded as beyond the domain of the registry enterprise for a number of reasons. First, the reduced data handled by registries which generate a survival statistic cannot be considered to measure the efficacy of any therapy, by any reasonable standard. Second, the data is normally unaudited, uncontrolled for omissions or lack of follow-up, and often comes from a multitude of centers with varying populations, immunosuppressive drug treatment regimens and care algorithms. Further, clear medically coherent definitions of clinical or treatment data entries are usually lacking. One would expect the medical community to be the formal interpreters of the registry information product.

One of the curious features of the international transplant registries is the penchant for continuing to analyze and reanalyze the constantly growing database over time. Often the graft survival curves will have such a large n factor that one can only surmise that the universe referred to is not reality-oriented, i.e., is larger than any waiting list. Thus, prescriptions, if based on some truth, may be irrelevant and ineffective, and the approach creates a false universe which can never exist over time, a universe which cannot be verified in a proper scientific way. The technical agenda seems to be large n, small p [1].

Recently, the use of retrospective registry data from Eurotransplant has been used in a more modern and sophisticated statistical way and has been prospectively verified. In these analyses, the reduced data could produce four sub-populations of the patient cohort, each with a different likelihood of having prolonged graft survival [16]. While this approach is laudable, it still does not answer fundamental questions of the justification for and accuracy of the reduced data which constructed the curves. It does not explain why a significant number of patients in the poorest prognostic group have a "good" prognosis if good is only measured by graft survival. Finally, it is unlikely that it reveals anything that medical observations and judgements have not already communicated in the literature. As an instrument of rationing policy-making, it is also weak. Because it does not relate to alternative cohort studies, little value can be placed on its therapeutic meaning. Even if those with the worst prognostic indices were denied an allograft, the shortage would not likely meet the needs of all appropriate candidates. Thus, what the prognostic index approach really pushes for in medical behavior is to narrow the referral gate, creating a new tension between patient and referring physician, one that merely substitutes the referring MD for the "referred-to" MD.

Moral authority

The earlier conclusion that was reached after considering the context and significance of the rhetoric about survival statistics and the graft survival curve iconography was that the claims represent the game of control between the immunologists and clinicians – the control of the rules of rationing, each justifying its own turf [1]. While this may seem obvious and it is useful to have such an inter-professional debate, one should question the moral authority of these self-interested groups to make policy. This policy-making role is being questioned in many ways now, since it has been recognized that the arguments for a particular rationing policy in a period of organ shortage are not necessarily genetic or medical. That the transplant establishment has empowered itself to make rationing rules is slowly becoming the focus of critical attention [17].

New rhetoric

Equally disturbing in the transplantation literature is the recent glib use of phrases such as *objective computer analysis, scientifically proven that, prospective, efficacy demonstrated, equity in access, fairness in access, fair distribution, medical utility and benefit, equitable allocation, cost-effectiveness,* etc., to promote the results of data analysis. The jargon of sophisticated statistics has also entered the arena with multivariate analyses. Often these analyses are repeated on the same or growing data base and are prepared on the limited scope of dichotomized data bits, ever changing. What is clearly technical is often referred to as scientific.

Conclusion

The influence of the visual presentations of the registries and rhetoric should not be underestimated. Data is presented, less often in the peer-reviewed medical journals than at congresses and in congress-associated publications. This vast exposure, as has been previously stated, can produce "computer-generated medicalization". Perhaps the statement by Veatch, made in another context is appropriate for this current prescriptive need which is believed to justify particular rationing rules. It is termed the "technical criteria fallacy" [18]:

> We may become so infatuated with our technical abilities to accumulate data and tally scores that we run the risk of seriously misunderstanding the nature of the difficult decisions that must be made.

It is my view that the precision of detail and accuracy of technical analyses, rather than the quality of information, has been seductive. It is a characteristic of an information society. The important descriptions of clinical care are elusive.

For those who think that a simple abstraction of the clinical setting or developing the proper policy on rationing life-improving and life-saving organs will be easy, we should be reminded of the way Mr. Palomar speaks of our natural tendencies [19]:

> A model is by definition that in which nothing has to be changed, that

which works perfectly; whereas reality as we see clearly, does not work and constantly falls to pieces; so we must force it, more or less roughly, to assume the form of the model.

It is important to continue to probe and reinterpret claims in the context of the transplantation field's primary purpose, the rehabilitation of patients selected by a rationing process in which the genetic and medical arguments are only part of a larger series of factors of personhood. Medical paternalism is an inappropriate attitude in health policy derivation and there are several other *interested parties* that need to be heard in the policy-making debate on organ rationing. Opening up the debate of this issue should not interfere with the medical profession's motivation to improve therapy.

References

1. Guttmann RD. The graft survival curve: ideology and rhetoric. Transplant Proc 1992; 24: 2407–10.
2. Medawar PB. The behavior and fate of skin autografts and skin homografts in rabbits. J Anatomy 1944; 78: 176–96.
3. Lowy I. Variances in meaning in discovery accounts: the case of contemporary biology. Hist Stud Phys Biol 1990; 21: 87–121.
4. Gjertson DW, Terasaki PI. The large center variation in half-lives of kidney transplants. Transplantation 1992; 53: 357–62.
5. Aswad S, Mann SL, Khetan U, et al. Omit HLA matching to attain shorter cold ischemic time? Transplant Proc 1993; 25: 3053–5.
6. Najarian JS, Gillingham KJ, Sutherland DER, et al. The impact of the quality of initial graft function on cadaver kidney transplants. Transplantation 1994; 57: 812–6.
7. Dausset J, Hors J, Busson M, et al. Serologically defined hl-a antigens and long-term survival of cadaver kidney transplants. New Engl J Med 1974; 290: 979–84.
8. Opelz G. HLA matching should be utilized for improving kidney transplant success rates. Transplant Proc 1991; 23: 46–50.
9. Kasiske BL, Neylan JF, Riggio RR, et al. The effect of race on access and outcome in transplantation. New Engl J Med 1991; 324: 302–7.
10. Koyama H, Cecka JM, Terasaki PI. Kidney transplants in black recipients. Transplantation 1994; 57: 1064–8.
11. Butkus DE, Meydrech EF, Raju SS. Racial differences in the survival of cadaveric renal allografts. New Engl J Med 1992; 327: 840–5.
12. Gjertson DW, Terasaki PI, Takemoto BS, et al. National allocation of cadaveric kidneys by hla matching. New Engl J Med 1991; 324: 1032–6.
13. Cecka JM, Cho YW, Terasaki PI. Analyses of the UNOS Scientific Renal Transplant Registry at three years – early events affecting transplant success. Transplantation 1992; 53: 59–64.
14. Wujcia T, Opelz G. A proposal for improved cadaver kidney allocation. Transplantation 1993; 56: 1513–7.
15. Thorogood DJ, Schreuder GMTh, Persijn GG, van Rood JJ. Organ sharing based on HLA matching saves dialysis years and patient lives. Transplant Proc 1993; 25: 3049–50.
16. Thorogood DJ. Statistical modelling of renal allograft survival and associated prognostic factors, The Hague, The Netherlands: Pasmans Offsetdrukkerij BV, 1992.
17. Veatch RM. Who empowers medical doctors to make allocative decisions for dialysis &

organ transplantation? In Land W, Dossetor JB, editors. Organ replacement therapy: ethics, justice and commerce. Berlin: Springer-Verlag, 1991: 331–5.

18. Veatch RM. The technical criteria fallacy. Hastings Center report 1977; August: 15–16.
19. Calvino I. Mr. Palomar. Toronto: Lester & Orpen Dennys Ltd., 1994: 109.

31. The nature of the selection of candidates for cardiac transplant

SUZANNE WAIT, R.D. GUTTMANN & J. JAIME CARO

Introduction

Over the past few years, the increasing gap between donor organ availability and transplant patient demand has prompted clinicians to carefully examine the process of selection of candidates for cardiac transplantation [1]. This selection actually involves several stages. First, the treating physician selects patients for referral to a transplant program. These patients are then assessed by the transplant selection team to determine who will go onto a heart transplant waiting list, who is not yet ready to be placed on the list, and who is unacceptable for the list. It is believed that this selection reflects those patients who might derive the greatest benefit from a heart transplant and whose current medical needs are most appropriate. A further selection occurs once a donor organ becomes available. The final recipient choice is based on a set of rationing rules, often derived locally, that take into account blood group, physical characteristics, and other criteria. By contrast, the initial selection of patients to be placed onto the active waiting list is left to the discretion of the transplant selection team. This pivotal step in the selection process also requires rationing of a scarce and valuable resource: a place on the waiting list.

Since the innovative early days of transplantation, clinical teams have sought to elaborate a medically justifiable protocol for the selection of patients for transplant [2]. In the hope of attaining this, clinicians periodically assess the reliability of criteria used for the selection of patients from the transplant list.

The purpose of our study was to determine which criteria were used by our program's selection committee for the assessment of 354 patients referred to our hospital for cardiac transplantation. We then derived a predictive model for acceptance of patients onto the cardiac transplant waiting list. We discuss the justification of this model with reference to the cardiac transplantation literature.

J.L. Touraine et al. (eds.), Organ Shortage: The Solutions, 243–252.
© 1995 *Kluwer Academic Publishers*.

Methods

Patients included in this study were referred for heart or heart-lung transplantation to the Royal Victoria Hospital (RVH) in Montreal, Canada, between April 1985 (the initiation of the heart transplant program) and January 20, 1990 (cutoff date). Also included were seven patients who had received transplants at another Montreal hospital between July 1982, and January 1985, and were transferred when their transplant surgeon moved to the RVH. Information on patients was obtained mainly from records kept in the RVH Heart Transplant Clinic and by the transplant surgeons. When necessary, these sources were supplemented by (i) referral letters from the patient's cardiologist, (ii) hospital medical records, and (iii) minutes from the transplant selection committee weekly meetings. Data on these patients, including those not accepted for transplant, were updated until May 1, 1991.

For all referred patients, data were collected on demographics, medical history, cardiac function and other laboratory tests as well as on the psychosocial evaluation performed during the patient's pre-transplant assessment. Data concerning post-transplant survival, readmissions and rejections were also obtained for all patients receiving transplants, but were not used in this analysis. Conflicts in the historical information were resolved by the transplant surgeon or the nurse clinician.

For analysis, information on all illnesses was reduced to a binary variable (presence/absence), and numerical variables were classified in ordinal scales. Primary diagnoses were classified into five categories for heart transplant candidates, and eight for heart-lung candidates. Actuarial analysis was used to obtain the distribution and mean of decision time (time from initial referral to final decision on candidacy), and of waiting time (from initial appearance on the waiting list until transplantation or death). When, at the cutoff date, no decision had been reached as to suitability for transplant or a patient was still waiting on the transplant active list, the cutoff date was used as the endpoint ("censored") for calculations of decision time and waiting time. For patients who died before a decision was made, their date of death was taken as the end-point for decision time.

To assess whether a feature was a determinant of patient selection for transplantation, the rate of acceptance onto the waiting list in patients with the feature was compared to that in patients without the feature, thus producing a rate ratio (RR) of acceptance. The statistical significance of this ratio was calculated using χ^2 analysis.

Using stepwise logistic regression (SAS™ software), a predictive model for acceptance onto the waiting list was sought. First, a correlation matrix was used to establish covariance between features. Correlated features were then grouped into single binary variables. All features pertaining to cardiac condition were grouped. Patients with either cardiac output above 5.0 l min^{-1}, or cardiac index above 1.5, or wedge pressure below 12 cm^2 H$_2$O, or left or right ejection fraction above 35% were considered to have a "good"

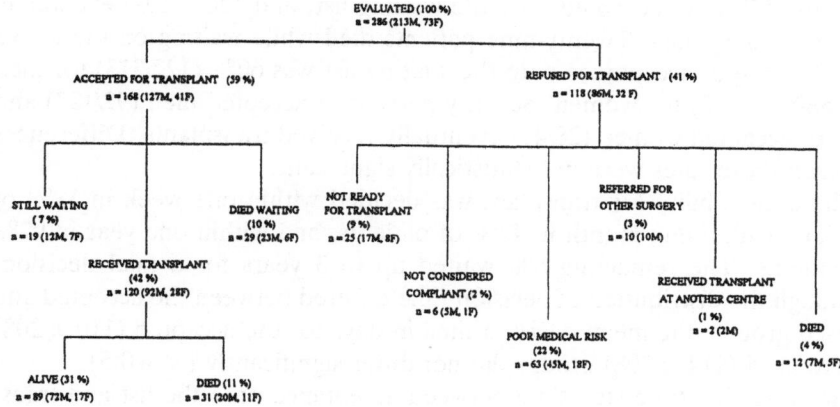

Fig. 1. Status on May 1, 1991 of all patients evaluated at the RVH for heart or heart-lung transplant, and referred between April 16, 1982 and January 20, 1990.

cardiac condition. All others were considered to have a "poor" cardiac condition. Both features pertaining to the patient's overall health status were grouped. Patients with a sickness status of 1 or 2 on an ordinal scale of 1 to 6, or a New York Heart Association status (NYHA) status of I or II were considered to be in "good" overall health status. All active pathologies considered relative contraindications by the local transplant selection committee (hypertension, hyperlipidemia and hypercholesteremia, hepatitis, renal disease, pneumonia or tuberculosis) were grouped as "other clinical contraindication." Perceived "absolute" contraindications, such as peripheral vascular disease (PVD) and previous serious infectious disease were considered separately.

Presence of psychosocial problems as determined by the social worker or psychiatrist in the patient's pre-transplant assessment, and continued substance abuse were grouped. All other features were considered individually in the construction of the regression model.

Results

During the time covered by this study, 354 patients were referred to the heart and heart-lung transplant program. Of these, 68 were not evaluated because of patient refusal or death before evaluation. In a few cases, the referral was not pursued because the assessing transplant clinician considered that the patient presented an obvious contraindication.

A classification flow diagram of the 286 evaluated patients as of May 1, 1991, is shown in Figure 1. Two patients eventually transplanted and followed at another center were excluded from further analysis. Of the remaining 284 patients, 168 were accepted onto the waiting list, and 120 (71%) eventually received transplants. Twenty-nine patients died while waiting on the active list. The rate of acceptance onto the waiting list was 60% (127/213) for men and 56% (41/73) for women. Seventy percent of accepted men (92/127) and 61% of accepted women (28/41) eventually received transplants. Differences between these rates were not statistically significant.

The acceptability for transplant was decided within one week in 18% of patients, within one month in 42% of patients, and within one year in 92% of patients. The remaining 8% waited up to 3 years for a final decision. Although the distribution of decision time differed between the accepted and refused groups, the mean decision time in days for the accepted (110 ± 208) and refused (114 ± 208) groups did not differ significantly ($p > 0.5$).

Mean waiting time (the time between acceptance onto the list and transplant) was 174 ± 21 days for men and 165 ± 29 days for women ($p > 0.5$). Patients over 60 years of age had a mean waiting time of 145 days, compared to 175 days for those under 60 ($p > 0.5$). Mean waiting times were significantly shorter ($p < 0.0001$) for patients in NYHA Class IV (80 ± 19 days) compared to NYHA Class III or II (219 ± 29 days). Waiting time was strongly correlated with decision time ($p < 0.0001$). Stated reasons for refusal of 111 of the 116 patients not accepted are shown in Figure 2. These reasons are documented both in the patient evaluation reports and in the minutes taken at the selection committee weekly meetings. For 5 patients, no documented reason for refusal was found.

Table 1 shows relative rates of acceptance onto the waiting list according to patient features. These rates are calculated only for patients with information available on the feature. Young age, poor sickness status, poor cardiac condition, absence of psychosocial problems, absence of peripheral vascular disease, presence of serious infectious disease, presence of other clinical contraindication and anergy were individually significantly associated with acceptance.

The most predictive model obtained by optimization suggests that a sicker heart, a worse health status (hospitalised or bed-ridden versus out-patient), absence of psychosocial problems, absence of CMV antibody, absence of previous cardiac surgery, and absence of diabetes mellitus are the factors which favour a patient's acceptance onto the waiting list. None of the other features achieved statistical significance on entry into the model.

Discussion

In the face of donor shortage, the method of selection of patients for transplantation is an issue of major concern. The availability of heart transplants at increasing numbers of centers, together with the shortage of suitable donor hearts, places enormous responsibility on those who make selection decisions. Moreover, the experience of many transplant centers appears to

Table 1. Rates of acceptance amongst evaluated patients according to specific clinical features*

| Feature at evaluation | Patients with feature | | Acceptance rate (%) | Relative rate of acceptance** | Null *p* value |
	n*	%			
Gender					
Female	73	25.7	56.2	0.93	0.547
Male	213	74.3	60.2	–	
Age					
<40	53	19.4	67.9	–	0.050
40–59	189	69.2	60.8	0.89	
≥60	31	11.4	45.2	0.66	
Sickness status					
Poor	222	78.2	62.2	1.29	0.051
Good	62	21.8	48.4	–	
Cardiac condition					
Poor	134	66.0	73.9	1.27	0.021
Good	69	34.0	58.0	–	
Psychosocial problems	51	18.0	33.3	0.51	0.000
History of:					
Diabetes	36	12.7	47.2	0.78	0.120
Peripheral Vascular Disease	32	11.3	37.5	0.61	0.008
Serious Infectious Disease	52	18.3	75.0	1.35	0.010
Other clinical contraindication[a]	181	63.7	65.7	1.58	0.003
Previous cardiovascular surgery	23	8.1	47.8	0.79	0.250
CMV Antibody Presence	59	39.3	83.1	0.93	0.296
PRA					
<30	233	95.5	62.2	–	0.054
≥30	11	4.5	90.9	1.46	
Anergy to skin-hypersensitivity tests	68	25.5	75.0	1.45	0.001

*All features excluded from this table (smoking history, blood group, peripheral vascular resistance (pvr), auto-antibody presence, creatinine and cholesterol levels) showed non-significant differences in acceptance rates onto the heart transplant list.
**Relative rate of acceptance = Acceptance rate in patients with clinical feature ÷ Acceptance rate in patients without clinical feature or with reference clinical feature
where reference features are: male, <40, good sickness status, good heart condition, no history of diabetes, pvd, previous surgery, or serious infectious disease, no other clinical contraindication, no psychosocial contraindication, negative CMV antibody presence, PRA under 30, and non-anergic on skin hypersensitivity tests.
[a]Hypertension, hyperlipidemia, renal disease, pneumonia, hepatitis, tuberculosis.

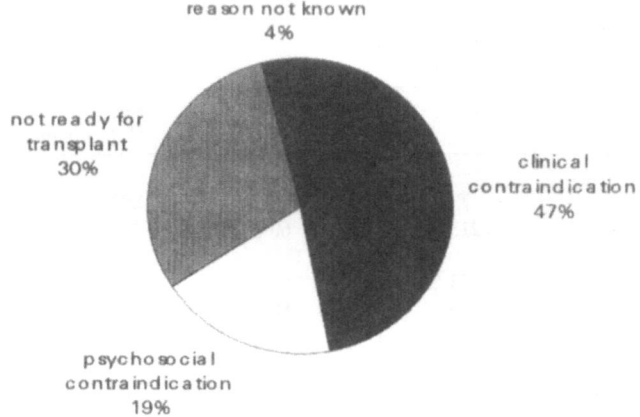

Fig. 2. Reasons for refusal onto the heart transplant waiting list.

Clinical contraindications: multisystem disease, Peripheral Vascular Disease, pathologies of high medical risk, other organ failure, age over 65, immunological contraindication, high pulmonary vascular resistance (pvr).

Psychosocial contraindications: social problems noted by assessing social worker, psychiatric problems noted by assessing psychiatrist, non-compliance with medical treatment feared by the transplant selection committee, patient refused transplant, continued substance abuse.

Not ready cases: not sick enough to warrant transplant, patient referred for other surgery, other reasons for not being ready for transplant.

challenge the established contraindications to cardiac transplantation [3, 5–14]. The answer to the question "who is a suitable candidate?" thus demands very close scrutiny of each patient's case and the consideration of all potential complications.

In the pioneering days of cardiac transplantation, physicians were guided by the motto "best chances for best patients" [4], the "best" patient being the person who needed a heart most urgently and yet presented the best odds of surviving the transplant surgery. Today, however, the transplant procedure has been elevated by successful clinical results to the ranks of a highly-acceptable treatment of end-stage heart disease. Its widespread use remains restricted by the limited availability of the needed resource, the donor heart, at a time when waiting lists are growing and many patients are dying without receiving a transplant. This situation calls for careful selection of patients to whom the procedure is offered, reflecting medical and ethical principles. Current selection criteria are meant to assess patients relative to their prognosis without transplantation (a poor prognosis being 6–12 months life expectancy [4]) versus their potential survival post-transplant. Many of the so-called contraindications to transplantation are thus diseases which are likely to be aggravated by immunosuppressive therapy or natural history

Table 2. Analysis of maximum likelihood estimates obtained in the Stepwise logistic regression analysis

	B Estimate	Standard error	Null p	Odds ratio
Intercept	+1.28	0.35	0.0002	–
Absence of psychosocial problems	+1.38	0.48	0.0040	3.6
Poor sickness status	+1.03	0.46	0.0257	4.0
Poor cardiac condition	+1.40	0.45	0.0020	2.8
Absence of diabetes	+1.55	0.57	0.0069	4.0
No previous cardiovascular surgery	+2.35	0.65	0.0003	4.8
CMV antibody absence[a]	+1.37	0.59	0.0207	4.0

MODEL: Acceptance onto the heart transplant waiting list = F_x [all clinical features].
Independent variables entered into the model: age, gender, heart condition, general sickness status, psychosocial contraindication, history of peripheral vascular disease, of diabetes, of serious infectious disease, other clinical contraindication, history of emboli, hypersensitivity to skin reactions (anergy), previous cardiovascular surgery, smoker, presence of cytomegalovirus (CMV) antibody, presence of auto-antibodies, pulmonary vascular resistance, blood type, cholesterol level, creatinine level.
[a]In order to correct for missing information, a presence/absence dummy variable was added for each clinical variable for which several patients had missing information. These dummy variables for CMV antibody presence and blood type were not removed from the regression model, but their regression coefficients are not shown above.

(malignancies, renal dysfunction, diabetes, concurrent infections) or which pose significant risks of post-transplant morbidity.

There have been numerous challenges to the Stanford list of contraindications. Patients with cardiac sarcoidosis [6, 7], Chagas' Disease cardiomyopathy [8], malignancies [9, 10], progressive muscular dystrophy, active infection at time of transplant [11] and both type 1 and type 2 diabetes mellitus [12] have been shown to survive cardiac transplantation at rates comparable to those attained by patients without these diseases. An age limit of 55 or 60 has also been challenged [13, 14], as has been the claim that men survive transplantation better than women. The possibility exists that the immunosuppressive therapy given by "protocol" post-transplant is too heavy for women and may thus induce lesser host resistance and lesser chances for survival [15, 16]. The conclusions derived from clinical experience with these patients, although tentative, do challenge the criteria used currently.

At the RVH, 59% of all referred patients were accepted onto the waiting list, 71% of these eventually received transplants during the study period. These figures are comparable to those obtained by Evans et al. [17] in their 1986 study of 1,102 referrals for cardiac transplantation in 5 American hospitals (34.6% overall acceptance, of whom 71.9% received transplants).

The univariate analysis results suggest the preferential selection of patients with a poor cardiac condition reflecting the priority given to patients with the sickest hearts. PVD was considered a relative contraindication by the selection committee and is not statistically significant in the regression model. The higher probability of acceptance onto the waiting list in patients with a history of infectious disease and anergy on skin testing is likely explained by the high correlation found between anergy, presence of infectious disease and a worse sickness status. Neither anergy nor infection remained in the regression model.

The regression model shown in Table 2 confirms that priority is given to patients partly according to medical urgency and perceived need. Patients with an overall health status indicative of CCU/ICU hospitalisation or of a bed-ridden condition are more likely to be accepted onto the active waiting list than out-patients or patients with limited physical disability. Similarly, patients with the sickest hearts are given higher priority to get onto the waiting list. These results are supported by the significantly shorter waiting times for patients in the highest compared to the lowest NYHA classes.

The priority given to patients in perceived critical status needs to be addressed in the current era of extreme donor shortage. One study using actuarial survival analysis, has shown that the expected improvement in survival after transplantation for patients waiting at least 6 months on the list (the average waiting time for out-patients in their center) is only in the order of 5% [18]. Whereas the improvement in survival post-transplant can be significant for critically ill patients, patients in "better" condition may forfeit any gain in life expectancy or quality of life by obtaining a late transplant. Their condition while on the waiting list may worsen and secondary complications of heart failure that may not necessarily be reversible post-transplant may set in. Thus, there may be a case to be made for more frequent updating of priorities within a given waiting list and a more precise quantification of the expected benefit to be derived from transplantation. Prolonged waiting times also evoke the emotionally charged issue of waiting list deaths, which are more obvious and tension-provoking in the hospitalised patient. This situation poses significant ethical and program control questions, and is of growing concern in the present state of donor organ shortages [19].

The role of psychosocial assessment in the selection of patients is an important finding of our analysis. As indicated in Figure 2, 19% of all evaluated patients were refused acceptance onto the waiting list primarily on psychosocial grounds. The high importance granted by our center to psychosocial 'soundness' conforms to the Stanford list of contraindications. A thorough assessment by a psychologist, psychiatrist and/or social worker is an inherent part of most transplantation candidate selection protocols. Although the subjectivity of these assessments could be criticized, it is the belief of the team that psychosocial stability is a primary determinant of post-transplant compliance and survival. Nevertheless, precise research should be done in this area to determine whether the importance attributed to patients' psychosocial stability is merely presumptive or whether significant differences in transplant outcomes are actually observed in patients based on particular psychosocial or psychiatric profiles. A survey conducted in 204 active transplant programs [20] found that the proportion of patients rejected for transplantation on psychosocial grounds varied from 0% to 37%, with an average of 5.6% in the United States and 2.5% in non-U.S. programs. The survey also reveals important lack of consensus among programs pertaining to the importance of behavioural (cigarette smoking, recent alcohol and drug abuse, criminality) and psychological factors (affective and personality disorders) and other factors such as a history of noncompliance. The survey supports the need for further research on the validity and appropriateness of psychosocial selection criteria.

The presence of CMV antibody status in the regression model may be due to the high correlation between previous cardiac surgery and positive CMV antibody, induced by higher exposure to transfusions and hospital-associated transmission. The importance granted to lack of previous cardiac surgery may be a consequence of a population of candidates seen to have fewer secondary complications, or other exclusion factors. With respect to diabetes mellitus, several studies discussed above have established that this condition is not necessarily a strict contraindication to cardiac transplantation.

Summary

We studied the criteria used in the initial selection of candidates to be placed onto the cardiac transplant waiting list at our center. A regression model of acceptance on to the list showed that it related mainly to the perceived urgency of the medical condition. Another significant factor was the presence of "psychosocial" problems. We conclude that the experience of the transplant selection process reflects a general flexibility and interdependence of selection criteria and emphasizes the need to re-examine the validity and reliability of selection protocols. The difficulty of selecting the "best candidates" for cardiac transplantation, in terms of present medical urgency and best expected survival, is complicated by the undoing of former beliefs about outcomes and the individual and committee subjectivity in evaluating individual cases. The problem of prolonged waiting time due to the increased shortage of donor hearts forces selecting personnel to contemplate candidates in view of both predictors of pre-transplant survival and post-transplant survival. The issue of patients dying while on the waiting list poses serious process dilemmas for those involved in selection decisions. This argues for the need to reconsider not only the rules of selection and priorities, but also the possibilities of changing individual priorities within a given waiting list over time. Development of the most sensible and transparent system of patient selection and priority criteria, given an extreme donor organ shortage, remains a significant challenge for the future of cardiac transplantation.

References

1. Copeland JG, Emory RW, Levinson MM, et al. Selection of patients for cardiac transplantation. Circulation 1987; 75: 2–9.
2. Clark DA, Stinson EB, Griepp RB, et al. Cardiac transplantation in man, vi. Prognosis of patients selected for cardiac transplantation. Ann Intern Med 1971; 75: 15–21.
3. Anthuber M, Kemkes BM, Schuetz Z, et al. Heart transplantation in patients with "so-called" contraindications. Transplant Proc 1990; 22: 1451–3.
4. Vagelos R, Fowler MB. Selection of patients for cardiac transplantation. Cardio Clin 1990; 8: 23–38.
5. McCarthy PM, Starnes VA, Shumway NE. Heart and heart-lung transplantation: the Stanford experience. In: Terasaki P, editor. Clinical transplants. Los Angeles, CA: UCLA Tissue Typing Laboratory, 1989: 63–71.
6. Billingham ME. Results of cardiac transplantation in active myocarditis. J Heart Transplant 1989; 8: 99.
7. Hardesty RL, et al. Mortally ill patients and excellent survival following cardiac transplantation. Ann Thorac Surg 1986; 41: 126–9.
8. Stolf NAG, Higushi L, Bocchi E, et al. Heart transplantation in patients with Chagas' Disease cardiomyopathy. J Heart Transplant 1987; 6: 307–11.
9. Armitage JM, Griffity BP, Hardesty RL. Cardiac transplantation in patients with malignancy. Heart Transplant 1989; 8: 89.
10. Edwards BS, Hunt SA, et al. Cardiac transplantation in patients with preexisting neoplatic diseases. Am J Cardiology 1990; 65: 501–4.
11. Anguita M, Arizon JM, et al. Influence on survival after heart transplantion of contraindications seen in transplant recipients. J Heart Lung Transplant 1992; 11: 708–15.
12. Rhenman MJ, et al. Diabetes and heart transplantation. J Heart Transplant 1988; 7: 356–8.
13. Amrein C, Vulser C, et al. Is heart transplantation a valid therapy in elderly patients? Transplant Proc. 1990; 22: 1454–6.
14. Olivari MT, Antolick A, et al. Heart transplantation in elderly patients. J Heart Transplant 1988; 7: 258–64.
15. Crandall BG, et al. Increased cardiac allograft rejection in female heart transplant recipients. J Heart Transplant 1988; 7: 419–23.
16. Esmore D, et al. Heart transplantation in females. J Heart Lung Transplant 1991; 10: 335–41.
17. Evans RW, Maier AM. Outcome of patients referred for cardiac transplantation. JACC 1986; 8: 1312–7.
18. Stevenson LW, Hamilton M, Tillisch IH, et al. Decreasing survival benefit from cardiac transplantation for outpatients as the waiting list lengthens. JACC 1991; 18: 919–25.
19. McManus RP, O'Hair DP, et al. Patients who die awaiting heart transplantation. J Heart Lung Transplant 1993; 12: 160–72.
20. Olbrisch ME, Levenson JL. Psychosocial evaluation of heart transplant candidates: an international survey of process, criteria, and outcomes. J Heart Lung Transplant 1991; 10: 948–55.

32. Should we review the indications for transplants because of the shortage of organs?

P. DETEIX

Introduction

Does the shortage of organs for transplants mean that we should review the indications for transplants? In other words, is it necessary to limit access to organ transplants so that all or nearly all of registered recipients can have their transplants? Of course this is not the most crucial question regarding organ transplantation. Of most importance is: how can we make our message clear to the general public to obtain more transplants?

Meanwhile, today the situation is still one of shortage. Considering the current trends in transplant indications and the extended, yet foreseen, time scale for developing efficient prevention of organ deterioration and novel therapeutic possibilities such as xenografts, this shortage is likely to continue into the future. Indeed, many experts think that demand will always be higher than supply for organ transplants. Therefore should registration on waiting lists be further restricted?

This paper will concentrate on the problem regarding kidney transplants but will also give some thought to other organs such as the heart and the liver. There is a big difference between the kidneys and the other organs: for heart and liver we obviously need organs but, further, we need organs at the right moment. We will first discuss the policy of limiting organ transplant waiting lists. Then we will summarise the results from a survey of French doctors working in the field of organ transplants. Finally, we will examine the arguments for and against limiting registration. The purpose of this paper is to suggest several relevant topics for further thought by those involved with organ transplants.

Why restrict registration?

Are there cases where medical care in Western Europe and North America is not freely available? In certain countries comprehensive medical care may be out of reach of patients with low income. In all countries delay in seeking

J.L. Touraine et al. (eds.), *Organ Shortage*: *The Solutions*, 253–260.
© 1995 *Kluwer Academic Publishers*.

medical care (sometimes with very serious consequences) can result from health education which is inadequate or not properly understood by the general public. Limited availability of medical care may not necessarily be associated with a patient's lack of resources but can stem from the techniques involved in medicine production. For example, beta interferon, proposed in the United States for treating multiple sclerosis, is not yet available in sufficient quantities. It has been suggested that the first patients to receive this treatment should be selected by drawing lots.

A general lack of resources means that the best treatment available is withheld from certain patients: during a recent trial called GUSTO, recombinant plasminogen activator (rTPA) was shown to be more effective than streptase in the treatment of coronary thrombosis fibrinolysis, but since rTPA is more expensive than streptase (FF 3630 compared to 660), rTPA is only given to the young while the elderly receive streptase. There have been recent cases where patients with chronic renal insufficiency who are aged, diabetic, or are carrying the hepatitis virus or suffering from a general syndrome with poor prognosis have been refused for dialysis [1]. Another example of limiting medical care is related to patient behaviour. Certain doctors suggest that patients with chronic ischemia who have not stopped smoking should not undergo peripheral bypass surgery. The reason supporting this argument is the lower rate of success of such operations with smokers [2]. Besides the above-mentioned restrictions of an economical, technical and socio-economical nature, there is also a shortage of material resources which are not primarily explained by a lack of financial means. Such is the situation which exists for organ transplants, where the number of potential recipients exceeds the number of donors, thus leading to considerable periods of delay, often fatal, for those on the waiting list.

Theoretically two options are possible regarding this shortage. The first is to accept all patients who need and want to receive a transplant on the waiting lists. The second option is to limit the waiting list so that most of those on it can receive transplants within a reasonable delay. This would also avoid too large a discrepancy between the number of patients on the waiting lists and the number of transplants performed. Patients never likely to receive transplants would not be placed on the waiting list, while those on it would be more often and more quickly treated. If this list is long in relation to the number of transplants performed in a particular category selection from the list (and not before registration) is problematic. Certain recipients are passed over for several years because they are either at low risk, and priority cases take precedence, or at high risk but never chosen because of the particular selection criteria used.

Generally the number of organs required for treating renal disease can be reduced by intervening at various stages in disease development. Prevention and treatment in renal disease should result in decreasing the frequency of chronic renal insufficiency. The prevention of fibrosis and alterations from nephron reduction should delay terminal renal insufficiency. Minimizing cases of first graft rejection should also decrease the number of patients needing transplants. Restricting numbers of patients on the waiting list is of course another method of reducing the quantity of organs required. Finally, the last limitation is immutable and only leaves the choice of the criteria free. This relates to the suitability between those organs available and the patients to receive transplants.

We will now discuss the criteria for registration which could be adopted if the waiting list is to be limited, for example, concerning kidney transplants. These criteria, most of which are open to discussion because they are not unconditional, are of a medical or statutory nature or decided by society. Medical criteria include the cardiovascular status, discipline as regards treatment, intellectual ability to understand treatment, evolving hepatic viral infections and of course evolving bacterial infections and cancers. Statutory criteria concern the financial status of non-residents in France (the Ministry has recently set a price for a kidney transplant performed in France, irrespective of place or methods) and nationality since a non-resident must be given official authorisation to be placed on the list. Social criteria consider the family situation, professional status and age.

Another obstacle to the inscription of a patient with renal insufficiency on the waiting list is the prolonged hemodialysis treatment given to such patients in certain places. A choice between two policies is already becoming apparent in relation to medical criteria: should one favour the optimal use of a transplant or the use of this transplant at an individual level for a given patient, whatever the risks of failure? These are often the same criteria which can be suggested for limiting inscriptions and for managing the distribution of organs to waiting patients. Limiting registrations does not affect renal insufficiency patients, who do have an alternative to transplantation, in the same way as potential heart and liver recipients do not have any other possible treatment available.

Survey of the opinions of transplant physicians

A questionnaire was sent to all French organ transplant teams to obtain the opinion of these doctors about waiting list registration. Seventy-six individual replies were received from 45 teams, of which 31 perform kidney transplants (kidney alone and multiorgans); 8, heart transplants; 5, liver transplants; and 1, lung transplants.

The first question asked doctors whether a group of "recipients at risk" existed, for which survival of both the patient and graft are statistically much lower. Of the 76 replies, 71 were positive; the large majority of practitioners believed that there are different groups at risk. The second question related to the shortage of transplants. Forty-five out of 74 doctors thought that there is a general shortage, 26 that the shortage only concerns certain organs (mainly kidneys and hearts), and 3 thought there is no shortage. The third question was "Do you think that limiting inscription on the list is an accept-able solution to managing this shortage?" Forty-nine replied that they did not consider this an acceptable solution and 26 acknowledged that this was a possibility. Sixty-six percent of doctors involved with kidney transplants are opposed to this solution as are 62% of liver and heart transplant doctors. The fourth question was directed at the current methods for selecting a recipient in France. Twenty-nine considered these satisfactory, 37 as unsatis-factory, and 10 did not have any opinion on the subject. The fifth question concerned the unconditional contraindications of a medical nature for regis-tering a patient apart from cancer (except for liver transplants) and evolving infections. Out of 72 replies, 51 suggested other unconditional contraindica-tions (cardiovascular status, previous non-observance of treatment during a first graft . . .), and 21 did not suggest any unconditional contraindications. Another question asked about the delays in kidney transplants. The replies indicated delays of 16 months for non-immunised recipients and 52 months for immunised recipients. Recipients waiting the longest had been registered, on average, for 96 months; for non-immunised recipients, the delay after registration on the list was 46 months. For heart recipients the mean delay for an organ transplant is 6 months.

Should inscriptions on the list be limited and, if yes, according to which criteria?

This question does not arise in the case of contraindications of an uncon-ditional medical nature which are acknowledged by the entire medical com-munity. It is a question which has to be faced for *conditional* contraindica-tions, which can be deliberately used as criteria for limiting the waiting list for an organ. The trend in the ratio of people with transplants to those patients awaiting an organ can provide initial insight into the need to limit lists. For kidneys, the number of transplants was increasing in France up to 1991, but is now stable and, since 1992, has lowered by about 10%. However, the number of waiting recipients has increased by around 14% between 1988 and 1993 (although there has been a decrease in potential recipients between 1991 and 1993). For kidneys, the number of patients awaiting an organ is much higher than the number of transplants performed each year; this is not the case for other organs. Waiting times on lists increase yearly, as shown in the United States [3] and this also reflects the shortage of kidneys. For organs such as the heart and liver, the death rate of patients waiting on the list is a good indicator of the shortage of organs.

All the teams practising liver or heart transplants stated in our survey that they had lost patients through a lack of donors. In 1993, in France, 320 patients died while waiting for an organ. For these organs, priority is in terms of emergency or super emergency. Theoretically, it is possible that several patients are classified as emergencies. When a donor becomes available, should the organ in question be transplanted where it has the greatest chance of success or according to which criteria? Should all potential recipients be registered? McManus et al., using the UNOS (United Network for Organ Sharing) data file have shown that the deaths of patients on the heart transplant waiting list have increased between 1988 and 1990 [4]. Stevenson et al. of UCLA call attention to the large number of patients waiting for a heart registered each month in 1994 on the waiting list, a number higher then the number of transplants performed [5]. He also adds that the patients receiving transplants will always be selected among hospitalised patients listed as emergencies.

Which criteria to adopt?

The decision to register a patient is a medical decision made when the doctor deems this to be the best treatment possible for a patient. Every medical decision includes considerations of an individual and economic nature and is ideally made in view of optimising the use of a graft. This decision should be carefully analysed so that future choices can be rationalized and the rules dictating distribution further developed. As already mentioned, collective interests aiming to make best use of the transplant with the greatest chances of success are in opposition to individual interests – those of a candidate at high risk, prepared to confront the danger involved, of which he is totally aware.

The restriction is evident when the potential recipient has a major risk, such as an evolving infection, neoplasm (except for liver transplants), very advanced cardiopathy and, in the case of heart transplants: raised pulmonary vascular resistance, recent pulmonary infarction, extensive cerebrovascular or peripheral disease, active peptic ulceration, psychosocial unsuitability [6].

However, most often, the criteria dictating non-registration are assessed differently from one team to another. For example, the age of patients. Tesi et al. have shown, as have other authors, that equally satisfactory results are obtained with kidney transplants after 60 years of age [7]. These results are even better if patients dying with a functional graft are not included in graft survival statistics (censored graft survival). However, mortality is higher and, as pointed out by Chang [8], 65% of deaths after age 60 are with a functional graft compared to 37% before age 60. In other words, deaths with a functional graft are three times more common (9.8%) after 60 years of age than before (2.8%). This author refers to the double tragedy when a patient dies with a functional graft [8]. Once again, an individual policy involving a possible choice of risk is in opposition to a collective policy which favours making the best use of a graft by proposing it to the patient with the best chances of survival. In other terms, is it ethical to use a graft with an immunological survival reckoned in decades in an elderly patient with a statistical probability of another 6 years of life?

Stevenson et al. suggest lowering the age limit for heart transplants to 55 years, which would reduce registrations by 30% each month and decrease the number of patients waiting in the United States to 1,490 instead of more than 3,700. He also raises the possibility of only registering those patients with an 80% risk of sudden death or deterioration in the coming year (52% currently) which would further decrease the list by 30% and allow a distribution of available hearts for 50% of non-hospitalised patients not classified as emergencies. Such patients would then have an 11% chance every month of receiving a transplant instead of 0% or practically 0% as is the present case [5].

Powelson et al. have analysed the impact, under conditions of shortage, of liver retransplants on the survival of all the patients waiting for liver transplants and the survival of patients on the waiting list [9]. The survival of all patients on the waiting list is reduced as soon as retransplants are performed and the survival of patients receiving transplants for the first time decreases as the rate of retransplants reaches 35%. This author suggests reducing the number of retransplants particularly when their rate of success is low, i.e. they are performed between D4 and D30 (24% survival).

Another remedy to uncontrolled growth of the kidney transplant list is restricting the registration of non-residents on the list. This question, much discussed in France today, has been thoroughly investigated by P. Michielsen [10] in Belgium, who gives the following figures: on the Belgian lists 42.5% were non-residents, and 37.6% on Austrian lists for kidneys. This percentage was 3.2% in Holland and 1.5% in Germany, countries also belonging to Eurotransplant but which do not accept non-resident recipients. This attitude differs radically from one country to another and can vary just as much from one centre to another within the same country. Such heterogeneity is not without problem as regards a national waiting list. The main problem in registering non-residents is the absence of grafts contributed from the non-resident's country. Several French transplant centre managers would like greater openness regarding this subject and see in the refused inscription of non-residents a way of reducing the uncontrolled growth of the list. It is currently difficult to know precisely the number of patients registered on the lists who are non-resident in our country. This data could not be provided by France Transplant. Certain practitioners are in favour of setting a quota which should not be exceeded – a quota for each transplant centre and not, of course, an overall quota for the national list.

Vulnerability of the policy of limitation

Renal insufficiency patients registered on the list are increasingly in a poor state of health, with aorto-iliac vascular prostheses, generalised coronary artery disease. It is important to know if there is a reduced chance of graft and, especially, the rate of survival for these groups before accepting these pathological states as dictating non-inscription.

Other non-inscription criteria can be suggested such as hyper-immunisation or a general disease. It seems difficult to exclude such patients from graft waiting lists. The argument is always that of the best possible use of a kidney which should be transplanted into a receiver least likely to lose it. Also, it does not seem particularly ethical to refuse registration for patients who do not have either professional or family responsibilities.

There is already considerable divergence of medical opinion concerning medical contraindications to registration. This is clearly shown by the data of Ramos et al. [11] in relation to cardiovascular and liver pathology in kidney transplants. The percentages with which the various criteria are accepted as criteria dictating refusal varies between 12 and 74% according to the different pathologies, i.e. no one criterion obtains more than three quarters of the votes in favour.

The theoretical problems of restricting waiting lists are multiple: is it possible to exclude a candidate who is aware of the statistical data which puts him or her at higher risk and is yet prepared to undergo surgery? Should such decisions be based on criteria difficult to define and which are modified as technological progress is achieved? What should one think about a national waiting list with centres which limit the number of recipients and others which continue to register all or nearly all of their candidates?

Another side effect of restricting the waiting list is the risk of refusing a heart or liver because there is no patient with the correct weight and size.

Conclusion

Throughout this paper the disagreement between the requirements of individual treatment and the necessity to make the best use of a limited wealth, expressed as the number of grafts available, has been made clear. Pichlmayr et al. [12] compares "the highest potential effect in the length and quality of graft function" to "the highest individual need of the human being". Of course no definite reply is given as to the choice between these two attitudes. This is more of a political than medical decision.

If the list is not limited, the question is only referred back to a prior stage, which is the distribution of organs, which can be governed by the very same criteria under review. Who should distribute the organs? According to which distribution rules? How much leeway is left to transplant centre doctors and surgeons? Wujciak and Opelz have set a computerised distribution centre for available kidneys based on HLA compatibility, waiting time, the importance of the transplant centre and the centre's import/export ratio [13]. Sanfilippo describes 6 factors to be taken into account for optimising kidney distribution: immunological interdictions (ABO and HLA), regulation interdictions, prognosis (function and rehabilitation), the difficulty posed by a recipient for finding a kidney, the costs, and the impact on the organ pool [14]. All of these questions are highly topical and one of the first tasks of the new "Etablissement Français des Greffes" in France will be to find an answer offering the maximum degree of consensus. It may be hoped, although this wish probably belongs to the realms of Utopia, that, in the future, a much greater availability of organs and more efficient medical treatment preventing kidney deterioration during the course of disease would make such questions redundant. Currently, the best solution could be to register all recipients, with the exception of those for which the medical risk is deemed too high, and to clearly define the criteria governing organ allocation. These criteria must follow rules which are known to everyone, including the patient, who must also be aware of the mathematical impossibility of satisfying everyone. My conclusion is no limitation of the waiting list but full transparency in the allocation.

References

1. Parsons V, Bewick M, Snowden S, Keogh A, Doherty A. The ethical problems of triage for renal failure in the United Kingdom. In: Land W, Dossetor JB, editors. Organ replacement therapy: ethics, justice, commerce. Berlin: Springer-Verlag, 1991: 373–6.
2. Powell JT, Greenhalgh RM. Arterial bypass surgery and smokers. BMJ 1994; 308: 607–8.
3. Ellison MD, Breen TJ, Guo TG, Cunningham PRG, Daily OP. Blacks and whites on the UNOS renal waiting list: waiting times and patients demographics compared. Transplant Proc 1993; 25: 2462–6.
4. McManus RP, O'Hair DP, Beitzinger JM, Schweiger J, Siegel R, Breen TJ, Olinger GN. Patients who die awaiting heart transplantation. J Heart Lung Transplant 1993; 12: 159–71.
5. Stevenson LW, Warner SL, Steimle AE, Fonarow GC, Hamilton MA, Moriguchi JD, Kobashigawa JA, Tillisch JH, Drinkwater DC, Lacks H. The impending crisis awaiting cardiac transplantation: modeling a solution based on selection. Circulation 1994; 89: 450–7.
6. Mullins PA, Schofield PM, Scott JP, Solis E, J Dunning, Avarot DJ, Large SR, Wallwork J. Cardiac retransplantation: is it an ethical use of scarce resource? In: Land W, Dossetor JB, editors. Organ replacement therapy: ethics, justice, commerce. Berlin: Springer-Verlag, 1991: 445–9.
7. Tesi RJ, Elkhammas EA, Davies EA, Henry ML, Ferguson RM. Renal transplantation in older people. Lancet 1994; 343: 461–4.
8. Chang RWS. Renal transplantation in older patients. Lancet 1994; 343: 801.
9. Powelson JA, Cosimi AB, Lewis WD, Rohrer RJ, Freeman RB, Vacanti JP, Jonas M, Lorber MI, Marks WH, Bradley J, Jenkins RL. Hepatic retransplantation in New England – a regional experience and survival model. Transplantation 1993; 55: 802–6.
10. Michielsen P. Unlimited admission of patients to the waiting list for transplantation. In: Land W, Dossetor JB, editors. Organ replacement therapy: ethics, justice, commerce. Berlin: Springer-Verlag, 1991: 364–7.
11. Ramos EL, Kasiske BL, Alexander SR, Danovitch GM, Harmon WE, Kahana L, Kiresuk TJ, Neylan JF. The evaluation of candidates for renal transplantation. Transplantation 1994; 57: 490–7.
12. Pichlmayr R, Kohlhaw K, Frei U. Organ transplantation: what are the limits? Transplant Proc 1992; 24: 2404–6.
13. Wujciak T, Opelz G. A proposal for improved cadaver kidney allocation. Transplantation 1993; 56: 1513–7.
14. Sanfilippo F. Organ allocation: current problems and future issues. Transplant Proc 1993; 25: 2467.

33. Can we select candidates for combined kidney and heart or liver transplantation?

J.L. GARNIER, A.C. MARRAST, C. POUTEIL-NOBLE,
X. MARTIN, G. DUREAU, G. CHAMPSAUR, J. NINET,
P. BOISSONNAT, J.P. GARE, P. CHOSSEGROS,
J.M. DUBERNARD & J.L. TOURAINE

A better understanding of diseases such as primary hyperoxaluria and multiorgan failure have led to the performance of combined organ transplantation. We present here the indications and results of combined kidney and heart or liver, and discuss whether we can select the candidates for combined organ transplantation.

Combined kidney-heart transplantation

As presented in Tables 1 and 2, ischemic heart failure and cardiomyopathy in chronic renal failure (hemodialysis or kidney transplant patients), represent the more frequent causes of heart failure: heart disease is the main cause of death in hemodialysed patients; hypertension and diabetes are both causes of renal and heart failure. Arteriolar nephrosclerosis due to hypertension and ciclosporine nephrotoxicity is the main cause of renal failure in heart transplant patients. The mean age of these patients is higher than other patients on kidney transplant lists; vascular diseases are progressing slowly and represent a risk factor increasing with age.

Rejection episodes do not occur more frequently than in isolated organ transplantation and can be dissociated (Table 3). Main causes of death are related to infections, hemorrhage, or heart graft failure (Table 4).

Combined kidney-liver transplantation

Combined kidney-liver transplantation is indicated in primary hyperoxaluria (PH) [1–3], HBV or HCV-induced cirrhosis in patients with chronic renal failure, most of them having recieved a kidney graft. Congenital diseases,

J.L. Touraine et al. (eds.), *Organ Shortage: The Solutions*, 261–265.
© 1995 *Kluwer Academic Publishers*.

Table 1. Etiology of heart failure

Cases	Dilated cardiomyopathy	Ischemic heart disease	Graft rejection
Literature 19 [1]	47%	47%	
Creteil 7 [2]	23%	57%	14%
Lyon 16	62%	31%	6%

Table 2. Etiology of renal failure

Cases	Chronic nephropathy	Ciclosporine toxicity	Graft rejection
Literature 19	63%	10%	5%
Creteil 7	85%	15%	
Lyon 16	50%	12%	12%

Table 3. Results

Cases	Rejection: kidney	Rejection: heart	Survival time of graft
Literature 13			
19	5	7	(3 months–5 years)
Creteil 5			
7	2	3	(17–64 months)
Lyon 8			
16	2	1	(1 month–5 years)

such as hepatic fibrosis with associated renal lesions, is another indication of combined kidney-liver transplantation [1].

Survival of isolated kidney transplants in PH is about 20% at 2 years [4]. Since the disease is due to hepatic enzyme amino-glyoxylate amino-transferase defect, combined kidney-liver transplantation is proposed to those patients; results of a European collaborative study show an 80% rate of patient survival at 2 years, and 75% graft survival [5]. However, the phenotypic expression is not related to enzyme deficiency [6] and other factors (genetic or renal), not yet known, may play a role in the progression of the disease. Only patients with familial form of PH, and patients with a previously rapid recurrence of oxalosis on kidney graft should be selected at present for combined kidney-liver transplantation.

Cirrhosis due to HBV or HCV infection is a frequent cause of mortality in patients with kidney graft. HBV infection prevalence was as high as 45% in hemodialysed patients, and is now around 15% after the development of

Table 4. Causes of death

Number: Cases	Time of graft	Infections	Hemorrhage	Heart non-function
Literature	4			
19	(15 days–6 months)	4		
Creteil	2			
7	(15 days)	2		
Lyon	8			
16	(1 day–4 months)	2	4[a]	2

[a]Cerebral hemorrhage, gastro-intestinal, intra-abdominal bleeding, kidney graft hematoma.

a vaccination [7]. Before transplantation, in 49% of patients HBV-DNA is present in serum; this frequency rises to 80% with immunosuppressive therapy [8]. HCV infection is present in 10–25% of patients undergoing renal transplantation [7]; replication of the virus, detected by PCR, is present in almost all patients [9]. Chronic active hepatitis is present in 43% of patients with HBV infection, and cirrhosis develops in 73% of these cases [8].

Recurrence of HVB or HCV infection on liver graft is a main complication. HVB recurrence is linked to the presence of HBV-DNA at the time of transplantation; it can be controlled by long-term therapy with anti-HBs immune globulins [10]. HCV recurrence on liver graft occurs in 50% of patients and can be controlled by Ribavirin and Interferon alpha [11]. In kidney transplant patients, Interferon therapy leads to rejection, and trials with anti-viral agents are currently performed; Ganciclovir is successful in clearing HBV-DNA during the treatment, but unfortunately, relapse occurs after the end of the treatment [12], and we will use oral Famciclovir for new protocols. Ribavirin therapy is also under study in our patients with HCV infection [9].

Unfortunately, data concerning recurrence of viral infection on liver graft in combined kidney-liver transplantation is scarce; Margreiter's group reports on 3 recurrences of HVB-infection in 3 patients [13]; in our experience, 2 patients with HBV infection recurred at 3 and 12 months after transplantation. It is possible that patients who received long-term immunosuppressive therapy for a previous kidney graft are more likely to have a large reservoir of infected cells and, as a consequence, undergo recurrence of infection on liver grafts.

Selection of patients

For a first combined kidney-heart transplantation, candidates can be selected according to their age, and the importance of atherosclerosis; for a first combined kidney-liver transplantation, the best candidates seem to be the patients with non-viral induced liver defect.

For a combined kidney-liver transplantation for viral-induced cirrhosis, replication of the virus needs to be treated by anti-viral agents before the graft; return to dialysis may help clearing HVB or HCV infection.

Patient candidates for a second graft have already been submitted to immunosuppressive treatment. Cirrhosis and its complications usually take more than 10 years to develop in kidney transplant patients [14, 15]; we must carefully check for infections, vascular diseases or cancer in these patients.

Chronic renal failure is due to chronic rejection in transplanted patients or to chronic nephropathy (some patients with heart or liver transplant, either due to arteriolar sclerosis, diabetes associated with drug nephrotoxicity, other related complications such as IgA, membranous or proliferative glomerulonephritis in patients with HBV, HCV infection and cirrhosis, or unrelated complications), and may develop in patients with heart failure and low cardiac output or in patients with cirrhosis and hepatorenal syndrome. We need to decide whether single organ transplantation can be safely performed without the risk of acute tubular necrosis or degradation of renal function due to nephrotoxicity of drugs.

The precise diagnosis of nephropathy is necessary. Renal biopsy can be performed; if signs of arteriolar sclerosis, diabetes or severe interstitial lesions are present, combined transplantation is probably preferred. Assessment of renal function needs to be performed; a glomerular filtration rate below 50 ml mn^{-1} should also help in deciding for combined transplantation.

We believe that there may be an immunological advantage in having the same donor for both organs.

Immunosuppressive therapy

Induction therapy rests on azathioprine, steroids and anti-lymphocyte globulins for 8–10 days; ciclosporine is introduced as soon as renal function starts and dosage is adapted to standard trough level. The frequency of rejection does not seem to be more significant than for single organ transplantation and patients do not need to be overimmunosuppressed. Starlz described a state of microchimerism that can be responsible for tolerance induced by the liver graft [16].

Conclusions

Improvement of multi-organ procurement and intensive care management have permitted combined organ transplantation.

Selection of patients can be based on age, vascular diseases, other debilities (infection, cancer).

We believe that there may be a higher risk of recurrence of HBV, HCV infection on liver graft in long-term immunosuppressed patients, and teatment with new anti-viral agents should be performed before transplantation.

Immunosuppressive therapy is based on the same protocols mostly used in single kidney, heart and liver transplantation.

References

1. Marrast AC. Transplantation combinée d'un rein avec le coeur, le foie ou le pancréas [thèse médecine]. Lyon-Nord, France: Université Claude Bernard-Lyon I, U.F.R., 1993.
2. Pineau B, Benvenutti C, Bourgeon B, et al. Transplantations cardiaque et rénale simultanées: Société Française de Transplantation, Paris, 3–4 décembre 1993. Transpl Proc. In press.
3. Watts RWE, Danpure CJ, De Pauw L, et al. Combined liver-kidney and isolated liver transplantations for primary hyperoxaluria type 1: the European experience. Nephrol Dial Transplant 1991; 6: 502–11.
4. Broyer M, Brunner FP, Brynger H, et al. Kidney transplantation in primary oxalosis: data from the EDTA registry. Nephrol Dial Transplant 1990; 5: 332–6.
5. Jamieson N, editor. Proceedings of the Second European Workshop on PH1, Cambridge, September, 1992.
6. Danpure CJ. Molecular and clinical heterogeneity in primary hyperoxaluria type 1. Am J Kidney Dis 1991; XVII: 366–9.
7. Hadengue A, Degos F. Prevalence and aspects of chronic hepatitis during hemodialysis and renal transplantation. Transplant Clin Immunol 1991; XXIII: 59–70.
8. Chossegros P, Caillette A, Pouteil-Noble C, et al. In kidney graft recipients chronically infected with HBV, the expression of low level replication, wild type and variants may be influenced by immunosuppression. Transplant Clin Immun 1991; XXIII: 71–3.
9. Daoud S, Garnier JL, Chossegros P, et al. Hepatitis C virus infection in renal transplantation; therapy with Ribavirin: Société Française de Transplantation, Paris, 3–4 décembre 1993. Transplant Proc. In press.
10. Samuel D, Muller R, Alexander G, et al. Liver transplantation in European patients with the hepatitis B surface antigen. N Engl J Med 1993; 329: 1842–7.
11. Trepo C, Ducerf C, Chevallier P, et al. Interêt de l'association Interféron– Ribavirine dans le traitement des réinfections virales C après transplantation hépatique. Revue Française de Gastro-entérologie 1994; avril: 11.
12. Chossegros P, Pouteil-noble C, Samuel D, et al. Ganciclovir in chronic hepatitis B after transplantation. Gastroenterology 1993; 104(S4): A888.
13. Vogel W, Steiner E, Kornberger R, et al. Preliminary results with combined hepatorenal allografting. Transplantation 1988; 45: 491–3.
14. Chossegros P, Lefrançois N, Chevallier P, et al. Influence of HBV and HCV infections on the survival of long-term follow-up kidney graft recipients. Transplant Clin Immun 1993; XXV: 440.
15. Chossegros P, Pouteil-noble C, Chevallier P, et al. Co-infection with HCV does not influence the outcome of chronic hepatitis B after kidney transplantation. Transplant Clin Immunol 1993; XXV: 441.
16. Starlz TE, Demetris AJ, Murase N, et al. Cell migration, chimerism, and graft acceptance. Lancet 1992; 339: 1579–82.

34. When to refer a patient for lung transplantation

IRVIN L. PARADIS, JAN D. MANZETTI, DANIEL E. FOUST,
GERENE S. BAULDOFF & BARTLEY P. GRIFFITH

Introduction

Lung transplantation has become a therapeutic option for selected patients with end-stage pulmonary parenchymal or vascular disease. This is primarily because survival has increased to 60% locally (Figure 1) and internationally at 2 years after lung transplantation [1, 2]. When heart and lung transplantation was the only procedure to treat such patients and waiting times were <6 months, the principle criteria to determine transplant candidacy was the presence of right ventricular failure. Because isolated lung transplantation has replaced heart and lung transplantation and the average waiting time for a donor has increased to 18–24 months, criteria requiring right heart failure for transplant candidacy are no longer viable. Thus the appropriate time to refer, list and perform a lung transplant is unclear.

The purpose of this study was to provide guidelines regarding the optimum time to refer and transplant patients with end-stage pulmonary parenchymal or vascular disease. Our approach was to compare the survival of patients with different types of diseases while waiting for a lung transplant, to examine clinical characteristics that might define those candidates who died waiting versus those who survived long enough to receive a lung transplant, and to compare the expected survival of patients with various forms of end-stage pulmonary parenchymal or vascular disease with the survival of the same types of recipients after a lung transplant procedure.

Methods

To accomplish these goals, we retrospectively reviewed the outcome and clinical characteristics of the 425 candidates who met our selection criteria (Table 1) and were added to the United Network for Organ Sharing (UNOS) list for lung transplantation between July 1990 and July 1993 (Table 1). Each candidate was assessed by age, gender, spirometry indices (% predicted FVC and FEV_1), diffusing capacity for carbon monoxide (% predicted DLCO),

J.L. Touraine et al. (eds.), Organ Shortage: The Solutions, 267–275.
© 1995 *Kluwer Academic Publishers.*

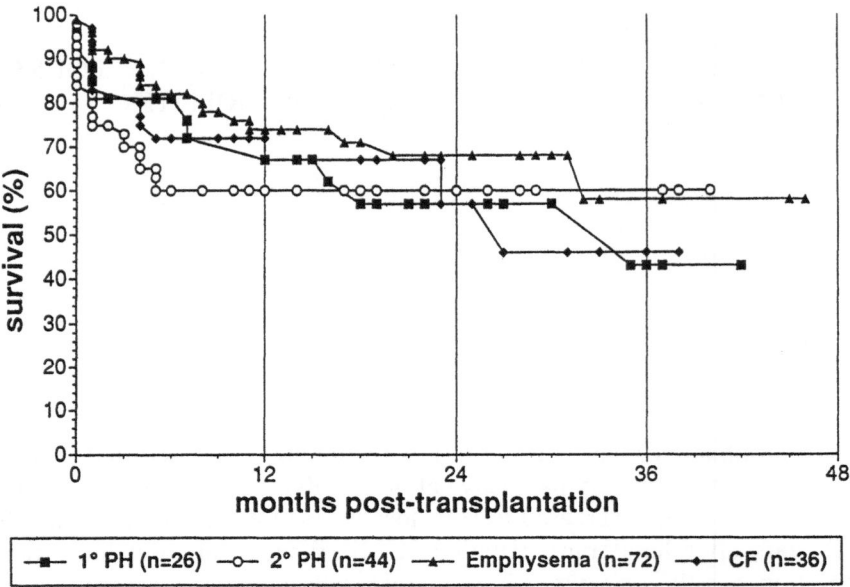

Fig. 1. Survival after lung transplantation between January 1, 1990 – January 1, 1994 at the University of Pittsburgh.

arterial blood gases at rest on room air, nutritional status as assessed by body mass index (BMI), 6–minute walk distance (6 MWD) and hemodynamic parameters of systolic, diastolic and mean pulmonary artery pressures, pulmonary capillary wedge pressure and cardiac output obtained by right heart catheterization. Males >40 years of age and females >45 underwent coronary arteriorgraph to exclude silent but significant coronary artery disease. Only candidates with primary pulmonary hypertension (PPH) (n = 35), idiopathic pulmonary fibrosis (IPF) (n = 34), cystic fibrosis (CF) (n = 78), and emphysema, including those with alpha-1–antitrypsin deficiency (E/A1a) (n = 101), were analyzed. This is because only those groups contained sufficient numbers of candidates to allow for statistical comparisons and because published data were available regarding the natural history of these types of diseases.

Comparisons between candidates who died waiting versus those who were transplanted (Tables 3 and 4) were made by the Mann-Whitney Rank Sum test. Actuarial survival for lung transplant recipients was calculated by the method of life table analysis. A *p* value of <0.05 was regarded as significant.

Results

Of these 425 candidates, 132 (31%) were transplanted, 82 (19%) died while waiting for a transplant and the remaining 211 candidates (50%) were still

Table 1. Selection criteria for lung transplantation

Indications	End stage pulmonary parenchymal and/or vascular disease with:
	Projected life expectancy <2 years
	NYHA Class III or IV
Relative contraindications	Weight outside ±10% predicted range
	Prednisone >10 mg qd or 20 mg qod
	Bilateral surgical pleurodesis
Absolute contraindications	Physiologic age
	>65 for SLT
	>60 for DLT
	>50 for HLT
	Psychosocial instability
	Inadequate financial resources
	Tobacco use within 1 year
	Mechanical ventilation
	Another life limiting illness such as
	HIV infection
	Recent malignancy
	Bone marrow failure
	Liver failure (T. bili >2 mg dl^{-1})
	Renal failure (S. Cr >2 mg dl^{-1})

waiting for a donor as of July 1, 1993 (Table 2). The risk of dying while waiting for a transplant was greatest for candidates with IPF (89%) or those awaiting retransplantation (70%), intermediate for candidates with restrictive diseases other than IPF (7/16 = 44%) or pulmonary hypertension (PH), either primary or secondary in etiology (38%), and lowest for candidates with CF (26%) or E/A1a (15%) (Table 2). For candidates with PPH and IPF, the mean time until death was only 70 and 120 days, respectively (Tables 3 and 4), while for candidates with E/A1a and CF the mean was 172 and 230 days, respectively (Table 4). During the same time period, the two-year actuarial survival after lung transplantation for recipients with CF was 57%; E/A1a, 68%; PPH, 58%; and Eisenmenger's, 60% (Figure 1).

Risk assessment for survival was analyzed by the relevant parameters of prognosis for the four major disease groups (Tables 3 and 4). For candidates with PPH (Table 3), although the PaO$_2$ was lower, the A-a oxygen gradient was wider, the mean right atrial (mRAP) and mean pulmonary artery pressure (mPAP) were higher, and the cardiac index (CI) was lower in those who died waiting versus those who were transplanted; only the percent predicted DLCO approached statistical significance ($p = 0.06$). For candidates with CF, although the percent predicted DLCO and 6–minute walk distance (6 MWD) were lower; only the percent predicted FVC and FEV$_1$ were significantly lower in those who died waiting as compared to those candidates who survived long enough to receive an allograft (Table 4). For candidates with E/A1a, there were no parameters distinguishing between

Table 2. Candidates with different types of diseases who were listed for lung transplantation and who were transplanted (Tx) or died waiting

Type of disease	Candidates	Tx	Died	
			n	%
Primary PH	35	11	7	(39)
Secondary PH				
Eisenmenger's	59	17	10	(37)
Thromboembolic	6	1	1	
Obstructive lung disease				
Nonseptic				
Emphysema/A-1-a	101	41	7	(15)
Bronchiolitis Obliterans	3	1	0	
Septic				
Cystic fibrosis	78	31	11	(26)
Bronchiectasis	12	4	0	
Restrictive lung diseases				
IPF	34	2	16	(89)
Sarcoidosis	12	5	3	
Silicosis	4	2	1	
Chemotherapy	12	2	3	
Other	1	0	0	
Other:				
Retransplants	34	7	16	(70)
Lymphangioleiomyomatosis	5	3	1	
CREST/Scleroderma	12	1	6	
Other	17	4	5	
Total	425	132	82	

those candidates who died waiting versus those who lived long enough to receive a transplant. For candidates with IPF, it was not possible to make meaningful comparisons between the candidates who died waiting versus those who received an allograft, because only 2 candidates with this disease lived long enough to receive an allograft during this 3–year time interval. The candidates who died waiting did have a severe restrictive impairment (FVC 48 ± 19% pred), a severe reduction in the DLCO (22 ± 11% pred) and a severe impairment in oxygenation with a mean A-a oxygen gradient of 38 mmHg when accepted as candidates.

Discussion

The most significant finding from our analysis was that the type of underlying disease affected the likelihood that a candidate would survive long enough to receive a transplant. Candidates with PH, either primary or secondary in etiology, and, especially, candidates with IPF were less likely to survive to receive a lung transplant as compared to candidates with emphysema and

Table 3. Comparison of prognostic indices of survival for candidates with primary pulmonary hypertension who were transplanted or died waiting

	Transplanted	Died waiting
mPAP (mmHg)	53 ± 20	60 ± 5
	n = 7	n = 6
mRAP (mmHg)	6 ± 6	17 ± 2
	n = 3	n = 2
CI (L min^{-1}/m^2)	2.0 ± 0.5	1.6 ± 0.7
	n = 7	n = 4
PaO$_2$ (mmHg)	75 ± 18	66 ± 19
	n = 7	n = 6
A-a O$_2$ grad	32	43
	n = 7	n = 6
DLCO (% pred)	90 ± 36*	58 ± 19
	n = 8	n = 6
Time to outcome in days:		
Mean	272	70
Range	14–543	3–235

Data expressed as mean ± 1 Standard Deviation.
*p = 0.06 by Mann Whitney Rank Sum test.

Table 4. Comparison of prognostic indices of survival for candidates with cystic fibrosis (CF), emphysema/alpha-1–antitrypsin deficiency (Emphysema) and idiopathic pulmonary fibrosis (IPF), who were transplanted (Tx) or died waiting

	Cystic Fibrosis		Emphysema		IPF
	Tx	Died	Tx	Died	Died
FVC (% pred)	44 ± 17	32 ± 8*	50 ± 18	43 ± 16	48 ± 19
FEV$_1$ (% pred)	25 ± 10	18 ± 5*	20 ± 7	18 ± 6	50 ± 16
FEV$_1$/FVC	49 ± 12	48 ± 12	31 ± 9	37 ± 18	85 ± 12
DLCO (% pred)	58 ± 25	38 ± 7	31 ± 15	29 ± 13	22 ± 11
PaCO$_2$ (mmHg)	50 ± 15	54 ± 9	50 ± 13	55 ± 11	42 ± 6
PaO$_2$ (mmHg)	56 ± 17	54 ± 6	59 ± 10	61 ± 14	56 ± 17
A-a O$_2$ grad	22	24	25	16	38
6 MWD	982 ± 280	780 ± 224	488	330	610 ± 390
	n = 8	n = 6			n = 6
BMI	18 ± 3	18 ± 3	22 ± 4	21 ± 5	
Time to outcome in days					
Mean	341	230	348	172	120
Range	18–1118	82–403	17–962	25–407	7–475

Data expressed as mean ±1 Standard Deviation.
PaO$_2$ measured on room air.
*p < 0.05 by Mann Whitney Rank Sum test.

CF (Table 2). These findings are similar to those reported by another lung transplant center, where 75% of the candidates with IPF and 40% of the candidates with PPH died waiting, whereas only 10% of the candidates with emphysema, 28% of the candidates with cystic fibrosis and 22% of the candidates with congenital heart disease died waiting [3].

This situation occurred either because patients with PPH and IPF declined more quickly or were referred for lung transplantation later in the course of their illness as compared to patients with emphysema or CF. Our data suggests the later possibility, as our candidates with PPH and IPF who died waiting were referred and listed when severe disease was already present. The candidates with PPH who died waiting were listed when significant cardiac compromise was already present as evidenced by a low cardiac index of 1.6 ± 0.7 L min^{-1}/m^2 and an elevated right atrial pressure of 17 ± 2 mmHg (Table 3). In the National Pulmonary Hypertension Registry, median survival was 1 month when the mRAP was ≥ 20 mmHg and 17 months when the CI was <2 L min^{-1}/m^2 [4]. The lower DLCO and wider A-a oxygen gradient among our non-survivors were probably also markers for more impaired cardiac function in this group. Similarly, the candidates with IPF who died waiting already had a severe restrictive impairment with an FVC of $48 \pm 19\%$ of predicted and a severe impairment of gas exchange with a DLCO of $22 \pm 11\%$ of predicted and a widened A-a oxygen gradient of 38 mmHg when listed for lung transplantation (Table 4). As the actuarial survival was only 50% at 2 years after diagnosis of IPF in patients whose initial FVC was $\leq 67\%$ of predicted [5], it is perhaps not surprising that our candidates with even more severe lung disease did not survive long enough to receive a transplant.

The central question is when to refer a patient with one of these diseases for lung transplantation. The simplest approach is to compare the survival of patients with a particular type of disease to the survival of these patients after lung transplantation (Figure 1). A patient should be referred for lung transplantation when his/her expected survival post-transplantation exceeds that of the underlying disease.

For patients with PPH, the National Registry reports overall survival at 50% at 2.5 years after diagnosis [4]. Since survival is also 50% at 2 years after lung transplantation (Figure 1), one could recommend that all patients with PPH should be referred for lung transplantation at the time that the diagnosis of PPH is made. However, survival for patients with PPH has been further stratified by mRAP, mPAP and CI. In the National Registry, median survival decreased from 46 months when the mRAP was <10 mmHg to 1 month when the mRAP was ≥ 20 mmHg; from 48 months when the mPAP was <55 mmHg to 12 months when the mPAP was ≥ 85 mmHg; and from 43 months when the CI was ≥ 4 L min^{-1}/m^2 to 17 months when the CI was <2 L min^{-1}/m^2. With an average waiting time for a donor now at 18 months at this center, most patients with an mRAP ≥ 20 mmHg, mPAP ≥ 85 mmHg and a CI of <2 L min^{-1}/m^2 would die waiting, while those with an mRAP of <10 mmHg, mPAP of <55 mmHg and a CI of ≥4 L min^{-1}/m^2 would have a predicted survival which exceeds that after lung transplantation. Therefore, the optimum candidate for lung transplantation with PPH would appear to have an mRAP between 10–20 mmHg, mPAP between 55–85 mmHg and a CI between 2–4 L min^{-1}/m^2. As our candidates who died waiting had evidence of severely impaired cardiac function with a mean mRAP of 17 mmHg and a mean CI of 1.6 L min^{-1}/m^2, our data (Table 3) supports these recommendations.

For patients with CF, the risk of death within 2 years has been about 50% when the FVC was less than 40% of predicted, the FEV$_1$ was less than 30% of predicted, the room air PaO$_2$ was less than 55 mmHg, the PaCO$_2$ was greater than 50 mmHg, and the height to weight ratio was less than 70% [6]. As the 2–year survival post-transplantation for CF is about 70%, one could recommend that patients with CF be referred for lung transplantation when they reach this profile. This is reinforced by our data (Table 4), where candidates with a mean FVC of 32% of predicted and a mean FEV$_1$ of 18% of predicted were significantly less likely to live long enough to receive a lung transplant as compared to the candidates with better preserved lung mechanics.

For patients with emphysema, the 2–year survival with an initial post-bronchodilator FEV$_1$ of <30% of predicted and age <65 years has been reported to be 60% [7]. However, this patient population was relatively small (n = 200) and hypoxemic patients did not receive supplemental oxygen, which does influence survival [8]. In a larger sample of 1,000 nonhypoxemic patients with emphysema, the 2–year survival in patients <65 years with an initial post-bronchodilator FEV$_1$ of <30 of predicted was 75% [9]. Since the expected survival 2 years post-transplantation for emphysema is about 70% (Figure 1), it appears appropriate to refer a patient for lung transplantation when the post-bronchodilator FEV$_1$ becomes <30% of predicted. Probably because all of our candidates fell well below this limit (Table 4) with a mean FEV$_1$ of 20% of predicted among recipients and 18% of predicted among those who died waiting, we were unable to observe differences between these two classes of candidates.

For patients with IPF, the overall mean survival at 2 years after diagnosis has been reported to be 80% [10]. When subsets of patients with IPF were examined, 2–year survival after diagnosis was lower for men (60%) than women (80%), lower with increasing age (60% for 60–69 years of age vs. 75% for <50 years age), lower with increasing radiographic infiltrates, and lower with more histologic fibrosis [11]. More importantly, the 2–year survival rate was only 50% in patients with an initial FVC ≤ 67% of predicted, who did not respond to treatment with immunosuppressant medications within 4–6 weeks as demonstrated by a >10% increase in the FVC that was maintained for at least one year [5]. As the 2–year survival after lung transplantation for IPF is 58% [2], one could recommend that patients with IPF be referred for lung transplantation when the FVC is <67% of predicted and there has been no response to immunosuppressant medications. Our experience supports this recommendation (Table 4). All of our candidates with IPF presented with far advanced disease, as evidenced by a mean FVC of only 48% of predicted in the candidates who died waiting. All (n = 16) but 2 (89%) of these candidates died while waiting for an allograft.

Our findings suggest that the timing of the referral for lung transplantation is a factor that predicts outcome. According to current UNOS policy, lung transplant candidates receive allografts in the order in which they are placed on the UNOS list without regard for severity or type of underlying illness [12]. Thus, candidates with very different diseases such as PPH and emphysema compete with each other for available allografts.

Based on current UNOS donor allocation policies and anticipated waiting times of 18–24 months, our results suggest that patients with PPH and IPF probably should be referred when the diagnosis is confirmed and definitely should be referred when they develop the clinical pictures just outlined. At present, these patients are being referred too late in the course of their disease and are unable to compete successfully with patients with emphysema and CF, whose clinical course may be less rapid or who are being referred at an earlier stage of their disease. Patients with cystic fibrosis should be referred when their FEV_1 is <30% of predicted and their FVC is <40% of predicted. Patients with emphysema should be referred when their post-bronchodilator FEV_1 is <30% of predicted. These findings should enable care givers to identify and refer candidates for lung transplantation before their medical condition becomes too tenuous for successful transplantation.

References

1. Griffith BP, Hardesty RL, Armitage JM, Hattler BG, Pham SM, Keenan RJ, Paradis IL. A decade of lung transplantation. Ann Surg 1993; 218: 310–20.
2. Kaye MP. The Registry of the International Society for Heart and Lung Transplantation: Tenth official report – 1993. J Heart Lung Transplant 1993; 12: 541–8.
3. Hayden A, Robert R, Kriett J, Smith C, Nicholson K, Jamieson S. Primary diagnosis predicts prognosis of lung transplant candidates. Transplantation. 1993; 55: 1048–50.
4. D'Alonzo G, Barst RJ, Ayres SM, et al. Survival in patients with primary pulmonary hypertension. Ann Int Med 1991; 115: 343–9.
5. Rudd RM, Haslam PL, Turner-Warwick M. Cryptogenic fibrosing alveolitis: relationships of pulmonary physiology and bronchoalveolar lavage to response to treatment and prognosis. Am Rev Resp Dis 1981; 1241: 1–8.
6. Kerem E, Reisman J, Corey M, Canny GJ, Levison H. Prediction of mortality in patients with cystic fibrosis. N Engl J Med 1992; 326: 1187–91.
7. Traver GA, Cline MG, Burrows B. Predictors of mortality in chronic obstructive pulmonary disease. Am Rev Resp Dis 1979; 119: 895–902.
8. Nocturnal oxygen therapy trial group – continuous or nocturnal oxygen therapy in hypoxemic chronic obstructive pulmonary disease: a clinical trial. Ann Intern Med 1980; 93: 391–8.
9. Anthonisen NR, Wright EC, Hodgkin JE (IPPB Trial Group). Prognosis in chronic obstructive pulmonary disease. Am Rev Resp Dis 1986; 133: 14–20.

10. Carrington CB, Gaensler EA, Coutu RE, Fitzgerald MX, Gupta RT. Natural history and treated course of usual and desquamative interstitial pneumonia. N Engl J Med 1978; 298: 801–9.
11. Turner-Warwick M, Burrows B, Johnson A. Cryptogenic fibrosing alveolitis: clinical features and their influence on survival. Thorax 1980; 35: 171–80.
12. Pierce G. UNOS: time waiting for thoracic organ candidates – amended policy 3.7.5. UNOS Memorandum 1993; April: 3–4.

16. ...

35. Must the choice of surgical procedure for lung transplantation be guided by organ shortage?

JEAN FRANÇOIS MORNEX, MICHÈLE BERTOCCHI, THÉRÈSE WIESANDANGER, and FABRICE THÉVENET

Pulmonary transplantation is peculiar in the sense that with the heart and lung from a single donor, multiple procedures can be performed. For instance, the heart-lung en bloc can be transplanted to a single recipient, a double lung and a heart transplantation can be performed in two recipients, two single lung and one heart transplants can be performed in three recipients. Thus, the number of recipients benefiting from a single heart-lung donor can vary according to the type of procedure choosen.

Initially, heart-lung transplants were mostly performed, then the lung and the heart were transplanted separately because of the following observations:

1. right ventricular dysfunction can recover after lung transplantation,
2. simple septal defect can be corrected at the time of lung transplantation, and
3. the incidence of chronic rejection is the same whatever the procedure is.

Furthermore, an unnecessary heart transplantation should be avoided, since the risk of accelerated coronary arterosclerosis exists; the results of heart transplantation alone are better than that of heart-lung transplantation, therefore the heart should be transplanted separately.

In this context, there has been an evolution in the type of pulmonary transplantation performed in the world, with a steep increase in the total number of pulmonary transplantations, a plateau in the evolution of the number of heart-lung transplantations, and a marked increase in the number of single and double-lung transplantations. It is now necessary to reassess this evolution, trying to answer the question: Are the results similar whatever the surgical procedure is?

Results can be assessed as survival rate or improvement in pulmonary function tests, in any case, they should be evaluated differently according to the underlying disease.

Based on various registries (St. Louis international lung transplant registry [1]) or single institution experiences [2, 3] there is no difference in the survival rate of the different procedures: survival rate of single lung vs. heart-lung transplant or single-lung vs. double-lung transplant are not different.

J.L. Touraine et al. (eds.), *Organ Shortage: The Solutions*, 277–280.

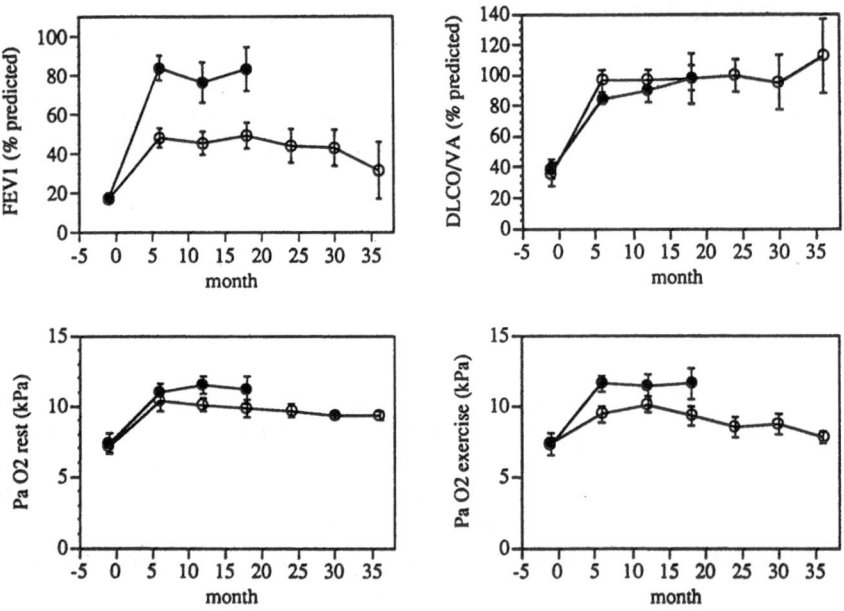

Fig. 1. Pulmonary function tests before and after single lung (n = 6; open circle) and double lung (n = 5; closed circle) transplantations performed for pulmonary emphysema at Hôpital Louis Pradel. Results shown as mean ±SEM.

Since the underlying diseases cause very different results, they should be assessed accordingly. The two major causes of transplantation are pulmonary emphysema and primary pulmonary hypertension. The survival rate for single-lung and double-lung transplantation in emphysema are not different [4, 5]. The pulmonary function test results (Figure 1) show a major improvement in most of the parameters, after both single-lung and double-lung transplantation. But the improvement in the FEV-1 is incomplete after single-lung transplantation. Similarly, the survival curves after single-lung or heart-lung transplantation in primary pulmonary hypertension are not different, nor is survival different after double lung transplantation [6]. The main pulmonary function test abnormalities (Figure 2) are also corrected similarly after single-lung and heart-lung transplantation. Therefore, the results are similar whatever the type of surgery, but some complications, such as bronchial, are more frequent in single- and double-lung than in heart-lung transplantation [7, 8]. Furthermore, acute graft dysfunction is difficult to manage after single-lung transplantation.

Since the numbers of donors and pulmonary transplantations are decreasing the maximum number of transplants should be performed for single donors. In this context, the type of surgical procedure should be guided by organ shortage, trying to benefit the maximum number of recipients. But

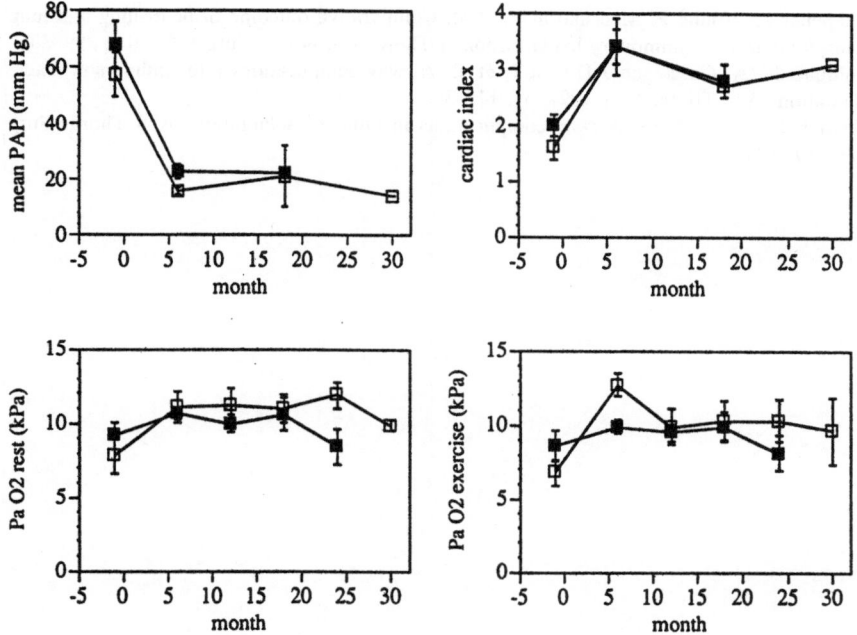

Fig. 2. Pulmonary function tests before and after single lung (n = 7; open square) and heart lung (n = 5; closed square) transplantations performed for primary pulmonary hypertension at Hôpital Louis Pradel. Results shown as mean ±SEM.

there is certainly a limit in trying to perform mostly single lung transplantations. This limit is shown by the decrease of FEV-1 in emphysema patients receiving single lung transplantation (Figure 1), which may result in bronchiolitis obliterans and decrease the rate of success.

References

1. The Registry of the International Society for Heart and Lung Transplantation: Tenth official report – 1993. J Heart Lung Transplant 1993; 12: 541–8.
2. Dromer C, Velley JF, Jougon J, et al. Long-term functional results after bilateral lung transplantation. Ann Thorac Surg 1993; 56: 68–73.
3. Cooper JD, Patterson GA, Trulock FP, et al. Results of single and bilateral lung transplantation in 131 consecutive recipients. J Thorac Cardiovasc Surg 1994; 107: 460–71.
4. Patterson GA, Maurer JR, Williams TJ, et al. Comparison of outcomes of double and single lung transplantation for obstructive lung disease. J Thorac Cardiovasc Surg 1991; 101: 623–32.
5. Low DF, Trulock EP, Kaiser LR, et al. Morbidity, mortality and early results of single versus bilateral lung transplantation for emphysema. J Thorac Cardiovasc Surg 1992; 103: 1119–26.

6. Chapelier A, Vouhé P, Macchiarini P, et al. Comparative outcome of heart-lung and lung transplantation for pulmonary hypertension. J Thorac Cardiovasc Surg 1993; 106: 299–307.
7. Colquhoun IA, Gascoigne AD, Au J, et al. Airway complications after pulmonary transplantation. Ann Thorac Surg 1994; 57: 141–5.
8. Shennib H, Massard, G. Airway complications in lung transplantation. Ann Thorac Surg 1994; 57: 506–11.

36. Is cardiac transplantation justified in patients over 60 years of age?

J. ROBIN, J. NINET, E. BONNEFOY, J. NEIDECKER,
P. BOISSONNAT & G. CHAMPSAUR

Introduction

Over the past few years, improvements have been made both in surgical techniques and post-operative treatments, allowing the growing development of heart transplantation (HTx). So many patients who would have been excluded as candidates a few years ago are now considered excellent for HTx. It is generally admitted (Aravot et al. 1989; Frazier et al. 1988) that the upper age limit for HTx is 60 years. However, an increasing number of elderly candidates are now accepted for HTx. In our institution, as in numerous centers, the age limit has expanded over 60 years. Using our experience, starting in 1987, our follow-up allows the study of long-term results and comparison with other teams.

Between January 1987 and August 1993, 250 patients underwent an orthotopic heart transplantation in our institution. Excluding 46 patients transplanted before 20 years of age, generally for complicated congenital heart defects, 48 patients were over 60 years of age at the time of HTx (Group I) and 156 between 20 and 59 years (Group II). We studied and compared retrospectively the two populations to see if the age of the recipient influences early or long-term results of HTx.

Patients and methods

The mean age was 62.9 ± 3 years in the first group (range 60–67.4) and 47.5 ± 8.8 years in the second (range 21–59). The gender ratio was similar in the two groups (89.6% Gr I vs. 85.8% Gr II).

There was no difference in the distribution of etiology (Table 1). The first cause of transplantation in the two groups was idiopathic cardiomyopathy (50% Gr I vs. 53.2% Gr II). Ischaemic cardiopathy was less frequent, with the same distribution in the two groups (29.2% Gr I vs. 27.5% Gr II). Finally, in the first group only one retransplantation was performed (2.1%)

J.L. Touraine et al. (eds.), Organ Shortage: The Solutions, 281–286.
© 1995 *Kluwer Academic Publishers*.

Table 1. Etiology

	Group I (n = 48)		Group II (n = 156)		
	n	%	n	%	(p = 0.05)
Idiopathic	24	50	83	53.2	NS
Ischaemic	14	29.2	43	27.5	NS
Valvular	9	18.7	22	14.1	NS
Chronic rejection	1	2.1	8	5.1	NS

Table 2. Risk factors

	Group I (n = 48)		Group II (n = 156)		
	n	%	n	%	(p = 0.05)
Smoking	11	22.9	5	3.2	NS
Overweight	7	14.6	12	7.7	NS
Dyslipidemia	4	8.33	6	3.8	NS
Diabetes	4	8.33	4	2.56	NS
High blood pressure	4	8.33	2	1.28	NS

Table 3. Haemodynamic data

	Group I (n = 48)	Group II (n = 156)	(p = 0.05)
PAPm (mmHg)	31.1 ± 11.8	32.2 ± 10.7	NS
PAOP (mm Hg)	20.1 ± 9.0	24.1 ± 9.1	NS
EF (%)	20.8 ± 7.3	24.3 ± 9.7	NS
CI (l mn^{-1}/m^2)	1.79 ± 0.51	1.86 ± 0.44	NS

PAPm: mean pulmonary artery pressure, PAOP: pulmonary artery occlusion pressure, EF: ejection fraction, CI: cardiac index.

for chronic rejection or graft degeneration versus 8 (5.1%) in the second group (NS).

The risk factors were analyzed in the two groups (Table 2): the most frequent factor was smoking in Group I (23%) and overweight in Group II (7.7%).

All the patients were in NYHA functional class III or IV before transplantation. Haemodynamic data were obtained for each patient. The distributions of pulmonary artery pressure and wedge pressure (Table 3) were not significantly different between the two groups. Ejection fractions (20.8% vs. 24.3%) and cardiac index (1.79 vs. 1.86 l mn^{-1}/m^2) were low, expressing the low cardiac output and the deterioration of the left ventricular function. Pulmonary resistances were similar in the two groups and compatible with an HTx.

In 14 cases, the patient required a mechanical support (Abiomed BVS System 5000) as a bridge to transplantation. All these patients were less than

Table 4. Causes of early death

	Group I (n = 48)		Group II (n = 156)		
	n	%	n	%	Stat (*p* = 0.05)
Graft dysfunction	5	10.4	5	3.2	*p* = 0.043
Acute rejection	1	2.08	4	2.56	NS
Sepsis	0	2	1.28	NS	
Non-cardiac death	24.16	4	2.56	NS	

60 years old (Group II). This device was implanted during 4.4 ± 3 days, range 1–10 days.

The study of operative data shows the only discriminative element between the two groups; donor age was significantly different: 42.3 ± 12.1 years in Group I (range 14–67) and 30.6 ± 10.7 years in Group II (range 11–56). On the other hand, technical data were similar: cold ischemia 138.1 ± 62.4 mn in Gr I (range 55–330) versus 147.3 ± 61.6 mn in Gr II (range 50–380), warm ischemia 74.4 ± 22.7 mn in Gr I (range 32–65) versus 49.7 ± 8.8 mn in Gr II (range 31–80).

After transplantation, all patients were treated with the same immunosuppressive therapy associating Cyclosporine, steroid and azathioprime. To detect a possible rejection during the hospital stay, patients were followed up by echocardiography and endomyocardial biopsy every week during the first post-operative month and every 2 months thereafter. Treatment varied with the class of rejection: steroid and antithymocyte globuline for rejection grade I or II, OKT3 (monoclonal antibody) for rejection grade III.

Early results (< 30 days)

Hospital mortality was 14.6% in Group I (7 patients) versus 8.97% in Group II (14 patients) without significant difference ($p = 0.13$). The most common cause of early death (Table 4) was the dysfunction of the graft (left or right ventricle) with a significant difference between the two populations: 10.4% Gr I versus 3.2% Gr II ($p = 0.043$). On the other hand, the rate of acute rejection was similar: 2.08% vs. 2.56%. Lastly, 2 sepsis were observed in patients less than 60 years old and 6 non-cardiac complications (neurological death) were encountered.

Early complications were equally frequent in the 2 groups: 14% in Gr I vs. 17.4% in Gr II. Rejection grade I or II were observed in 8.33% in Gr I versus 10.25% in Gr II (NS). Only 2 patients presented a rejection grade III, which was treated with success.

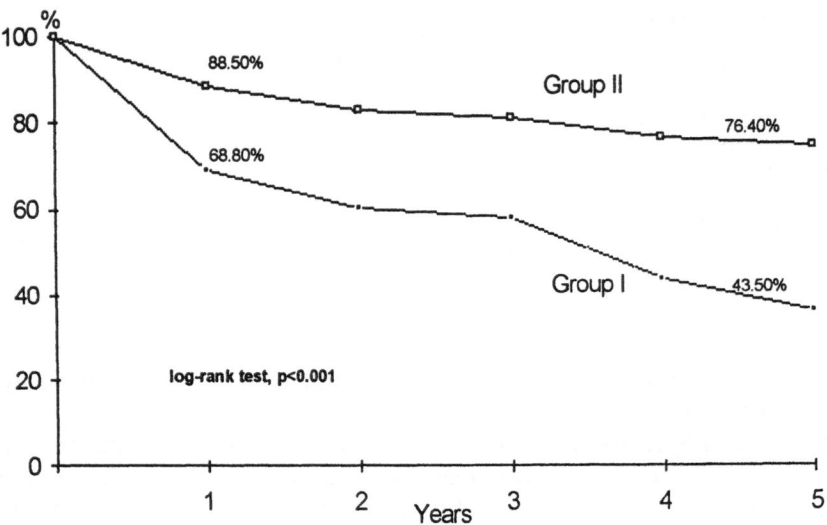

Fig. 1. Actuarial survival showing a significant difference between the two groups.

Table 5. Causes of late death

	Group I (n = 48)	Group II (n = 156)
Rejection	3	3
Acute death	2	9
Malignancies	4	1
Others	2	3
Total	11	16

Late results

Patients were followed up from May 1987 to September 1993, and none were lost during this period. The mean follow-up for the patients over 60 years of age at the time of transplantation was 20.4 ± 19.3 months (range 1–73) and 35.4 ± 23 months (range 1–77) for patients less than 60 years of age.

The actuarial survival (Figure 1) shows a significant difference between the two populations: at 1 year, the actuarial survival rate was 68.8% in Group I versus 88.5% in Group II. This difference increased with time as shown on the survival curves: 43.5% in Group I versus 76.4% in Group II (Log rank test, $p = 0.001$ at 1 year, $p = 0.008$ at 5 years).

The causes of late death were also different between the 2 populations (Table 5). In Group I, 11 late deaths were observed versus 16 in Group II. If the rate of fatal rejection was similar, acute deaths were less frequent in Group I (2 patients) than in Group II (9 patients). Conversely, malignancies were most often observed in patients over 60 years of age (4 cases) than in younger patients (1 case).

Comments

Is cardiac transplantation justified after 60 years of age? This study was performed retrospectively between two groups matching for etiology, haemo-dynamic and surgical data. Donor age was the only distinctive data between the two populations. Early results were similar in the two groups concerning hospital mortality and the causes of early death. However, the rate of early graft dysfunction was more important in patients transplanted after the age of 60, without significant difference in the age of donors in the 2 groups (38.4 years Gr I vs. 30.3 years Gr II). The rate of fatal early rejection was similar. Previous studies (Copeland 1988; Frazier et al. 1988) emphasized the strong early results of HTx in recipients over 60 years of age.

The long-term results showed a faster deterioration of the survival in patients transplanted after 60 years of age. Other teams (Aravot et al. 1989; Frazier et al. 1988; Rendlund et al. 1987) considered that there is no differ-ence in the 12- or 24-month actuarial life survival, and similar or reduced numbers of rejection in this age group. However, follow-up of the earlier studies did not exceed 1.5-2 years and our study showed an increasing difference between the two curves after 1 year of follow-up. If the one-year survival rate in patients over 60 years of age was comparable to that of younger patients, the five-year rate was extremely different.

Moreover, the causes of late death were also different. Acute deaths were more frequent in patients less than 60 years; in these cases, the age of the donors was the same in the two groups (39 years Gr I vs. 35.8 years Gr II), eliminating this data as a risk factor of mortality. This could be a determining element of graft degeneration, because graft coronary lesions seemed to be more frequent in this group. Otherwise, malignancies were most often ob-served in patients transplanted after 60 years of age. A non-cardiac disease could be frequent in this age group, but non-diagnosed at the time of pre-transplant check-up. These data could explain a deterioration of long-term results in this group.

Conclusion

Heart transplantation is justified in patients over 60 years of age, if we consider the early results during the first post-operative year. The long-term results observed in this study, however, show that heart transplantation should be considered with care in this age group. The present organ shortage increases the duration of the waiting list for transplantation; for this reason, our team favours like-aged donors for recipients over 60 years. Otherwise, non-cardiac diseases are frequent and must be carefully researched before HTx, according to the number of malignancies observed in these patients treated with immunosuppressive therapy.

References

1. Aravot DJ, Banner NR, Khaghani A, Fitzgerald M, Radley-Smith R, Mitchell AG, Yacoub MH. Cardiac transplantation in the seventh decade of life. Am J Cardiol 1989; 63: 90–3.
2. Copeland JG. Cardiac transplantation after 60 years of age. Ann Thorac Surg 1988; 45: 115–6.
3. Frazier OH, Macris MP, Duncan JM, Van Buren CT, Cooley DA. Cardiac transplantation in patients over 60 years of age. Ann Thorac Surg 1988; 45: 129–32.
4. Rendlund DG, Gilbert EM, O'Connell JB, Gay WA, Jones KW, Dewitt CW, Menlove RL, Bristow MR. Age-associated decline in cardiac allograft rejection. Am J Med 1987; 83: 391–8.

37. The media and organ shortage

B. CUZIN & J.M. DUBERNARD

The relationship between the media and organ shortage and, more precisely, between the media and organ shortage is complex. First, examples illustrating the different ways in which the media can influence organ donation will be examined. Secondly, the general effects of and laws regarding the media and society will be exposed and, thirdly, suggestions will be considered regarding how these laws permit to explain population's attitude toward organ donation and transplantation and how to improve organ shortage.

The facts

France: Press review

Daily papers are collected by the documentation department of the Lyon hospitals. The articles concerning organ transplantation and harvesting have been extracted and analysed for the years 1991, 1992 and 1993 and the results have been summarized (Table 1). They are classified as "technical" and "polemic" articles. The increase of items in the category "miscellaneous" in 1992 is due to xenografts, and increase of items in the category "liver transplantation" is due to living donors and split livers. A balance between the number of "technical" and "polemic" articles existed in 1991. In 1992, many items about organ procurement were written corresponding mainly to the "Amiens" problems. In 1992 and 1993, the increase of polemic articles was linked to organ shortage: Is it true? Is it wrong? It is difficult to conclude because of the complexity of the laws governing public opinion.

Spain and England: Press review

This combined newspaper review, using a different item classification system, was compiled for articles appearing in 1991 (J.L. Piero Ibanez 1993, unpubl. data) (Table 2). In these countries, interest in transplantation has been mainly concerned with the political-judicial point of view and discussions

J.L. Touraine et al. (eds.), Organ Shortage: The Solutions, 287–293.

Table 1. Press review in France: 1991, 1992, 1993

	1991	1992	1993
Technical articles			
Heart transplantation	1	5	2
Lung transplantation	2	1	2
Bone marrow transplantation	2	1	0
Kidney, pancreactic transplantation	1	2	0
Liver transplantation	2	3	15
Miscellaneous	10	20	7
TOTAL	18	32	26
Polemic articles			
Traffic in organs	8	5	6
Organ procurement:			
–Information	3	3	3
–Controversies	3	29	11
Organ allocation	5	21	22
Brain death	1	0	0
TOTAL	19	56	42

have concerned individual cases, donors and donations. As intensive care progresses, Spain has increased its number of organ donors, which explains the importance of items classified as "donations, global statistics, organization" in technical articles.

According to these two reviews, in France, Spain and England, the public's and journalists' preoccupations regarding organ allocation and donation seem to be closely related.

Australia: Television advertisements

The following was reported in 1992 [1].

In 1987, an Australian national survey was undertaken by the Australian National Foundation (AKF) to determine the population's knowledge about and attitude toward organ donation and transplantation:

– 98% agreed with organ transplantation
– 34% were prepared to donate their own organs
– 17% were prepared to donate the organs of their next of kin

In 1989, the AKF produced television advertisements highlighting the need for organ donation; these were screened over a period of 6 to 12 months. A national follow-up survey, undertaken in 1990, showed unchanged opinions among the community.

In my mind, this example illustrates the difficulty in changing public opinion about any issue by the exclusive means of television, even with well-

Table 2. Press review in Spain and England

1991 Subjects	"El Pais"% items	"The Times"% items
Technical articles		
Heart	15	60
Kidney	11.5	20
Liver	11.5	20
Bone marrow	7.7	0
Lung	3.8	0
Pancreatic islets	3.8	0
Cornea	1.9	0
Donations, global statistics, organization	45	0
TOTAL	100	100
Polemic articles		
Official declarations and political-judicial implications	20	27
Figures and ranking	16.6	4
Donors and donations	16.6	15
Individual cases	15	42
Hospital infrastructures	13.3	4
Economic aspects	11.6	4
Scientific innovations in congresses	3.3	4
Traffic in organs	3.3	0
TOTAL	100	100

(J.L. Piero Ibanez 1993, unpubl. data).

done advertisements in a country where people have a long historic past with a particular subject (in this case, cadaveric renal transplantation, which began in Australia in 1965). The Australian example will be returned to later in this article.

Saudi arabia: *Mass media educational program*

The results of a mass media educational program in Saudia Arabia were published in 1992 [2]. In 1986, a program was started by the National Kidney Foundation (NKF), including:

- television – movies, posters, sharp messages, interviews (religious authorities and physicians)
- newspapers – one article per week on such topics as brain death, organ donation, social and religious aspects of organ donation, benefits offered to the donor's family
- radio – interviews, sharp messages

Two years after the media focus on the issues of transplantation a public survey was conducted:

- 82% were aware of the existence of the NKF
- 88% agreed to the idea of organ donation
- 14% had signed a donor card
- 88% were aware that Islam accepts kidney donation
- 92% were aware that humans can live with only one kidney
- 33% understood what brain death meant

This educational program seems to have been promoted by the media and the results are considered very encouraging. Nevertheless, many imprecisions in the article cause one to be cautious in drawing conclusions.

The Saudi Arabian example concludes a review of experiences in different countries where the media has been used to change public opinion toward transplantation. This illustrates the general and well-known law regarding the difference between expected and real effect.

The media and society

General effects

Relationships between the media and society have been studied, and the general effects are stereotypical and, often, foreseeable [3].

The image of the media
People have an image of a given medium which has an influence on their gullibility. This image presents two different aspects: on one hand, it concerns intrinsic qualities that an audience attributes to a medium as technique (the press, the television) or as a social institution ("the Times", the " C"); on the other hand, the image of an instrument of information concerns the capacities of influence which are attributed to a particular medium, considered in turn as a technique and an institution.

- The *intrinsic qualities* attributed to the media: each group or individual assigns a level of value, of reliability, of power, of impartiality to a given medium.
- The *"powers" attributed to the media*: a subjective appreciation about the capacity of influence, the nature or the aim of the media actions. The real impact of the media is the opposite of expected impact. For example: the most favorable situation for a public man is when the media is thought to be hostile to him, but is in reality kind.

"mosaic" culture according to Abraham Moles
In 1965, Abraham Moles [4] described a sociocultual cycle, giving a representation of ideas renewal and circulation, conveyed by the media (Figure 1). In this cycle, the first actors are creators (artists, researchers). They create

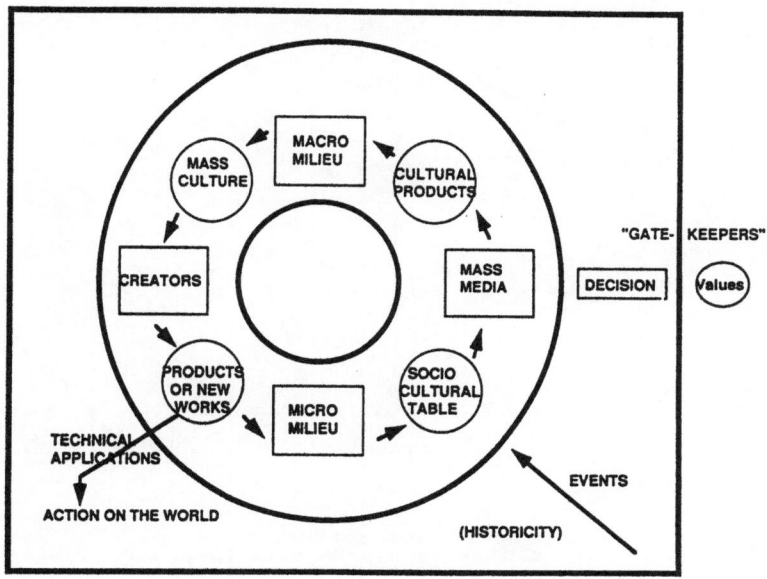

Fig. 1. Sociocultural cycle according to A. Moles.

new ideas, then local intelligentsia and intellectuals focus on fragments of these new ideas. The media, in their turn, take these fragments of ideas, and shake them up with current events. They exert a selection, depending on the politics they want to promote (gate-keepers).

The consequences of this "mosaic" culture are:

– a half-random culture: each individual discovers the world in which he lives according to trials and errors
– a reversed cognitive act: in classical thought or "humanism", a cognitive act proceeds with deductions on the basis of general concepts, stages and logic. "Mosaic" culture induces a total reversal of these processes.

Principal influence networks and their respective stakes
Several levels of action are possible to influence the public (Figure 2) [3]. The first is *sensitization*, which corresponds to the first initiation of a given question or subject. The second level is *information*, where the elements of knowledge and assessment are organized. The most important level is the level of the *opinion leaders* (general or specialised). During his famous survey in 1940, the "People's Choice", Lazarsfeld [5], individualized a go-between group: the opinion leaders. The superiority of personal contacts explains how this group can influence public opinion more deeply than the media. The final level, *socialisation*, points out the group of individuals adopting the progressively received ideas.

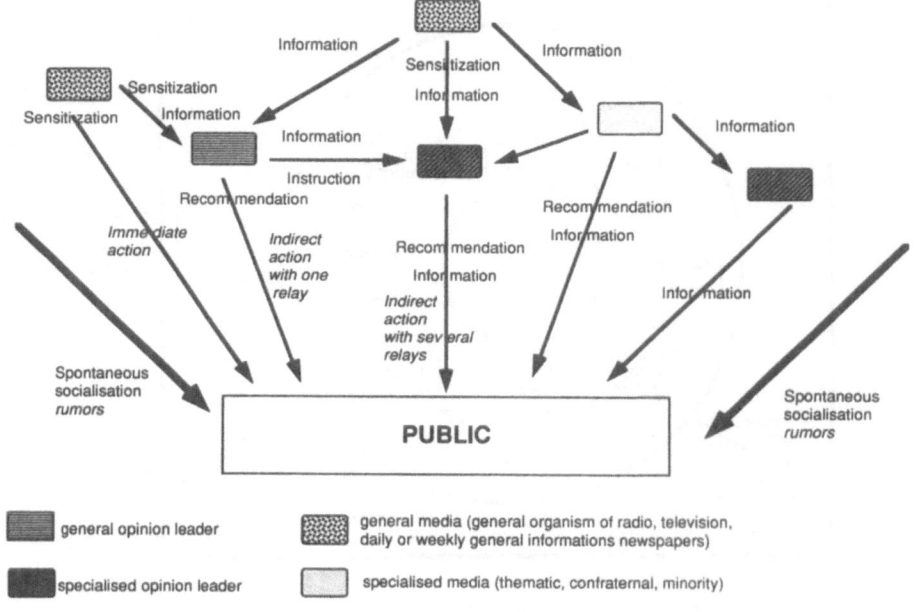

Fig. 2. Principal influence networks and their respective stakes.

General effects applied to transplantation

The general principles expressed above permit us to better understand the population's knowledge about and attitude toward organ donation and transplantation. The half-random and chaotic "mosaic" culture encourages feelings of wonder, uncertainty, fear or even horror by the public toward transplantation. This reaction could take a long time to emerge in the collective mind and, very likely, is not present in a country where transplantation is relatively new.

Popular culture, inherited from newspapers and movies, has acquired a use of language, which is unsuited to ideas underlying transplantation and organ donation (e.g. unpleasant connotation of "harvest", confusion induced by "brain death"). Popular culture's concept of death, the main idea related to transplantation, is exclusively inherited from the media and strikes the mind at a preconscious or unconscious level. The concept of death in a "mosaic" culture also opposes classical humanism, inherited from school, family, and ancient ways of life.

The efficiency of "opinion leaders" in promoting ideas and information could be used for transplantation education. Direct contact with individuals or groups, using their language, could deeply influence public opinion. Such is the current experience in Australia as regards the Australian cross-curriculum program for secondary schools. The first results are encouraging [1].

Conclusion

The media can be both a useful and confusing tool in promoting organ transplantation. The most effective system would be a social program including both the media and the opinion leaders, who could create direct contacts with individuals.

At least in my opinion, the polemic discussions around transplantation have not been created by journalists only to promote scandals or sensationalism: they are asking real questions but are often reporting the wrong or imprecise answers.

Transplantation Team ought to realize that transplantation is a choice of society, but a choice of adult society. A real culture of transplantation should be created, using education, family and rehabilitating the idea of Death in the Life.

References

1. Thomson NM, Sculy G, Knudson R, Wragg F, Angus J, White G, Marshall A. Transplantation – the issues: a cross curriculum programme for secondary schools. Transplant Proc 1993; 25: 1687–9.
2. Aswad S, Souqiyyeh MZ, Huraib S. The role of the media in cadaver transplantation in a developing country. Transplant Proceed 1992; 24: 2049–50.
3. Balle F. Médias et sociétés: presse, audiovisuel, télécommunication. 6th ed. Paris: Montchrestien Editors, 1992.
4. Moles A. Sociodynamique de la culture. Paris: Mouton, 1971.
5. Lazarsfeld P. The people's choice. New York: Free Press, 1948.

PART FIVE

Alternatives to human organ transplant

38. Gene therapy as an alternative to organ transplantation?

H. GILGENKRANTZ

Being a therapeutic tool appears to be the new status for DNA in the end of this century. The first example of gene therapy assay in humans consisted of transferring the adenosine desaminase gene in two little girls affected by a deficiency of this enzyme. This approach, therefore, could constitute an alternative possibility to marrow transplantation in this genetic disorder. Will gene therapy be the alternative to organ transplantation? Before answering this question, it is important to define what this new therapeutic approach covers.

Two different strategies

In the somatic gene therapy strategy, two different approaches have to be considered: (1) autografts of genetically modified cells or (2) direct transfer of the therapeutic gene. The principle of the first approach is to remove some cells from the patient, introduce the gene of interest into these cells and, finally, reinfuse the genetically modified cells in the patient. In some hematopoietic disorders, for example, hematopoietic stem cells constitute an excellent target for gene therapy since their longevity allows a prolonged therapeutic effect. In contrast, direct gene transfer will be proposed if the affected cells are disseminated or unable to be cultured ex vivo and/or reimplanted as tracheobronchial cells, for example.

How to transfer a gene?

Probably the most efficient tool to transfer DNA into cells either ex vivo or in vivo remains viruses. Until now, the most studied vectors have been retroviruses and adenoviruses. However, other non-immune vehicles are currently being developed, such as liposomes or DNA/polylysine complexes

J.L. Touraine et al. (eds.), Organ Shortage: The Solutions, 297–299.

linked to empty adenoviral particles. Each possesses advantages and disadvantages, which will be discussed.

What kind of gene?

Usually, the real therapeutic tool will not be the cDNA brought into the cells but the protein encoded by it. For genetic recessive disorders, the addition of one normal version of the altered gene in the affected cells could be sufficient to correct the phenotype by the expression of the corespondent protein in a sufficient amount. In some cases, however, the messenger will constitute the active molecule, as in the antisense approach for cancer, or to avoid stenosis after arterial dilatation, for example. In any case, the DNA of interest has to be known and cloned. This point can consititute a limitation of this approach since the molecular basis of some disorders are still not understood.

What kind of disorders?

Some recessive genetic disorders could be the first target of gene therapy: cystic fibrosis, hemophilia, ADA deficiency, have been among the first candidates. The deficiencies in one circulating enzyme or affections in which the correction of a limited number of cells could allow the diminution of the symptoms probably constitute the best candidates for a somatic gene therapy.

Besides genetic diseases, severe viral infections and some types of cancer have also been proposed for this kind of therapeutic trial.

Gene therapy as an alternative to transplantation?

Provided that the organ to be treated by one of these two approaches is not yet destroyed by the disease, somatic gene therapy could constitute, in some cases, an alternative to organ transplantation. However, two elements have to be considered:

1. the inheritance mode of the genetic disorder.
    - In dominant hereditary diseases, somatic gene therapy will probably have no place. In this case, the deleterious effect is produced by a function gain which will not a priori be replaced by an additional copy of the normal gene. In contrast, organ transplantation could be required and have a therapeutic effect.
    - In recessive disorders, where organ transplantation is an efficacious treatment, both approaches could be proposed.
2. the status of the defective organ

- If the organ to be replaced is unaffected by the defect, for example in urea cycle defects, both strategies will probably give positive results.
- If the organs is affected by the disease, as in the $\alpha 1$ antitrypsine deficiency, for example, especially if this disorder constitutes a cancer predisposition, transplantation will probably remain the only therapeutic possibility.

39. Xenochimerism and tolerance

MEGAN SYKES

Introduction

It has long been known that specific transplantation tolerance can be induced by transplanting hematopoietic cells across allogeneic histocompatibility barriers in lethally irradiated animal recipients [1–7]. This potent tolerance-inducing capacity of bone marrow results, in large part, from the ability of bone marrow-derived cells in the thymus to induce clonal deletion of developing thymocytes with T-cell receptors that recognize antigens they express [4, 8–10]. Thus, the regenerating T-cell repertoire is tolerant of the marrow donor. However, the use of this approach to the induction of transplantation tolerance is not practical in man, since successful bone marrow engraftment cannot reliably be achieved across major histocompatibility barriers, even after toxic myeloablative conditioning [11, 12], and because toxicity of preparative regimens which involve lethal whole body irradiation (WBI) [13, 14] and the risk of graft-vs-host disease (GVHD) [15–17] would not be justified in patients with non-malignant diseases. Therefore, the development of specific, relatively non-toxic methods of overcoming host resistance to allogeneic marrow engraftment will be necessary for the application of bone marrow transplantation to tolerance induction for organ allografts.

Protocols involving lethal WBI and bone marrow transplantation (BMT) have similarly been shown to permit marrow engraftment and induction of transplantation tolerance across xenogeneic barriers in rodent models [2, 18–21]. For similar reasons as those discussed above, it will be necessary to replace myeloablative conditioning regimens with regimens that specifically target those host elements which resist marrow engraftment, if BMT is to be a useful method of inducing specific transplantation tolerance across xenogeneic barriers in the clinical setting. Successful elimination of host elements that resist xenogeneic marrow engraftment should allow xenoengraftment to be achieved without a requirement for donor T-cells with the potential to cause GVHD. Development of a state of mixed lymphohematopoietic chimerism would be most desirable because of the improved immunocompetence that exists when host-type antigen-presenting cells are present

J.L. Touraine et al. (eds.), *Organ Shortage: The Solutions*, 301–308.
© 1995 *Kluwer Academic Publishers.*

in the peripheral tissues to allow optimal antigen presentation to T-cells that have developed in the host thymus, and which are therefore skewed toward recognition of peptide antigens in the context of host MHC.

A non-myeloablative conditioning regimen allowing xenogeneic marrow engraftment and the induction of mixed chimerism

Mixed chimerism and transplantation tolerance can be induced across complete allogeneic MHC barriers in mice using BMT after conditioning with a relatively non-toxic, non-myeloablative preparative regimen. This regimen involves specific elimination of host T-lymphocytes that resist engraftment using depleting doses of monoclonal antibodies (mAbs) against CD4–positive and CD8–positive T-cells [22]. Tolerance induction in these animals results primarily from initial ablation of the existing T-cell repertoire, followed by intrathymic generation of a new T-cell repertoire that is rendered tolerant by a clonal deletion mechanism. This deletion probably results from the presence of donor dendritic cells or macrophages, which can be detected in small numbers in the host thymus as early as 10 days following BMT, when host thymocytes begin to recover and show complete deletion of mature thymocytes with T-cell receptors that recognize donor antigens [23]. In addition, a small population of residual host T-cells that escapes antibody-mediated depletion in the periphery may be tolerized by an anergy mechanism when donor marrow is transplanted [23].

We have now extended this model to a xenogeneic rat/mouse strain combination [24]. Although mixed chimerism was not achieved using precisely the same preparative regimen which was successful in allogeneic combinations, the addition of host pretreatment with mAbs against natural killer (NK) cells and Thy1–positive cells permitted induction of mixed chimerism and specific tolerance after transplantation of T-cell-depleted rat BMC. The conditioning regimen includes administration of anti-CD4, CD8, NK1.1, and Thy1.2 mAbs on days −6 and −1, followed by a non-myeloablative dose of whole body irradiation (3 Gy) and a higher dose of local irradiation to the thymus (7 Gy) on day 0. T-cell depletion of rat marrow is necessary in order to avoid the complication of GVHD [24]. Recent studies have shown that similar levels of rat marrow engraftment can be achieved without thymic irradiation [37].

Donor-specific transplantation tolerance in mixed xenogeneic chimeras

Mixed xenogeneic rat→mouse chimeras prepared as described above demonstrate markedly prolonged acceptance of donor-strain rat skin grafts, with rapid rejection of non-donor strain third party rat skin grafts. Therefore, these chimeras are immunocompetent and are specifically tolerant of the xenogeneic donor strain. This tolerance has recently been confirmed by in vitro studies demonstrating long-term specific unresponsiveness to donor antigens in mixed lymphocyte reactions (MLR) and cell-mediated lympholysis (CML) reactions with normal anti-third party allo- and xeno-responses. This donor-specific skin graft tolerance and in vitro tolerance is still present up to at least one year following BMT. Although donor-specific skin grafts are eventually chronically rejected in these animals, we believe this rejection reflects recognition of skin-specific antigens, since, even after this rejection has occurred, we have observed specific unresponsiveness to donor antigens expressed on lymphohematopoietic cells in MLR and CML studies (L.A. Lee and M. Sykes, manuscript in preparation). Studies of recipient T-cell families using particular Vβ genes suggest that clonal deletion is a major mechanism of tolerance induction in these mice [37]. Consistent with the possibility that rat marrow-derived cells participate in negative selection in the thymus, preliminary studies have demonstrated the presence of rat cells with dendritic morphology in the thymi of chimeric mice (L.A. Lee and M. Sykes, unpub. data).

Stem cell competition as a factor limiting xenogeneic reconstitution

The level of rat hematopoietic reconstitution gradually declines in our chimeras, and rat cells are sometimes undetectable by 6 months following BMT [24]. Despite this decline, donor-specific skin graft prolongation and MLR and CML unresponsiveness were observed when skin grafting or in vitro studies were performed as late as one to one and a half years post-BMT (L.A. Lee and M. Sykes, manuscript in preparation). Because of these and other studies indicating that tolerance is maintained while chimerism is declining in these animals, we believe that donor-specific T-cell tolerance is maintained during the period when donor-type reconstitution declines. This loss of chimerism most likely reflects a competitive advantage enjoyed by host hematopoietic cells over xenogeneic ones. This advantage could be due to species differences in cytokines, adhesion molecules and their ligands, and other components of the marrow stromal environment. Since this environment is probably of host origin, it is not surprising that host hematopoiesis would gradually supercede donor rat hematopoiesis after recipient stem cells have recovered from the initial myelosuppressive irradiation dose.

Natural antibody tolerance in mixed xenogeneic chimeras

No evidence for an induced antibody response has been detected in mice rendered tolerant of rat antigens by BMT, even following the gradual decline in rat chimerism and the eventual rejection of rat donor skin grafts discussed above. However, when primarily vascularized organs are grafted between so-called "discordant" species [25], pre-formed i.e. "natural" antibodies (nAb), which are present despite the absence of prior known exposure to the donor antigens, are a major impediment to successful engraftment. We were therefore interested in the question of whether or not induction of mixed xenogeneic chimerism might be associated with a state of "natural antibody tolerance" in addition to the observed T-cell tolerance.

We have recently demonstrated that sera from normal, untreated mice contain nAb which bind to rat BMC but not rat lymphoid cells [26]. We used the mixed rat mouse chimera model to address the question of whether or not induction of mixed chimerism would be associated with suppression of donor-reactive nAb formation. A significant decrease was observed in the level of mouse nAb binding to rat BMC in rat BMT recipients compared to similarly-treated non-BMT control groups. This decline in nAb is unlikely to be due to adsorption of the mouse nAb on rat cells in the chimeras, since no mouse antibody bound to rat cells was detected at late times when the BMT recipients continued to show significantly reduced anti-rat nAb levels [27]. These results suggest that induction of mixed chimerism can lead to a state of tolerance among host nAb-producing B-cells.

Since swine are excellent potential xenogeneic organ donors for humans, we are interested in the potential of swine marrow to induce nAb tolerance for determinants expressed on swine endothelial cells. Absorption studies indicated that most human nAb target antigens expressed on swine endothelial cells are also shared by swine BMC and their progeny [28], suggesting that successful engraftment of swine marrow and induction of mixed chimerism in man might not only induce cellular tolerance, but could also induce tolerance among nAb-forming B-cells, and might therefore obviate the risk of hyperacute rejection when solid organ transplantation from swine donors was subsequently performed.

Swine BMT in immunodeficient mice

We next attempted to extend our results to a more disparate species combination, namely pig to mouse. To determine whether or not there were physiologic barriers to swine marrow engraftment in mice, we first performed studies in severe combined immunodeficient (SCID) mice, which lack T- and B-cell-mediated immunity [29]. Sublethal irradiation of SCID recipients permitted engraftment of swine marrow, resulting in partial, low level repopulation of blood, spleen and marrow by swine myeloid cells and in the presence of swine Ig in the serum. The levels of swine Ig gradually declined, and were undetectable by about 5 months following BMT. Swine hematopoietic progenitors were present in the marrow for at least 20 weeks post-BMT in some mice, suggesting that pluripotent hematopoietic stem cell engraftment may have been achieved [30]. However, long-term multilineage peripheral reconstitution by swine cells was not observed [30]. Since immune resistance was not a limiting factor in these mice, these results suggest that, in this extremely disparate species combination, non-immune species-specific environmental factors such as cytokines and adhesion molecules may limit reconstitution by xenogeneic marrow, so that the host hematopoietic cells enjoy an overwhelming advantage over the discordant donor. These results suggest that the addition of donor cytokines and/or genetic engineering to make swine marrow more "human-like" in its responsiveness to human environmental stimuli might be necessary for the successful use of this approach to the induction of xenotolerance in human recipients.

Swine thymus/liver grafts in SCID mouse recipients

We considered the possibility that improved swine reconstitution might be achieved if a swine stromal environment could also be provided. In an attempt to provide such an environment, we implanted second trimester fetal swine thymus and liver fragments under the kidney capsule of 4 Gy irradiated SCID mice. We also injected fetal liver cells from the same swine donors intraperitoneally as a source of swine hematopoietic stem cells [31, 32]. These fetal swine grafts grew markedly and survived for at least 4 months post-transplant. Histologically, these appeared to be normal thymi, and they contained swine T-cells and/or immature thymocytes. In these mice, swine T-cells appeared in the peripheral lymphoid tissues, and swine hematopoietic progenitor colonies were detected in the bone marrow of some of the recipients. Thus, primitive stem cells may have migrated from swine fetal liver fragments or cell suspensions to the marrow of these mice and survived long-term. Fetal liver cell suspensions were required in this model to maintain large numbers of swine T-cells in the grafts long-term, probably as a source of stem cells.

Swine fetal thymus/liver transplantation to immunocompetent mice

Because studies reported in the literature have demonstrated the capacity of thymic epithelium to induce T-cell tolerance, we evaluated the potential of swine fetal thymus/liver grafts to induce tolerance in immunocompetent mice. Euthymic or adult thymectomized (ATX) B10 mice were treated with T- and NK cell-depleting mAb's prior to treatment with 7 Gy mediastinal irradiation and 3 Gy WBI. Fetal pig thymus/liver grafts were placed under the kidney capsules and pig FLC were given i.p. Results of these studies showed that:

1) Murine T-cells that recovered in the host thymi of euthymic mice after conditioning therapy were not tolerized to pig antigens, and rejected pig thymus/liver grafts. Presumably, tolerance to pig antigens was not induced in these mice because mouse T-cell progenitors matured in the host

thymus, which lacked the pig antigens necessary to tolerize developing mouse thymocytes [33];

2) When mouse T-cells were continually depleted by repeated injections of anti-T-cell mAbs, the grafts grew markedly and swine thymopoiesis occurred continually in the swine thymus/liver grafts, but swine cells were not detectable in the peripheral lymphoid tissues. Mouse T-cells did not recover [33];

3) When mice were thymectomized but not given any additional anti-T-cell or anti-NK cell mAb's after two to six weeks post-transplantation, normal mouse thymopoiesis occurred in the grafted pig thymi. Thymocyte populations in the grafts were phenotypically almost indistinguishable from normal B10 thymocytes. Mature $CD4^+/CD8^-$ mouse T-cells were detected in peripheral blood and spleen and increased over time to normal levels. Peripheral $CD8^+$ T-cell numbers did not recover to the same extent as $CD4^+$ cells. The grafted pig thymi were required for the appearance of mouse $CD4^+$ cells in the periphery, and these cells appeared to be functional, as evidenced by normal alloresponsiveness in vitro and in vivo. Continued growth of the swine thymus/liver grafts in the presence of these mouse T-cells, coexistence of swine cells with mouse T-cells in some of the grafts, in vitro studies showing unresponsiveness to donor-type pig antigens, and the lack of IgG antibody responses to pig antigens all indicate that these mouse T-cells are tolerant of the swine donor (33).

These studies demonstrate that discordant xenogeneic thymic stroma is capable of supporting mouse thymopoiesis, and that $CD4^+$ mouse T-cells which are released into the periphery are phenotypically normal, functional and tolerant to donor xeno-antigens, and to host antigens. The lack of $CD8^+$ T-cell repopulation in the periphery may be due to failure of mouse CD8 to interact with pig MHC class I molecules [34], as has been demonstrated for mouse anti-human responses [35], thereby preventing efficient positive selection of $CD8^+$ thymocytes by swine thymic epithelium. Since human $CD8^+$ T-cells are able to interact with pig MHC class I directly [36], human $CD8^+$ T-cells might mature more effectively in swine fetal thymus grafts if this model were to be applied clinically to induce donor-specific tolerance to xenoantigens for clinical organ transplantation. Studies are currently in progress to extend these new approaches to inducing specific tolerance to large animal primate models.

Acknowledgements

This work was supported in part by a Sponsored Research Agreement from BioTransplant, Inc., and by NIH grant #HL49915.

References

1. Billingham RE, Brent L, Medawar PB. "Actively acquired tolerance" of foreign cells. Nature 1953; 172: 603.
2. Ildstad ST, Sachs DH. Reconstitution with syngeneic plus allogeneic or xenogeneic bone marrow leads to specific acceptance of allografts or xenografts. Nature 1984; 307(5947): 168.
3. Sykes M, Sheard M, Sachs DH. Effects of T cell depletion in radiation bone marrow chimeras: evidence for a donor cell population which increases allogeneic chimerism but which lacks the potential to produce GVHD. J Immunol 1988; 141: 2282.
4. Marrack P, Lo D, Brinster R, et al. The effect of thymus environment on T cell development and tolerance. Cell 1988; 53: 627.
5. Slavin S. Total lymphoid irradiation. Immunol Today 1987; 3: 88.
6. Pierce GE. Allogeneic versus semiallogeneic F1 bone marrow transplantation into sublethally irradiated MHC-disparate hosts: effects on mixed lymphoid chimerism, skin graft tolerance, host survival, and alloreactivity. Transplantation 1990; 49: 138.
7. Mayumi H, Good RA. Long-lasting skin allograft tolerance in adult mice induced across fully allogeneic (multimajor H-2 plus multiminor histocompatibility) antigen barriers by a tolerance-inducing method using cyclophosphamide. J Exp Med 1989; 169: 213.
8. van Ewijk W, Ron Y, Monaco J, et al. Compartmentalization of MHC class II gene expression in transgenic mice. Cell 1988; 53: 357.
9. Ramsdell F, Fowlkes BJ. Clonal deletion versus clonal anergy: the role of the thymus in inducing self tolerance. Science 1990; 248: 1342.
10. Schonrich G, Strauss G, Muller K-P, et al. Distinct requirements of positive and negative selection for selecting cell type and CD8 interaction. J Immunol 1993; 151: 4098.
11. O'Reilly RJ, Collins NH, Kernan N, et al. Transplantation of marrow depleted of T cells by soybean lectin agglutination and E-rosette depletion: major histocompatibility complex-related graft resistance in leukemic transplant recipients. Transplant Proc 1985; 17: 455.
12. Anasetti C, Amos D, Beatty PG, et al. Effect of HLA compatibility on engraftment of bone marrow transplants in patients with leukemia or lymphoma. New Engl J Med 1989; 320: 197.
13. Deeg HJ, Storb R, Thomas ED. Bone marrow transplantation: a review of delayed complications. Br J Haematol 1984; 57: 185.
14. Freirich EJ, Gehan EA, Rall DP, Schmidt LH, Skipper HE. Quantitative comparison of toxicity of anti-cancer agents in mouse, rat, hamster, dog, monkey, and man. Cancer Chemotherapy Rep 1966; 50: 219.
15. Sullivan KM, Witherspoon RP, Storb R, et al. Chronic graft-versus-host disease: recent advances in diagnosis and treatment. In: Gale RP, Champlin R, editors. Bone Marrow Transplantation: Current Controversies. New York: Alan R. Liss, Inc., 1989: 511.
16. Clift RA, Storb R. Histoincompatible bone marrow transplants in humans. Ann Rev Immunol 1987; 5: 43.
17. Makinodan T. Circulating rat cells in lethally irradiated mice protected with rat bone marrow. Proc Soc Exp Biol Med 1956; 92: 174.
18. Ildstad ST, Wren SM, Sharrow SO, Stephany D, Sachs DH. In vivo and in vitro characterization of specific hyporeactivity to skin xenografts in mixed xenogeneically reconstituted mice (B10+F344 rat→B10). J Exp Med 1984; 160: 1820.
19. Santos GW, Cole LJ. Effects of donor and host lymphoid and myeloid tissue injections in lethally X-irradiated mice treated with rat bone marrow. J Natl Cancer Inst 1958; 21: 279.
20. Bau J, Thierfelder S. Antilymphocytic antibodies and marrow transplantation. Transplantation 1973; 15: 564.
21. Muller-Rucholtz W, Muller-Hermelink HK, Wottge HU. Induction of lasting hematopoietic chimerism in a xenogeneic (rat→mouse) model. Transplant Proc 1979; 11: 517.
22. Sharabi Y, Sachs DH. Mixed chimerism and permanent specific transplantation tolerance induced by a non-lethal preparative regimen. J Exp Med 1989; 169: 493.

23. Tomita Y, Khan A, Sykes M. Role of intrathymic clonal deletion and peripheral anergy in transplantation tolerance induced by bone marrow transplantation in mice conditioned with a non-myeloablative regimen. J Immunol. 1994; 153: 1087.

24. Sharabi Y, Aksentijevich I, Sundt III TM, Sachs DH, Sykes M. Specific tolerance induction across a xenogeneic barrier: production of mixed rat/mouse lymphohematopoietic chimeras using a nonlethal preparative regimen. J Exp Med 1990; 172: 195.

25. Calne RY. Organ transplantation between widely disparate species. Transplant Proc 1970; 2: 550.

26. Aksentijevich I, Sachs DH, Sykes M. Normal mouse serum contains natural antibody against bone marrow cells of a concordant xenogeneic species. J Immunol 1991; 147: 79.

27. Lee LA, Sergio JJ, Sachs DH, Sykes M. Mechanism of tolerance in mixed xenogeneic chimeras prepared with a non-myeloablative conditioning regimen. Transplant Proc. 1994; 26: 1197.

28. Latinne D, Vitiello D, Sachs DH, Sykes M. Tolerance to discordant xenografts: human natural antibody determinants are shared on miniature swine bone marrow cells and endothelial cells. Transplantation 1994; 570: 238.

29. Schuler W, Weiler IJ, Schuler A, et al. Rearrangement of antigen receptor genes is defective in mice with severe combined immunodeficiency. Cell 1986; 46: 963.

30. Gritsch HA, Glaser RM, Emery DW, et al. The importance of non-immune factors in reconstitution by discordant xenogeneic hematopoietic cells. Transplantation 1994; 57: 906.

31. Gale RP. Development of the human immune system in human fetal liver. Thymus 1987; 10: 45.

32. Surh CD, Sprent J. Long-term xenogeneic chimeras: full differentiation of rat T and B cells in SCID mice. J Immunol 1991; 147: 2148.

33. Lee LA, Gritsch HA, Sergio JJ, et al. Specific tolerance across a discordant xenogeneic transplantation barrier. Proc Natl Acad Sci USA. 1994; 91: 10864.

34. Moses RD, Winn HJ, Auchincloss Jr H. Evidence that multiple defects in cell-surface molecule interactions across species differences are responsible for diminished xenogeneic T cell responses. Transplantation 1992; 53: 203.

35. Irwin MJ, Heath WR, Sherman LA. Species-restricted interactions between CD8 and the α3 domain of class I influence the magnitude of the xenogeneic response. J Exp Med 1989; 170: 1091.

36. Lucas PJ, Shearer GM, Neudorf S, Gress RE. The human antimurine xenogeneic cytotoxic response. I. dependence on responder antigen-presenting cells. J Immunol 1990; 144: 4548.

37. Tomita Y, Lee LA, Sykes M. Engraftment of rat bone marrow and its role in negative selection of murine T-cells in mice conditioned with a modified non-myeloablative regimen. Xenotransplant. In press.

40. Transgenic pigs and xenotransplantation

C.A. CARRINGTON, E.C. COZZI, G.A. LANGFORD,
A.C. RICHARDS, A. ROSENGARD, N. YANNOUTSOS
& D.G. WHITE

Introduction

The current shortage of donor organs for transplantation has led many groups to consider the use of animal organs as an alternative to human organs (xenotransplantation). Although, at first sight it would seem more reasonable to choose an animal phylogenetically closely related to man as a source of donor organs, such as one of the larger primates, for practical and ethical reasons the pig is a better candidate. Both pig and primate hearts and kidneys are similar, anatomically and physiologically, to the equivalent human organs, pig heart valves are currently used in cardiac surgery, and diabetics have been using porcine insulin for many years. However, pigs grow more rapidly than primates and achieve a size comparable with even the most over-fed human adult; and, unlike primates, pigs have large litters. So providing sufficient numbers of organs to meet the current, and predicted, demand would not be a problem. However, probably the greatest advantage in using pigs as organ donors is that they are already bred and slaughtered in large numbers to provide food. It will, therefore, be easier for the public to accept their use as organ donors. The use of more closely related species, such as baboons, is less likely to be acceptable to Western culture with its tendency to anthropomorphism.

There are also disadvantages in using pigs. First, the normal life-span of the pig is about 15 years. There is no way of knowing how long pig organs, successfully transplanted into humans, could remain viable. However, with a large supply of donor organs, it would theoretically be easy for a recipient to have more than one transplant. The initial xenograft could be used simply as a "bridge" to enable the patient to survive until a suitable human organ was available, or the patient could receive a second xenograft. Secondly, pigs are susceptible to atherosclerosis, and patients needing a transplant because of arterial disease could be at risk of developing the condition again. However, the same would be true of an allotransplant. The greatest problem is that a pig heart, transplanted into a human being, or perfused ex vivo with human blood, is subject to hyperacute rejection and usually ceases to function

J.L. Touraine et al. (eds.), Organ Shortage: The Solutions, 309–316.
© 1995 *Kluwer Academic Publishers*.

within 20–120 min. This extremely rapid rejection is mediated by complement [1].

Role of complement and regulators of complement activation

Complement can be activated either by the "classical pathway" which is initiated by the binding of antibody, or it can be activated by the "alternative pathway" which does not require antibody. Whichever pathway is most important in hyperacute rejection, both lead to the formation of C3 convertases which generate C3b. This then leads via C5–C9 to the formation of membrane attack complexes. These multi-peptide structures literally make holes in cell membranes and hence lyse them.

Complement is activated constitutively by the alternative pathway at a low rate all the time, but we are not gradually dissolved by our own immune system. The reason for this is that our cells are protected by regulators of complement activation (RCAs). Two members of this group are: Decay-Accelerating Factor (DAF, CD55) and Membrane Cofactor Protein, (MCP, CD46). These proteins are related structurally: they each have four short consensus repeats of sixty amino acids, and an O-glycosylated region. DAF has a glycosyl-phosphatidyl inositol (GPI) anchor, whereas MCP has a trans-membrane tail. They act on both the classical pathway and the alternative pathway of complement activation. Decay-accelerating factor, as its name implies, accelerates the decay of the C3 convertases, and MCP acts as cofactor to Factor I in the breakdown of the C3 convertases to the inactive form [2]. These molecules are species-specific; human DAF does not inhibit the activation of rabbit complement, and porcine DAF will not protect pig cells from the action of human complement. The work described here was based on the premise that organs from pigs transgenic for human RCAs would not be subject to hyperacute rejection.

Pigs transgenic for human DAF have been produced. These animals have been tested for hDAF DNA, expression of the transgene at the RNA and protein level, and for the complement regulatory function of the human protein.

Methods

Molecular biology

In order to produce pigs transgenic for human DAF, 2432 fertilised oocytes were micro-injected with a 6 kb DNA construct. This construct contained 4 kb of genomic DNA, incorporating the 5′ untranslated and signal peptide sequence of the DAF gene and the first exon and intron of the gene, linked to a 2 kb fragment that included the remaining exons of the gene (Figure 1). The piglets resulting from this procedure were screened for human DNA by

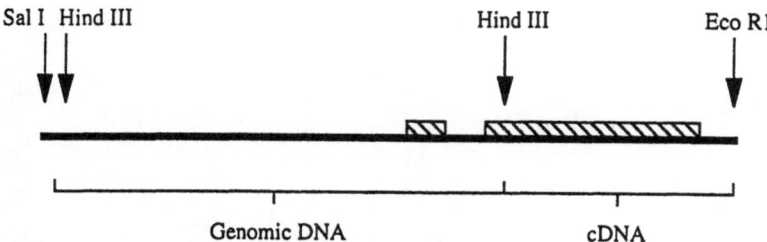

Fig. 1. The human DAF minigene construct. The human DAF minigene construct consisted of approximately 4 kb of genomic DNA between the two Hind III sites and 2 kb of cDNA between the Hind III site and the EcoR1 site. The genomic fragment which included 5′ untranslated and signal peptide sequences, the first exon and intron, extended to the Hind III site of the second exon. The Hind III to EcoR1 fragment included 41 adenosines constituting the mRNA poly-A tail.

slot-blot analysis of DNA extracted from ear biopsy samples. The samples were reacted with a radio-labelled cDNA probe for the human DAF gene and the signal detected by auto-radiography, the intensity of the signal being proportional to the number of copies of the gene incorporated. Blood samples from pigs positive for hDAF DNA were then screened by RT-PCR for expression of the human DAF gene. Tissue samples from a number of pigs, sacrificed during the course of the study, were assayed for expression by Northern blot (White et al. unpubl. data).

As the initial site of attack by complement in hyperacute rejection is the endothelium, endothelial cell cultures from normal pigs were transfected with hDAF. The hDAF construct used to produce the transgenic pigs was cloned into a plasmid which also contained a neomycin resistance gene as a selection agent. Several lines were isolated which were G418 resistant and which produced RNA for human DAF. These lines were then characterised by FACS analysis using an antibody specific for human DAF (BRIC 216) (Carrington et al. unpub. data).

Immunochemistry

Transgenic pigs were screened for expression of the hDAF protein on the cell surface of their peripheral blood mononuclear cells (PBMC) using a two-site immunoradiometric assay. Expression of hDAF protein in the tissue homogenates from sacrificed animals was also analysed by ELISA (White et al. unpubl. data).

Immunohistochemical analysis was performed on sections of tissue frozen in liquid nitrogen. Serial sections were stained with haematoxylin and eosin, an antibody for von Willebrand's Factor (an endothelial cell marker) and an antibody (BRIC 216) for human DAF (Rosengard et al. unpub. data).

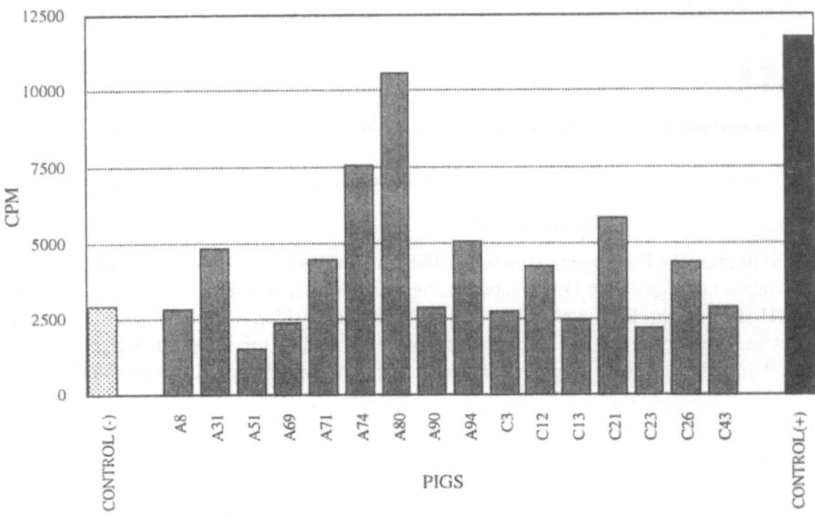

Fig. 2. Human DAF expression on the Cell Surface of Peripheral Blood Mononuclear Cells. The cell surface expression of hDAF by PBMC of transgenic pigs was determined by immunora-diometric assay. Negative control = PBMC of normal pig (5×10^6), PBMC from individual transgenic pigs indicated by number (5×10^6), positive control = human PBMC (1×10^6).

Complement lysis assay

Lymphocytes from normal or transgenic pigs, or endothelial cell cultures, were labelled with ^{51}Cr, and then incubated for 30 min with heat-inactivated human serum as a source of natural anti-pig antibodies. This was followed with a 2 h incubation with serial dilutions of human serum and the released radioactivity determined. Negative controls were incubated with medium alone, or with serial dilutions of pig serum. Positive controls were incubated with baby rabbit complement, or Tween 80 (Carrington et al. unpub. data).

Results

Using the micro-injection technique, 49 pigs transgenic for human DAF were produced, of which 45 were live births. The number of copies of the human DAF gene incorporated into the genome of these pigs varied from 1 to more than 30.

Approximately 67% of the founder transgenic generation showed detectable expression of RNA for hDAF. The level of expression varied between pigs, and also between tissues within the same pigs. There was no correlation between copy number and expression levels. This is because expression

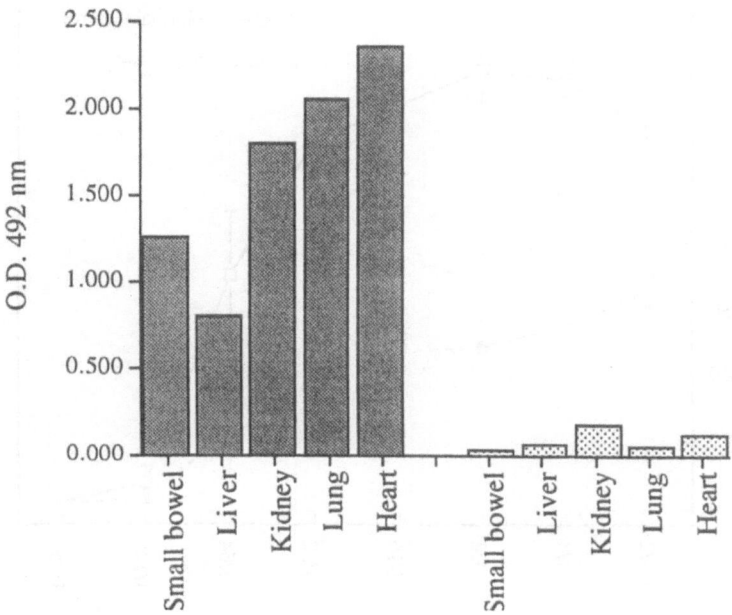

Fig. 3. Human DAF expression on different tissues of transgenic pig C46 and a normal control pig. Cell surface expression of hDAF in cell lysates from tissues of normal and transgenic pig (C46) was determined by ELISA. All lysates were present in the assay at the same concentration of protein.

depends on the site of integration, since there may be enhancer regions upstream or downstream from the insertion.

Expression of the hDAF protein on peripheral blood mononuclear cells, unsurprisingly, showed variation between pigs, but a number were clearly expressing hDAF on their PBMC (Figure 2). Similarly, with tissue homogenates, the level of expression varied from pig to pig, and from tissue to tissue within each pig (Figure 3). In some cases the level of protein detected is equivalent to that in the corresponding human organ.

Variation was also found at the histological level: between pigs, between tissues, and between different cell types within tissues. For example, hDAF has been demonstrated in the endothelial cells, or in the smooth muscle cells, or in both cell types in the arteries of different transgenic pigs.

Lymphocytes from both normal and transgenic pigs were lysed by rabbit complement and showed no significant degree of lysis with autologous sera. However, while lymphocytes from normal pigs were lysed by human complement, those from transgenic pigs exhibited a significant degree of protection from lysis (Figure 4).

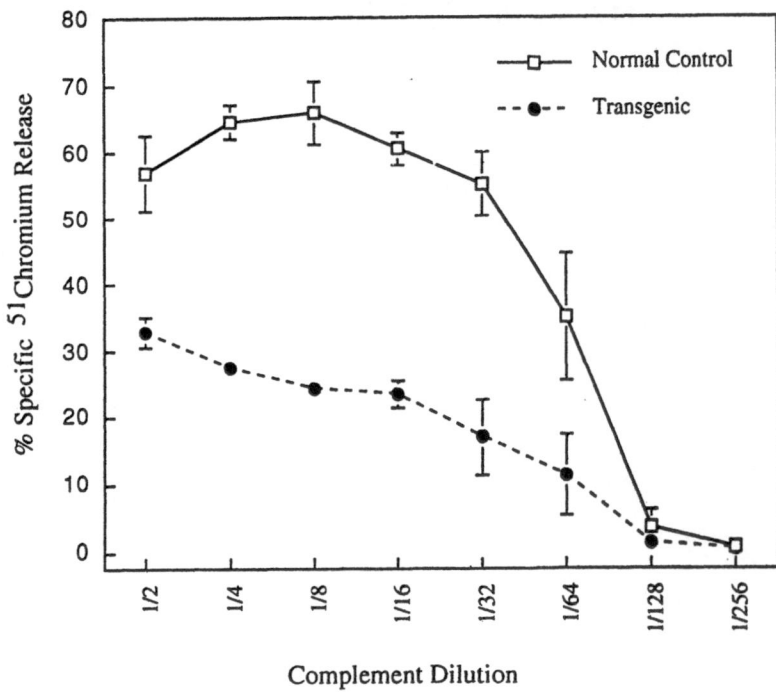

Fig. 4. Human complement mediated cytotoxicity of porcine lymphocytes from normal or hDAF transgenic pigs. Protection of transgenic pig A80 PBMC from lysis by human complement. Specific lysis was expressed as $[(cpm_{exp} - cpm_{ctrl}) / (cpm_{total} - cpm_{ctrl})] \times 100$, where cpm_{ctrl} is the non-specific release.

FACS analysis of the parent pig endothelial cell line, PAE-26a, showed no reaction with the anti-DAF antibody (BRIC 216), and a negative transfectant, PAE-26a9, which had incorporated the neomycin resistance gene but not the hDAF gene, was also not bound by the anti-DAF antibody. However, the positive transfectants, (such as PAE-26a8), exhibited a similar mean shift to that of human endothelial cells (HUVECs).

In Cr-release assays (Figure 5), all the pig endothelial cell lines were lysed by baby rabbit complement, and the untransfected cells, PAE-26a, and the negative transfectants, PAE-26a9, were also lysed by human complement. However, PAE-26a8, the hDAF positive cells were almost completely protected from lysis by human complement (Carrington et al. unpub. data).

The transgenic pigs grow and develop normally, and are now producing piglets of their own. Unfortunately, breeding homozygous transgenic pigs is not a simple case of mating a male transgenic pig with a female transgenic pig. As the site of insertion of the human construct is not controlled, each of the founders is unique: they have different numbers of copies of the gene, inserted into different sites in the genome. Therefore, female pig A and male pig B may not even bear their human transgene on the same chromosome.

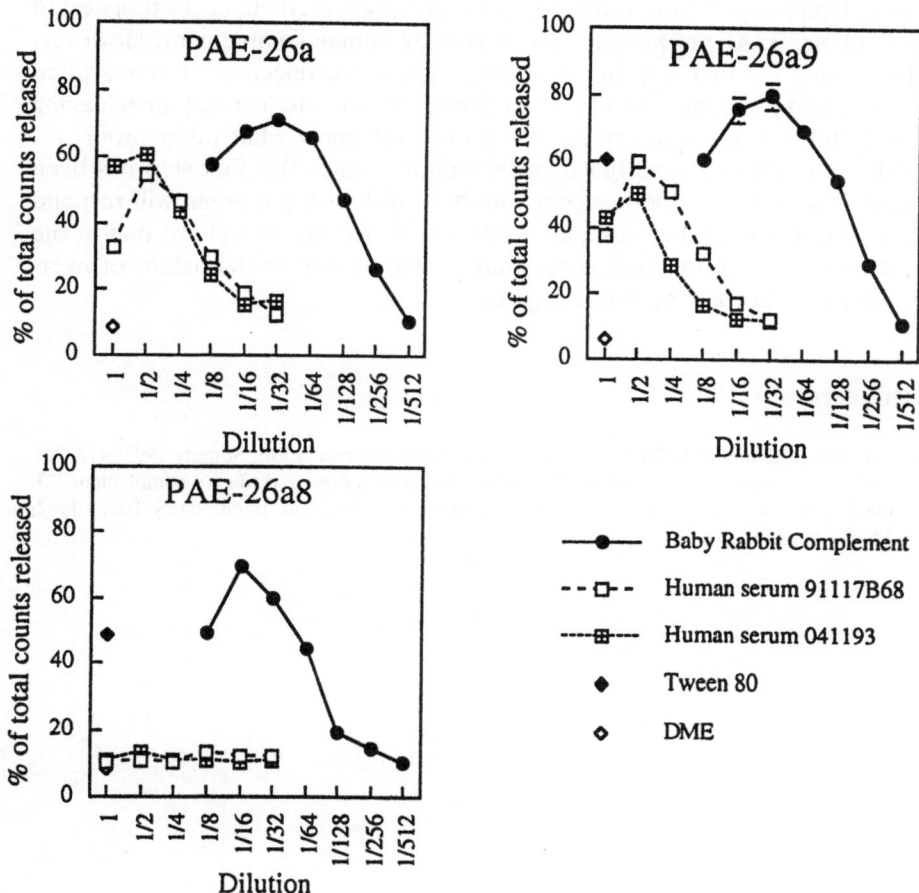

Fig. 5. Lysis of pig endothelial cells by human and rabbit complement. Protection of hDAF positive transfected pig endothelial cells from lysis by human complement. Specific lysis was expressed as (cpm_{exp} / (cpm_{total}) × 100.

Therefore, litters of f1 heterozygotes are being produced by crossing the best founder transgenics with normal pigs. Transgenic male and female siblings will then be bred to produce pigs homozygous for hDAF. These f2 homozygotes will have twice the number of genes for DAF as the parent generations, and in theory could exhibit twice the expression of hDAF protein.

Conclusions

In summary, we have shown that pigs can be made transgenic for human DAF, and that such pigs develop, grow, and breed normally. Peripheral blood lymphocytes from transgenic pigs, and pig endothelial cells transfected with human DAF are protected from lysis by human complement. However, this is only the first step in preventing hyperacute rejection of xenografted organs; and preventing hyperacute rejection is only the first step in achieving successful xenotransplantation. We do not yet know what other problems, both immunological and biochemical will arise once this first step has been taken. For instance, there is some doubt as to how a pig organ will respond in vivo to human cytokines and hormones. However, we believe that in the relatively near future, transgenic animals will be one of the means of overcoming the shortage of donor organs.

References

1. Braidley P, Dunning J, White D, Wallwork J. Xenotransplantation. Surgery 1993; 477–80.
2. Holers VM, Kinoshita T, Molina H. The evolution of mouse and human complement C3-binding proteins: divergence of form but conservation of function. Immunology Today 1992; 13 231–6.

41. The endothelial cell as a target of xenogeneic hyperacute rejection

Y. CALMUS, J. CARDOSO, L. GAMBIEZ, CH. CHÉREAU,
D. HOUSSIN & B. WEILL

For several years, our group has been interested in experimental models of discordant xenografts. The pig-to-human donor-recipient combination could have some clinical relevance in the future but experimentation is limited to in vitro and ex vivo models. In contrast, the guinea pig-to-rat combination also allows in vivo experimentation, but the data provided by such transplantations cannot easily be extrapolated to any clinical condition. In these experimental models, hyperacute rejection occurs within several minutes or hours, according to the combination or organ considered [2, 14]. This rejection is primarily mediated by the activation of the recipient's complement through its direct and alternative pathways which are simultaneously involved [4, 11]. The graft endothelial cells are the first targets encountered by the recipient's blood as soon as it bursts into the graft. Natural (preformed) antibodies [17, 18] bind to xenoantigens borne by the graft endothelium and engage the direct pathway [3, 6, 8], while the alternative pathway is activated by the contact with some unknown foreign molecules present on the endothelial surface [10, 15].

An ex vivo model of xenogeneic hyperacute rejection of pig liver: Role of complement [13; Cardoso et al., in press]

Liver xenotransplantation has been chosen as an experimental model because it is related to the clinical activity of our department. Isolated pig livers perfused with human blood were used to analyse the features of hyperacute rejection in the pig-to-human combination. Perfusion of pig livers was performed through portal vein and hepatic artery by warmed and oxygenated diluted human blood. Hyperacute rejection, determined by the occurrence of hemorragic necrosis, occurred in 4–5 hours. However, three successive phenomena preceded this end-point: first, a sinusoidal ectasy progressively increasing from the first hour on; then a heterogeneous hepatocyte necrosis; finally, a thrombosis of the micro- and macro-vascular beds invariably occurred when anticoagulants were omitted. Immunoglobulins (Ig) and comple-

J.L. Touraine et al. (eds.), *Organ Shortage: The Solutions*, 317–321.
© 1995 *Kluwer Academic Publishers.*

ment deposition was observed by immunohistochemistry as early as 10–30 min. Linear deposits of IgG, IgM, C1q, C3b, and factor B along the sinusoids confirmed that human complement had been activated through both pathways. Taken together, these data suggest that the endothelial cell is an essential target of hyperacute xenogeneic rejection in the pig-to-human model, and that the activation of complement plays a role in the appearance of endothelial lesions.

An ex vivo model of xenogeneic hyperacute rejection of guinea pig heart: Role of natural antibodies [6, 7]

In order to determine the role of natural antibodies in the occurrence of hyperacute xenogeneic rejection, we designed a model of isolated guinea pig heart perfused with rat serum using a Langendorf apparatus. Isolated guinea pig hearts were perfused through their coronary vessels with warmed and oxygenated buffer. Hyperacute rejection, determined by the cessation of heart beats, occurred 15 min after xenogeneic serum had been introduced into the circuit. In addition, rat IgG and IgM deposits were observed by immunohistochemistry after a few minutes.

We attempted to inhibit the fixation of natural rat anti-guinea pig antibodies by perfusing either rat $F(ab')\mu$ or $F(ab')_2\gamma$ prior to transplantation. Perfusing the guinea pig heart with rat $F(ab')\mu$ induced a significant delay in the rejection time (29 min vs. 14 min in the control group), whereas perfusing rat $F(ab')_2\gamma$ had no effect.

These data suggest that IgM, but not IgG, are responsible for the induction of hyperacute rejection in the guinea pig-to-rat model. Extrapolation of these results to other combinations remains elusive.

An in vitro model of xenogeneic hyperacute rejection in the pig-to-human combination: Mechanism of complement activation [16, 20]

In order to determine the mechanism of complement activation in the pig-to-human combination, we designed an in vitro model using pig aortic endothelial cells as targets and human serum as source of xenogeneic natural antibodies and complement. The cytotoxic activity of human serum was evaluated by means of a colorimetric assay using MTT. The rate of complement-dependent cytotoxicity oberved was 50% with undiluted human serum and 8% with syngeneic serum. The cytotoxic activity of C1q- or factor B-deficient xenogeneic sera was significantly less than that of normal sera, while the cytotoxicity of a mixture of both deficient sera was of the same order of magnitude as that of normal sera. These data suggest that complement activation is essential to the appearance of cytolytic lesions observed during hyperacute rejection, and that the two pathways of activation are involved.

Target antigens

Target antigens of hyperacute rejection were analysed in the rat-to-guinea pig and guinea pig-to-rat combinations using an immunoblotting technique [1]. Various tissular preparations (crude organ extracts, purified liver cell membranes, isolated endothelial cells and hepatocytes) were used; after electrophoresis, antigens were transferred onto nitrocellulose membranes and incubated with xenogeneic sera. Enzyme-linked anti-Ig (IgM or IgG) antibodies were then added to reveal natural antibodies combined with xenoantigens. Our results showed that, in the rat-to-guinea pig combination, proteins of 55 kD were the target of natural IgM; these antigens were present on the various organ preparations studied and also on the endothelial cells. However, they were absent from hepatocytes. In the guinea pig-to-rat combination, the molecular weight of the main target antigens was 110 kD. These data confirm that the target antigens of hyperacute xenogeneic rejection are present on endothelial cells, and suggest that they are ubiquitous.

Similar results have been obtained by Platt et al. in the pig-to-human combination [11, 12]: three main bands of 115, 125 and 135 kD are the targets of natural human IgM. The disappearance of those bands after pretreatment of the nitrocellulose membranes by glycosidases suggests that at least some antigens are glycoproteins, and that oligosaccharidic epitopes are recognized by human natural antibodies. Actually, natural antibodies are very heterogeneous and some of them probably recognize the protein core of these glycoproteins [19]. Indeed, an attempt to sequence these molecules suggest strong homologies with integrins.

Characterization of the target epitopes

The nature of the carbohydrate moiety of the xenoantigens recognized in the pig-to-human combination has been recently studied by several groups. Cooper et al. (1988) [3] have shown that di- or trisaccharides bearing the Gal (α1,3) Gal sequence significantly inhibited hyperacute rejection in in vitro and in vivo models. Data from our group, using in vitro models of cytotoxicity, indicate that the disaccharide GlcNAc (α1,4) Gal is also a major target epitope in the same pig-to-human combination [19].

Comparison between the antigenic properties of aortic endothelial cells and those of liver sinusoidal endothelial cells [Cottan et al., in press]

Most teams currently use aortic endothelial cells for in vitro studies, since they are much easier to isolate and culture than endothelial cells from organs. However, it has been established that endothelial cells from large vessels have morphological and physiological characteristics that differ from those of organ endothelial cells. In particular, sinusoidal endothelial cells in the liver have large fenestrae, weak intercellular adhesion structures, no real basal lamina and strongly express von Willebrand factor, compared to vascular endothelial cells.

In order to investigate whether aortic endothelial cells were appropriate target cells for in vitro models of hyperacute rejection, we have used aortic endothelial cells and sinusoidal endothelial cells isolated from pig liver in complement-mediated cytotoxicity tests, immunoblotting, and flow cytometry experiments. Aortic cells have been obtained from aortic intima according to conventional methods. Sinusoidal endothelial cells have been purified from liver cells obtained by collagenase perfusion of pig livers. Purity of this cell population was 80%. Our results indicate that aortic and sinusoidal endothelial cells were similar in terms of in vitro cytotoxicity and antigen expression, suggesting that both cell types can be used indifferently to study the mechanisms of xenogeneic hyperacute rejection in the pig-to-human combination.

Conclusion

The above data indicate that endothelial cells are the main targets of hyperacute xenogeneic rejection in several discordant combinations, namely in the pig-to-human combination. In vitro lysis of endothelial cells by human sera involves complement activation through both alternative and direct pathways, and requires the presence of natural antibodies.

However, in addition to cytotoxicity, which has been largely reported as a mechanism of hyperacute rejection, other phenomena are probably involved in the rejection process. Indeed, in vivo and ex-vivo, the graft necrosis is not due to endothelial cytolysis which is a delayed phenomenon. It is the consequence of an extensive thrombosis resulting from a loss of anticoagulant components and production of procoagulant substances by activated endothelial cells. However, in isolated hearts perfused with sera (devoid of fibrinogen and cells), hyperacute rejection occurs without thrombosis and obvious necrosis. The earliest phenomenon occurring in those models is a strong vasoconstriction [5, 9]. Therefore, the hyperacute rejection of xenografts results from complement activation, vasoconstriction and thrombosis, which are the three main mechanisms that therapeutic regimens should abrogate [5].

References

1. Calmus Y, Ayani E, Cardoso J, Chéreau C, Kahan A, Houssin D, and Weill B. The target antigens of hyperacute xenogeneic rejection in the rat/guinea pig and guinea pig/rat discordant combinations. Transplantation 1993; 56: 778–85.

2. Calne R. Organ transplantation between widely disparate species. Transplant Proc 1970; 2: 550–3.
3. Cooper DKC, Human PA, Lexer G. Effects of cyclosporine and antibody absorption on pig cardiac xenograft survival in the baboon. J Heart Transplant 1988; 7: 238–46.
4. Dalmasso AP, Vercellotti GM, Fischel RJ, Bolman RM, Bach FH, Platt JL. Mechanism of complement activation in the hyperacute rejection of porcine organs transplanted into primate recipients. Am J Pathol 1992; 140: 1157–66.
5. Filipponi F, Michel A, Houssin D. Prologation of guinea pig-to-rat xenograft survival with BN 52063, a specific antagonist of platelet-activation factor. Ital J Surg Sci 1989; 19: 325–9.
6. Gambiez L, Weill BJ, Chéreau Ch, Calmus Y, Houssin D. The hyperacute rejection of guinea pig-to-rat heart xenografts is mediated by preformed IgM. Transplant Proc 1990; 22: 1058–9.
7. Gambiez L, Salamé E, Chéreau C, Calmus Y, Ayani E, Houssin D, Weill BJ. Role of natural IgM in the hyperacute rejection of discordant heart xenografts. Transplantation 1992; 54: 577–83.
8. Hammer C, Chaussy C, Brendel C. Preformed natural antibodies in animals and man: outlook on xenotransplantation. Eur Surg Res 1973; 5: 162–5.
9. Massault PP, Calmus Y, Carayon A, Cherruau B, Legendre C, Weill B, Houssin D. Early endothelin production during hyperacute xenogeneic rejection of the liver. Transplant Proc 1994; 26: 1078.
10. Miyagawa S, Hirose H, Shirakura R, Naka Y, Nakata S, Kawashima Y, Seya T, Matsumoto M, Uenaka A, Kitamura H. The mechanism of discordant xenograft rejetion. Transplantation 1988; 46: 825–30.
11. Platt JL, Bach FH. The barrier to xenotransplantation. Transplantation 1991; 52: 937–47.
12. Platt JL, Lindman BJ, Chen H, Spitalnik SL, Bach FH. Endothelial cell antigens recognized by xenoreactive human natural antibodies. Transplantation 1990; 50: 817–22.
13. Platt JL, Fischel RJ, Matas AJ, Reif SA, Bolman RM, Bach FH. Immunopathology of hyperacute xenograft rejection in a swine to primate model. Transplantation 1991; 52: 214–20.
14. Tavakoli R, Devaux JY, Nonnenmacher L, Louvel A, Weill B, Houssin D. Discordant lung xenograft rejection in the rat. Transplantation 1991; 53: 235–7.
15. Tavakoli R, Michel A, Cardoso J, Ayani E, Maillet F, Fontaliran F, Crougneau S, Weill B, Houssin D. Prolonged survival of guinea pig-to-rat heart xenografts using repeated low doses of cobra venom factor. Transplant Proc 1993; 25: 407–9.
16. Termignon JL, Calmus Y, Chéreau Ch, Kahan, Houssin D, Weill BJ. In vitro analysis of complement activation in xenogeneic hyperacute rejection. Transplant Proc 1990; 22: 1060–1.
17. Turman MA, Bach FH, Casali P, Platt JL. Polyreactivity and antigen specificity of human xenoreactive monoclonal and serum natural antibodies. Transplantation 1991; 52: 710–7.
18. Van de Stadt J, Vendeville B, Weill B, Crougneau S, Michel A, Filipponi F, Icard P. Renoux M, Louvel A, Houssin D. Discordant heart xenografts in the rat: additional effect of plasma exchange and cyclosporine, cyclophosphamide or splenectomy in delaying hyperacute rejection. Transplantation 1988; 45: 514–8.
19. Zhao Z, Michalski JC, Chéreau C, Calmus Y, Houssin D, Weill B. An approach to the structure of carbohydrate epitopes recognized by human natural antibodies on porcine endothelial cells. Proceedings of the Second International Congress on xenotransplantation; 1993 Sept 26–29; Cambridge, UK.
20. Zhao Z, Termignon JL, Cardoso J, Chéreau C, Gautreau C, Calmus Y, Houssin D, Weill B. Hyperacute xenograft rejection in the swine to human donor-recipient combination: in vitro analysis of complement activation. Transplantation 1994; 57: 245–9.

PART SIX

Posters

ORGAN DONATION

The Follow up of the French Grafts.

Philippe Romano, M.Busson, J.Hors.

France-Transplant, 75475 PARIS Cedex 10

From 1985 to 1994, the 103 french transplantation teams have operated 19910 grafts. We present the follow up of these organs from the data base of France Transplant which is an exhaustive registry of grafted patients.

3663 heart transplantations [30 teams] .
At seven years, 49% patients are alive.
There is a difference, 59% versus 27% at four years between first and second graft.

360 heart-lungs transplantations [18 teams].
At five years 30% are alive.

301 lungs transplantations [15 teams], The first one took place in France in 1987. At four years 37% are alive.

3223 liver grafts [26 teams].
All together 66% are living at one year and 53% at seven years.
At the fifth year there are a difference between :!
    * emergency transplantation 41% and non urgent 58%.
    * first transplantation 57% and second transplantation 34%.

21705 kidney grafts [40 teams].
From the total 53% grafts are functional at seven years.
There is no a significant difference between first and second graft.
At six years there is a difference between cadaveric 59% and relatives living donors 85%.

Conclusions
* These results have to be examined center by center and for each etiology.
* Second transplantations, for liver and particularly for heart, are ethical problems regarding the scarcity of available organs.

Acknolewdgements :   We   thank   all   intensive   care   units   members,   coordinators   and transplantation teams of France-Transplant for their participation in collecting data.

OUTCOME OF 490 KIDNEYS PROCURED FROM BRAIN DEAD DONORS IN ONE CENTER

G. BENOIT[1], P. BLANCHET[1], D. DEVICTOR[4], H. BENSADOUN[1], C. RICHARD[2], J. DEPRET[2], A. DECAUX[3], J. DECARIS[5], B. CHARPENTIER[6]

[1]Department of Urology, [2]Medical ICU, [3]Surgical ICU, [4]Pediatric ICU, [5]Nurse coordinators, and [6]Nephrology department, Hopital de Bicêtre, 78 rue du Général Leclerc, 94270 BICETRE FRANCE

The role HLA compatibility, antibody level and age have been clearly demonstrated.
We compared in a group of 490 procured kidneys in one center the effect of brain death causes, multiorgan procurement, hemodynamic unstability, external cardiac massage, epinephrine, lasix, age, sex and the preservation solution on the graft outcome 1 month after transplantation.

	N	creatininemia before procurement (µmo/l)		creatininemia 1 month after translantation (µmo/l)	
cranio encephalic trauma	178	116 ± 46		165 ± 93	
vascular hemorrhage	146	110 ± 53	p= 0.01	187 ± 149	NS
cranio encephalic wound	73	122 ± 36		206 ± 183	
anoxia	63	132 ± 52		196 ± 151	
multi-organ procurement +	387	115 ± 46	p=0.02	170 ± 116	p= 0.007
multi-organ procurement -	102	127 ± 58		221 ± 184	
stable hemodynamics	331	111 ± 44	p= 0.0001	165 ± 107	p= 0.006
unstable hemodynamics	154	133 ± 56		215 ± 178	
external cardiac massage +	116	134 ± 54	p= 0.0003	205 ± 164	NS
external cardiac massage -	363	113 ± 46		174 ± 124	
Epinephrine +	124	142 ± 59		202 ± 162	
Epinephrine -	318	108 ± 41	p= 0.001	176 ± 124	NS
Lasix +	79	138 ± 63		190 ± 99	
Lasix -	388	113 ± 45	p= 0.002	180 ± 143	NS
Age < 15 years	49	87 ±30		165 ± 122	
Age 16 to 55 years	403	122 ± 49	p= 0.001	180 ± 136	NS
age > 55 years	37	113 ± 56		211 ± 134	
male	364	123 ± 48		184 ± 144	
female	126	102 ± 47	p= 0.001	170 ± 100	NS
UW solution	267	114 ± 49		173 ± 124	
Eurocollins solution	95	120 ± 57	NS	220 ± 171	p= .006

This study shows that under these conditions 3 others factors unvolve a 50 µmol/l creatininemia increase at 1 month posttransplantation, so they must also be taken into account in kidney sharing.

ORGAN SHORTAGE AND A LOCAL WAITING LIST ALLOW A LOCAL KIDNEY ALLOCATION POLICY TO ENSURE BOTH SHORT ISCHEMIA TIME AND GOOD HLA-A,B,DR MATCHING.

Bertoni E., Tosi P.L., Bandini S., Rosati A., Pradella F., Mattiuz P., Taddei G., Nicita G., Salvadori M., Rindi P.*, Rizzo G.*, Carmellini M.**, Mosca F.**.

Dept. of Transplantation – Careggi Hospital and University of Florence.
*Division of Nephrology – Santa Chiara Hospital Pisa
**Institute of Experimental and General Surgery – University of Pisa

Organ shortage in our country is the main limiting factor to the transplant activity and generates a long waiting list, anyway the quality of transplant is as good as in foreign countries.Delayed graft function (DGF) defined as need of dialysis during the first week after transplantation,causes a worse outcome of renal grafts.DGF is related ,among other factors,to cold ischemia time that is certainly shorter in local sharing programs.However local organization could not assure an optimal HLA-A,B.DR matching because of short waiting lists. This seems not to be our case where severe organ shortage, long waiting list and local sharing ensures both short ischemia time and optimal HLA-A,B,DR matching.

Our Kidney Transplant program based on Tuscany, an Italian region 22.292 square Km wide and 3.5 x 10^6 inhabitants, started with two centers on 1991.We reviewed the charts of 93 primary, not immunized renal allografts performed from 01-01-1991 to 30-06-1993 for donor and recipient clinical data as well as for the data collected from the waiting list.

Due both to the increasing number of pts. waiting for a kidney graft in our program (303, 289, 342 respectively in 1991, 1992, 1993) and better clinical results obtained with a good HLA-A,B,DR match in large series of pts. treated with Cyclosporine A we assumed the histocompatibility as major criteria for organ allocation (a minimum of 1B + 1DR antigens match required).Over the period of the present study only 6 kidneys (6.3%) were not locally allocated and were sent outside the program.The histocompatibility of the transplanted kidneys has been very high. Looking at HLA-A,B,DR mismatches we had respectively 13.4%, 29.1%, 36.3%, 17.9% transplants with 1,2,3,4 mismatches. Looking at HLA-B,DR mismatches we had respectively 16.2%, 44.1%, 39.1% transplants with 0,1,2, mismatches.These results were better than those reported by the Collaborative Transplant Study (CTS).

Mean cold ischemia time was 17 hours over 93 transplants,ranging from 6 to37 hours. 30.1% of the kidneys were transplanted in 12 hours;51.6% between 12 and 24 hours and only 18.3% after 24 hours of cold storage.The overall results of our renal transplant activity were good with an incidence of DGF of 22.6%.The actual patient survival at one year was 97.8%.The actual graft survival at one year was 86%.Actual graft survival at one year in the group of the 21 patients experiencing DGF was 71.4% vs. 90.3% out of the 72 patients that didn't have DGF.

In the case of organ shortage and a wide waiting list a local organization allocates the vast majority of the retrieved organs allowing low costs,short ischemia times,reduced DGF,good HLA matching and a good graft survival.In such conditions national allocation policies should be reserved to hyperimmune patients, urgencies, pediatrics, etc.

FRANCE TRANSPLANT REGIONAL TRANSPLANT COORDINATION UNIT °3
JJ COLPART, B GUILLOT, G SAURY, B MAILLEFAUD, B BOUTTIN, A MARION,
D MINARRO, C MICAUD, JF MOSKOVTCHENKO - FRANCE TRANSPLANT
REGIONAL COORDINATION Lyon

1. France Transplant Organization
France is divided with seven regions. One each region is managed by
intensivist MD as regional transplant coordinator. Transplant coordinators
have to respect national and regional rules.
2. France Transplant region n°3 organization
This region is compound of Auvergne, Bourgogne, Rhône Alpes and La
Réunion island. The surface is 101 468 km2 and the population is 8 281 568
inhabitants.
3. France Transplant region n°3 functionning
    3.1. human means an 1 MD, 1 chief nurse, 4 nurses, 2 secretaries
    3.2. materiel means an telecom and computer networks, rent road and
air services
    3.3. 2 nurses are on duty H/24 one for multiorgan procurement
regulation and the other one for coordination and technical help in general
hospitals
        3.3.1. M.O.P. regulation
        In 1993, a 512 organ proposals were managed by regional
transplant coordination unit. 250 potential donors were referred and 167
donors were harvested. The percentage of multiorgan donor was 83,2 %, 72
organs per million population were procured, 19,6 % of refusals were noted
but only 9,83% in general hospitals versus 26,20% in University hospitals
        3.3.2. Technical Aid
        In 1993 regional transplant coordinator nurses participated in 45
multiorgan procurement inside general hospital that specific activity
procured 158 organs which 26% of global regional activity

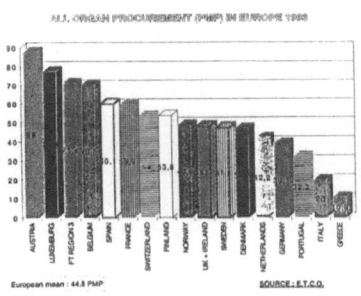

THE ORGANIZATIVE TRANSPLANT MODEL IN CATALONIA: THE O.CAT.T
Fernandez, E.; Aguayo, M.T.; Viedma, M.A.; Via, J.M. : BARCELONA

HISTORY

Forty years have passed since the first successful kidney transplant was performed in Boston, USA; the year was 1954. Eleven years after this significant event, in 1965, the first ever kidney transplant was performed in Spain; precisely by a transplant team from the Clinic Hospital in Barcelona, Catalonia. Indeed, Catalonia has continued to be a pioneer within Spain in numerous transplants. In 1983, the Clinic Hospital performed the first kidney-pancreas transplant; in 1984, the Hospital of Bellvitge performed the first liver transplant and the St. Paul Hospital the first heart transplant; and in 1990, the Vall d'Hebron Hospital performed the first pulmonary transplant.

As experiment gave away to routine, and as more hospitals opened up new transplant programs, there was a need to create an organization capable of coordinating organ interchange. In this aspect, Catalonia has also been pioneer within Spain in creating an organizative transplant model. In 1982, PAIR(Renal Insuficiency Attention Program) was created and assumed the task of coordinating renal transplant. Two years later in 1984, the hospital transplant coordinator was established to promote organ donation and procurement of organs. At the same time, the first protocols for organizing and planning transplants were carried out. In 1987, the Transplant Coorinating Center of Catalonia was created. Its function was to coordinate the interchange of organs within Spain and between Spain and Europe. In 1989, with the ever increasing number of transplant programs opening throughout the major cities of Spain, the ONT (National Transplant Organization) was established in Madrid, responsible for coordinating organ interchange between all autonomous communities except within Catalonia, where it was then necessary to restructure its transplant program to what today is called O.CAT.T (Catalan Transplant Organization).

PRESENT SITUATION

According to the last census of 1991, Catalonia has a population of aproximately 6 million inhabitants spread over an area of 31.930 km2 situated in the northeastern part of Spain, bordering with France to the north.

In terms of transplant activity, Catalonia surpasses the spanish mean rate for renal, pancreas, lung, and liver transplant; only heart transplant was slightly lower than in the rest of the country. Catalonia also surpasses the spanish mean in terms of donation pmp.
The O.CAT.T is a program being run by the Catalan Health Service and primarily deals with organ transplant, tissue transplant, and bone marrow transplant. It forms an integral part in the functioning of an organizative structure which includes: 8 extraction and transplant centers, 18 procurement centers, hospital coordinators, a laboratory of histocompatibility, and a tecnical committee that elaborates protocols. Concretely, the UCIO (Organ Interchange Coordinating Unit), which is a branch of the O.CAT.T, is responsible for the following fuctions: waiting list management distribution of organs, and logistic support for the coordination of organ interchange, for heart, liver, lung and pancreas. It also offers a public service to promote organ donation.

The ambit of coordination include: coordination of all hospitals within Catalonia, cooordination of the rest of Spain with Catalonia, and coordination of all of Spain with Europe.

P. H. S. P. O.

Christine BOISRIVEAUD* et Philippe ROMANO**.

Le **P**rogramme **H**ospitalier de **S**ensibilisation aux **P**rélèvements d'**O**rganes et de tissus is the French equivalent of the European Donor Hospital Educational Programme (E.D.H.E.P.) .

History.
Sremmed from an initiative by the Eurotransplant Foundation, questionning how best to motivate the transplant personnel working within geographical area covered by this organisation.

Once documented, the program, which was conceived by a group comprising an english coordinator nurse, two university psychologists, a man and a woman, and a competent english health care consultant, was presented to the entire transplantation community.

The French adaptation was realised by a team comprising a local coordinator, a clinical psychologist, three regional coordinators and the medical director of France-Transplant.

Having followed an english based initiation and training course in the use of the EDHEP guidelines, performed at Leiden, these six persons translated the texts and modified them in line with french legislation and a non anglo-saxon population.

The goals of the P.H.S.P.O. are :
* To help service personnel who are dealing with subjects in a severely critical state, to meet with families and inform them of the impending death of their relative.

* Sensibilize these personnel to the idea of organ donation and guide them to a position where, in conjunction with the relatives, the process of decision making regarding organ donation can be embarked upon.

The Means.
The principal element is the participation of 14 to 18 professionnals, in a 2 days residential seminar during wich numerous informational documents are disributed ta attendees.

The first day is used to inform about tranplantation, rememorisation of the various puases of organ donation, brain death diagnosis, intensive cares and reporting on these factors in the event of brain death. Regulation and legislation, religious knowledge pertinent to these situations, administration of the organ removal processz and the distribution of organs in line with existing regulations.

The second day called « information for the bereaved family «, is aimed principally at presenting the different techniques which can be employed when communicating distressing news and how to adopt an appropriate manner in relation to the reaction of the bereaved. The rehearsal of diverse situations allows participants to consider how best to attribute their personal and professional intervention in such circumstances.

Conclusion.
This program is the first which target is to help physicians in charge of harvesting organs.

*   Psychologue Clinicienne. - Unités de transplantations.
        Pavillon P : Département de Néphrologie, Médecine de Transplantation et Immunologie clinique ;
        Professeur J-L. Touraine.
        Pavillon V : Urologie et Transplantations ; Professeur J-M. Dubernard.
        Hôpital Edouard Herriot
        69374 LYON Cedex.

**   Directeur Médical de France-Transplant.
        75475 PARIS Cedex 10.

HEALTHCARE ON THE WORKSITE : A STRONG MEANS OF COMMUNICATION TO PROMOTE ORGAN DONATION

(Préliminary results of an original experiment)

J.C DROUET* and coll. - J. BORSARELLI ** and coll. - M. BLANGERO*** - G. BOTTI**, * SIMTPA 450 rue A.
Einstein 13852 Aix en Pce Cedex 3 - ** Regional coordinator FRANCE TRANSPLANT ** Medical Information service TIMONE
Adults University Hospital 13385 Marseille Cedex 5 - ***(ADOT 13) ZAC Notre Dame 13120 GARDANNE

The number of organs transplanted has dropped over the last two years in France, whereas the figures concerning patients on waiting lists are constantly on the increase (1). This shortage of grafts is mainly due to the growing opposition from the next of kin concerning the removal of organs. Lack of and/or faulty information is the main cause of this opposition, quite apart from any cultural or religious reasons. The organisations in charge of promoting donation need relays to help make the maximum number of persons aware of needs. Industrial healthcare on the worksite is one of these relays, because 13 million salaried workers have a medical check-up per year.

An original experiment was carried out over a 12 month period by the Inter Professional Worksite Medical Committee of the Aix Area (SIMTPA). We report the results for the first three months concerning 5 819 persons seen for medical check-ups by 17 physicians on the worksite.

METHOD : Posters are put up in the centres and mobile units to attract people's attention, then brochures are handed out by the medical secretaries "yes to organ donation" (ADOT) at the beginning of the visit. The message is got over at the end of the examination by the physician concerned who hands out donor cards.

The investigation concerns "YES", "NO" and "UNDECIDED" answers to organ donation. Data is collected once a month by the same person on an ACCESS database. The answers are studied with respect to sex, age (< 30 years, 30 to 45 years, > 45 years), of social and professional categories, family status, number of children (< 3 children, > 3 children). The statistical method used was the CHI2 test for comparing frequency. The threshold of significance chosen was 0,05.

RESULTS : The first results show a very high proportion of indecision (about 60 %), greater generosity in women, married subjects with more than three children and at executive level.

CATEGORIES	Nomber	YES	NO	+ or -
Population	5 849	31 %	9 %	60 %
Males	2 950	30 %	9 %	61 %
Females	2 776	34 %	7 %	59 %
< 30	2 197	31 %	8 %	61 %
Age 30 à 45	2 564	33 %	9 %	58 %
* > 45	966	32 %	9 %	59 %
Married	3 773	33 %	8 %	59 %
Single	1 970	29 %	9 %	62 %
O children	2 186	29 %	9 %	62 %
1 to3 child.	3 130	32 %	9 %	59 %
> 3 child.	123	46 %	4 %	50 %
Executive	513	41 %	8 %	51 %
Employee	3 026	34 %	7 %	59 %
Worker	2 139	25 %	11 %	64 %
Commerce	2 422	25 %	7 %	68 %
Industry	675	37 %	12 %	51 %
Healthcare	990	40 %	6%	54 %
Services	1 760	32 %	11 %	57 %

* Non Significant

ADVANTAGE: : This experiment permitted us to attract the attention of a large number of persons (5 849) in a short period of time (3 months) through physicians who had previously been informed on this subject. It will be carried on until the end of October 1994 ; from November 1994 onwards, the population will be consulted once again to assess the impact of the information on the evolution of behaviour.

(1) France Transplant Annual Report 1993 Hôpital st Louis - Pavillon Lugol - 75475 Paris Cedex 10

TITLE: Aspects of the Legal Regulation of Living Donor Transplantation within Europe
AUTHORS: Austen Garwood-Gowers, David Price, Alison Lea and Peter Donnolly
CITY: Leicester. UK.

The purpose of this study is to provide an up to date study of national laws within the wider European area relating to living donor transplantation (LDT). This work is being undertaken as part of the EUROTOLD project in Leicester, England. The project has been funded by the European Commission and aims to study the legal and ethical dimensions of living donor organ transplantation within Europe. This study has been carried out with the collaboration of Mr Sev Fluss from the World Health Organisation in Geneva who allowed us access to files of national transplant laws and correspondence with lawyers across Europe.

The study indicates that the majority of countries with the wider European area have legislation containing specific regulation of LDT. However a few countries have laws that deal only with cadaveric donation and a small percentage have no laws containing specific transplant provision at all. In these situations the legal position of LDT and transplantation as a whole will be regulated by general law. Legislation has been created very recently in some countries, the Human Organ Transplants Act 1989 in the United Kingdom and the Russian Federation Transplant law of 1992. New law appears likely in the Netherlands where a transplant bill is currently passing through the national legislative assembly. This study looks at these and other European laws under categories of regulation. These are:
Clinical criteria that must be met for LDT to become a legal possibility,
The limitation of risk to the donor that will be legally tolerated,
The formalities and detailed content that is required before a valid legal consent can be given,
Legal restrictions on the class of person who can donate in terms of their relationship with the recipient,
The use of minors as donors
Provisions relating to the buying and selling of organs.

In the LDT laws of some countries there are gaps in terms of their being legal regulation on only some of the above points or only some organs. This may be deliberate in a few instances but more often it is a consequence of legal draftspersons not anticipating some of the legal concerns or the law being passed in response to a specific problem. An example of the latter is the United Kingdom's Human Organ Transplants Act 1989 that was passed in response to fears of an organ market developing and does not go far beyond commercial prohibition and prevention measures in the scope of its transplant regulations.

With regard to European community countries the increasing legal integration of member states will undoubtedly bring pressure for a European community wide policy on legal regulation of organ transplantation including living donor transplantation specifically. The beginnings of this have already been seen in the passing of a Council of Europe resolution in 1978, which was adopted by the Committee of Ministers of the Council of Europe in the same year. We have found a high degree of similarity in the laws of different European jurisdictions, but have also found that the use of living donors varies widely both between countries, and between regions in the same country and over periods of time. One possible danger of a European wide law is that it may suppress national or regional policies that are based on national or regional needs. Several countries appear to be working successfully without national transplant laws and it may be that legal regulation even when not highly restrictive of LDT has the effect of dissuading clinicians from using certain types of living donor or living donors as a whole.

All countries are experiencing organ shortages and if the number of organs is to be increased either from cadaveric or living donors then these legal factors need to be considered.

TITLE: A European Multicentre Study of Transplantation from Living Donors
AUTHORS: Alison Lea, David Price, Austin Garwood-Gowers, Peter Donnolly
CITY: Leicester U.K.

The demand for organs continues to outstrip supply. "Spare capacity" (cadaver organs not currently harvested for transplant) has been tackled within Europe by many strategies, medical, social, legal and educational with varying degrees of success. An alternative is to look for other sources of organs, one such alternative is to make use of living donors.

To look more closely at the use of living donors within Europe the European Commission has funded this project.

Our first task was to thoroughly review the extent to which live donors are used as a source of kidneys for transplantation in Europe. We have found that the use of living kidney donors within Europe is markedly different both between countries and between centres within the same country. Reviewing the most recent data available we found that in Turkey 80% of renal donors are living and in Greece living donors account for 42% of renal donors, Scandinavian countries use living donors for 11-40% of their renal transplants. In contrast the percentage is far more modest in countries such as Spain (1%), France (2.5%), Switzerland (6%) and Ireland who at present do not use living donors. In the UK the use of living donors nationally ranges between 0-20% between different centres. We have also found that most European countries are experiencing a decline in the numbers of living donors used despite rising numbers of patients on waiting lists and the inability of cadaver organs to meet the demand.

Having identified these differences in living donor use this project will go on to look more closely at the interaction between ethical values, social customs and cultural traditions with national laws and legislation together with public and professional attitudes towards living donation. The work programme will involve in depth interviews with medical staff at each participating centre to evaluate their practice and attitudes towards living donation, this will be followed up with interviews with past living donors and recipients and a community survey of attitudes towards living donation in each country.

Another aspect of the project has been to develop a database of European laws and legislation relating to transplantation and living donation. Many European countries are currently reveiwing their legislation that governs transplantation and in particular living donation. Many Eastern and Central European countries such as the Czech Republic, Slovak Republic, and Estonia are legislating for the first time and it is hoped that this database will allow them access to review current European legislation.

As a result of initial interviews with past donors we have started to develop a protocol that will enable centres to keep a registry of their previous living donors health. This protocol includes an in-depth interview using a semi-structured questionnaire with the Living Donor together with the completion of the General Health Questionnaire and a thorough physical health check. It is hoped that allowing past donors to express freely their thoughts and experiences of donating a kidney that this information together with a careful monitoring of their health will enable a protocol to be developed that will allow living donors of the future to experience kidney donation with minimal risk to both their physical and psychological health.

The current remit of the project includes all countries of the European Union along with Austria, Finland Norway, Sweden and Turkey. We have recently applied for funding to include Central and Eastern European countries and countries of the Former Soviet Union. It is envisaged that the project will produce a comprehensive review of living donation throughout the wider European area and will serve as a useful source of information that will allow clinicians and researchers to access contacts and collaborators throughout Europe.

KIDNEY TRANSPLANTATION FROM LIVING RELATED DONORS.

C. MOUQUET*, H. BENALIA**, B. BARROU**, J. LUCIANI*, M.O. BITKER**, P. VIARS*.
* Department of Anesthesiology, ** Kidney and Pancreas Transplantation Unit,
CHU Pitié-Salpêtrière, University Paris VI, Paris, France.

Kidney transplants with living related donors (LRD) could be an alternative to the shortage organ of cadaveric donors (CD). Patients and graft's survival are better in LR with HLA-identical or haploidentical donors than in CD recipients (1), without any risk for renal function's donor. **The aim** of this retrospective study is 1) to determine incidence of LRD transplants during the last 20 years in our unit, 2) to evaluate the risk of acute tubular necrosis (ATN), acute rejection, patients and graft survival vs recipients of CD. Postoperative outcomes of donors are also presented.

Patients and methods : 38 chronic renal failure patients and their LRD were included between 1973 and 1993. Transplants were performed only with healthy, volunteering and related HLA-identical or haploidentical adults donors. Mean age of donors was 38 ± 11 years. The recipients with cardiovascular, hepatitic, or pulmonary disease were excluded for LRD transplantation. Thirty eight recipients (28 men, 10 women) received the kidney from LRD parents (16 cases) or sibling (22 cases). Mean age of recipients was 31 ± 9 years. Mean duration of dialysis was 23 ± 28 months. The incidence of sensitization of recipients was 20 ± 30 % (range : 0-100%). The patients were divided into 2 groups according to pretransplant blood transfusions and immunosuppressive regimen. In Group 1 (1973-1981), 15 patients had neither donor specific transfusion (DST) nor antilymphocytes globulins (ALG), in Group 2 (1985-1993), 23 patients received deliberate transfusions with DST or not, according to the red cells phenotype. All patients received ALG and 11 received cyclosporine. These results have been compared in term of ATN, acute rejection and survival rates, with a group of 167 CD recipients transplanted between 1983 and 1993 and prepared with systematic blood transfusions and receiving the same immunosuppressive regimen given in Group 2.

Results : The rate of LRD graft increased from 3 % before 1993 to 13%. In the postnephrectomy period, a transient and moderate increase in creatinine level (30%) of the donor was noted. No complication (especially pulmonary or thromboembolic) was observed in LR donors. No recipient developed ATN vs 4.2% in CD recipients. The incidence of early acute rejection is higher in Group 1 (66.7 % vs 28.6% in Group 2, p<0.05), while the incidence of this complication was 60 % in CD recipients. Patient survival rate was 100% in LRD vs 87% at 5 years and 75% at 10 years in CD patients. Graft survival rate in LRD was 88% (vs 89% in CD) at 1 year, 84% (vs 83% in CD) at 2 years, 84% (vs 68% in CD) at 5 years and 84% (vs 42% in CD) at 10 years. In LRD recipients, the mean follow up was 61 ± 72 months (range : 3 months to 21 years), 5 patients had returned in dialysis and 4 others were lost of follow up at 4 months, 4.5 years, 10.5 and 12 years respectively.

Discussion : The incidence of acute tubular necrosis is even lower in LRD than in CD recipients. The frequency of acute rejection is significantly less in LRD than in CD recipients since deliberate blood transfusions and ALG use. The main advantage of LRD transplantation remains the better long term results in recipients without deleterious consequence in the donors. Our experience is consistant with the literature (1). The satisfying results of this series should lead to increase the indications of LRD transplantation in response of the organ shortage like in US or Scandinavian countries.

Reference : 1) Albrechtsen D et al. In Clinical Transplants 1992. pp 207-213, Terasaki PI, Cecka JM Editors, Los Angeles, California

ROLE OF THE DONOR IN THE POST TRANSPLANT RENAL FUNCTION

L Dubourg[1,2], P Cochat[1], A Hadj-Aïssa[2], B Parchoux[1], X Martin[3], L David[1]

1. Unité de néphrologie pédiatrique ; 2. Service d'explorations fonctionnelles rénales ; 3. Service d'urologie et chirurgie de la transplantation. Hôpital Edouard Herriot, Lyon, France.

Introduction. The donor - i.e. cadaver (CD) or living related (LD), large or small size - might influence the outcome of the graft function.

Patients and methods. The GFR of 78 patients (age : mean±SD 10.4 ± 4.9, range 0.7-23.3) has been prospectively assessed for an average 4.4 ± 2.2 [0.7-10.9] years period. The patients were divided into 2 groups according to the donor : LD (n=17) and CD (n=61) ; the CD group was further divided into 2 subgroups regarding the donor size to recipient size ratio : CD1 (ratio<1, n=30) and CD2 (ratio>1, n=17). The GFR was assessed by Cin at 3 (M3, n=59), 6 (M6, n=68), 12 (M12, n=64), 24 (M24, n=55), 36 (M36, n=44), 48 (M48, n=31) and 60 (M60, n=17) months post transplant.

Results. The mean±SD GFR (ml/min.1.73m^2) was 68.9 ± 25.6 at M3, 70.8 ± 23.2 at M6, 73.9 ± 23.1 at M12 and 73.0 ± 22.9 at M24. The GFR was not different between LD and CD at M3 (78.2 ± 22.2 and 66.6 ± 26.1, respectively). The GFR of CD improved significantly between M3 and M6 (66.6 ± 26.1 and 73.5 ± 22.1, respectively, p=0.01) and was higher than that of LD after M12 (76.7 ± 23.5 and 62.1 ± 17.2 at M24, respectively, p=0.02). The GFR was lower in CD1 compared to CD2 at M3 (59.3 ± 20.6 and 79.4 ± 30.4, respectively, p=0.01) but there was no longer any difference at M6 and afterwards. The absolute GFR was comparable in both subgroups at M3 and became significantly higher in the CD1 subgroup at M6, suggesting a functional adaptation of the graft to the recipient's condition.

Discussion. These results show that the GFR of kidney transplant children is independent from the type of donor - cadaver or living related - during the early postoperative period. In the long term, 1) a progressive decrease in GFR was noted in living donor recipients ; 2) it is suggested that the small size of the graft in cadaver transplant recipients has no deleterious effect since GFR improves more rapidly in those patients and reaches adjusted GFR comparable to patients who received a graft from cadaver donors of larger size.

OLDER LIVING RELATED AND CADAVERIC DONORS IN RENAL TRANSPLANTATION

D. Gakis, V. Papanikolaou, A. Papagiannis, G. Imvrios, D. Takoudas and A. Antoniadis
Transplantation Dept, Hippocration Hospital,University of Thessaloniki,GREECE

Recent reports suggest that older donors (>50years) are an important source of kidneys for transplantation but their use could lead to poorer results compared to younger donors [1,2]. Age is not a criterion in our selection of suitable donors. We accept kidneys from older donors, cadaveric and living related, provided there is no evidence of renal impairment. We have reviewed our experience with 168 kidneys transplanted from donors aged 50 years or greater to assess the effect of donor age on graft and patient survival.

Patients and methods. Between January 1987 and December 1993 168 kidneys from older donors (>50 years of age) were transplanted in our department. 137 grafts were from living related (LRD) and 31 from cadaveric donors (CD).During the same period 119 kidneys were transplanted from donors aged between 20 and 50 years and this group served for comparison (52 LRD and 67 CD). All recipients were adults first time transplanted, blood compatible with negative cytotoxic cross-match. Triple immunosuppression was used for LRD and quadruple sequential for CD. The incidence of primary nonfunction, technical failure and 1,2, and 5 year graft survival were examined. Data were analyzed with Students t-test, Fisher's exact test, Kaplan-Meier survival analysis and Log rank sum test.

Results. The results have been summarized in table 1.

Table 1. Results

	LIVING RELATED DONOR			CADAVERIC DONOR		
	20-50y	>50y	p-value	20-50y	>50y	p-value
n	52	137	-	67	31	-
donor age	43±6y	63±8y	-	33±9y	62±7y	-
range	30-50y	51-84y	-	20-47y	52-76y	-
recipient age	25±11y	35±9y	<0.001	42±14y	43±15y	NS
HLA mismatch	2.2±1.1	2.5±0.7	NS	2.2±1.7	2.4±1.4	NS
prim. nonfunction	2	3	NS	1	4	<0.03
1 y graft survival	94%	93%		93%	77%	
2 y graft survival	90%	89%		86%	73%	
5 y graft survival	66%	75%	NS	81%	73%	NS

Discussion. Despite the shortage of available organs for transplantation and the increasing gap, between the available organs and the number of patients awaiting transplantation, there is some reluctance to use kidneys from older donors [3]. This is based on reports of inferior graft survival and bigger technical problems due to the necessity to perform anastomosis involving diseased vessels which are more prevalent in older donors [4,5]. In particular age related decline in functioning renal tissue, leading to limited functional reserve that may be further reduced by cyclosporine nephrotoxicity, acute tubular necrosis and acute or chronic rejection are possible reasons for poorer results reported with older kidney donors [6,7]. In this series results achieved using donors >50 years were comparable to those seen with kidneys from younger donors. There was significant difference of the mean recipient age with living related donor because older recipients have older relatives.There were no statistical differences of the HLA mismatching. The older cadaveric group had significantly more primary nonfunctions but there were no statistical differences between graft survival of younger vs older groups, both CD and RLD. Especially in cadaveric donor there is a trend towards worse survival rate in the older group that could be statistically significant with bigger numbers. It is concluded from these data that kidneys from older donors are suitable for renal transplantation and there is no upper age limit, provided there is no evidence of renal impairment.

References
1. *Creagh TA, Mclean PA, Donovan MG, Walshe JJ, Murphy DM. Older donors and kidney transplantation. Transpl Int;1993; 6:39-41*
2. *Sakellariou G, Alexopoulos E,Kokolina E, Daniilidis M, Gakis D, Papadimitriou M. Impact of donor age in relation with graft survival and quality of the remaining kidney of donor, in: Andreucci VE, Dal Canton A,eds Current therapy in nephrology.Kluwer Academic 1988:449-52*
3.*Ploeg RJ, Visser MT, Stijnen T, Persijn GG, Schilfgaarde R. Impact of donor age and quality of donor kidney on graft survival. Transplant Proc 1987; 19: 1532-4*
4. *Foster MC, Wenham PW, Rowe PA, et al. Use of older patients as cadaveric kidney donors. Br J Surg 1988; 75: 767-9*
5. *Georgehan T, Digard N, Leppington L, Harris KR, Slapak M. Functional and other parameters in assessment of cadaveric kidneys for transplantation. Transplant Proc 1984; 16: 64-66*
6. *Anderson S, Brenner BM. Effects of aging on renal glomerulus. Am J Med 1986; 80: 435-442*
7. *Foster Mc, Wenham PW, Rowe PA. The late results of renal transplantation and the importance of chronic rejection as a cause of graft loss. Ann R Coll Surg Engl 1989; 71: 44-7*

THE HIGH RISK DONOR IN KIDNEY TRANSPLANTATION.
EFFECT OF SEX AND AGE ON THE LONG TERM GRAFT OUTCOME.

Ed P. van Steenberge, Paul P. Mulder, Jan N. IJzermans and W. Weimar.

Department of Internal Medicine I, Department of Epidemiology and Biostatistics and Department of General Surgery, University Hospital, Rotterdam, The Netherlands.

The current exchange policy of kidneys for transplantation is predominantly based on HLA matching, without taking into account other donor characteristics. We examined the influence of other donor factors on the transplant survival rates, like age, sex, bloodgroup, cause of death, first and second warm ischemia times, cold ischemia time, method of kidney preservation, together with mismatch for the HLA ABDR-loci, and type of primary immunosuppression, making use of the Cox proportional hazards method, without the heterogeneity of a center effect. All 591 consecutive first cadaveric kidney transplantations performed between july 1972 and july 1992 at our center, were included in the analysis. The outcome measures were the relative risks (RR) of the covariates associated with functional graft survival (where patient death with functioning graft is censored), patient survival and overall graft survival. Factors having no influence on any outcome included: cause of death of the donor, warm and cold ischemia times and the method of kidney preservation. The factors significantly associated with functional graft failure were: female sex of the donor (RR 1.48), and azathioprine as primary immunosuppression (RR 1.57). The female sex of the donor also provided the highest risk of patient death (RR 1.78) and overall graft failure (RR 1.56). Each additional mismatch on the HLA ABDR-loci increased the risk of overall graft failure with 12% (RR 1.12), and azathioprine as primary immunosuppression increased the risk with 52% (RR 1.52). When we extended the Cox regression model with the covariates recipient sex, recipient age and donor-recipient age difference, the recipient age became the most significant factor associated with patient failure (RR 1.07 for each year increase in recipient age). The recipients of donor kidneys with a positive donor-recipient age difference, had an 68% increase in the risk of overall graft failure (RR 1.68 p=0.02) compared to the recipients of relatively younger donors. The recipients of relatively older female donor kidneys had significantly more delayed graft function (44% versus 28% respectively, p=0.001 chi-square test), and had significantly inferior graft function at three months post transplant compared to the recipients of relatively younger male donors (creatinine 177 μmol/l versus 133 μmol/l respectively, p<0.001 chi-square test). It is likely that the number of functioning nephrons, which is lower in female compared to male donor kidneys, is responsible for the donor sex effect. The vulnerability to ischemia and aging factors of the older kidneys could be responsible for the donor-recipient age difference effect. We conclude that donor kidneys from relatively older donors and kidneys from female donors have a higher risk of transplant failure. Matching for age could improve the graft outcome of the high risk older and female donors.

THE LACK OF DONOR OR LACK OF UNDERSTANDING AND COOPERATION RESULTS OF THE ATTITUDE SURVEY AMONG PUBLIC MEDICAL AND NURSING PROFESSION.

WALASZEWSKI JANUSZ, ROWINSKI WOJCIECH, LAO MIECZYSLAW, MICHALAK GRZEGORZ, BARCIKOWSKA BOZENA.

WARSAW MEDICAL SCHOOL,   UL.NOWOGRODZKA 59   02-006 WARSAW, POLAND

The demand for renal replacement therapy in our country has been similar to that of countries in Europe. However the actual number of such treated patients is much lower and approaches only 60/million inhabitans/year. Despite that the average number of cadaveric kidney transplantation in Poland has been low (10/million inhabitans/year) in recent two years we have noticed even further decline of that number (380/in 1990, 370/in 1991, 310/in 1992, 320/in 1993).

The study of the prospective donor availability in central Poland (5 million inhabitants) based on the analysis of the records all cases of hospital death in two consecutive years showed that if in all medically suitable cases organ procurement took place the actual number of donors per year would be increased from 6 to 25/million of inhabitants.

The oppinion survey was conducted among the public, general practitioners, ICU and neurological departments medical and nursing personell and the students of the Medical Schools in Poland. The questionaire prepared for the nurses and the students included the knowledge and the attitude questions. The results showed that approximately 70% of the questioned public supported on the theoretical ground the idea of donation but most of them expressed the strong oppinion that the family consent should be searched for. In practice organ procurement takes place however only in 20% of potential donors. The survey among the physicians showed that 40% of them are lacking detailed knowledge or willingness to cooperate with the transplant centers. 20% of the doctors would not notify the transplant center about the possibility of harvesting beeing afraid of the oppinion of their collegues, nurses and the local society.

Conclusions. Despite the law regulation in Poland permits the organ procurement basing on the presumed consent of the deceased the progress in that field is not only slow, but shows some decline of the actual procurement rate. This is not due to the lack of donors but due to the lack of understanding and lack of willingness for cooperation from the medical society. Special educational program are being instituted.

ORGAN PRESERVATION, SURGICAL TECHNIQUES AND IMMUNOLOGICAL PROTOCOLS

JUGULAR OXYMETRY AND BRAIN DEATH
DURING INTENSIVE CARE OF COMATOSE PATIENTS

B. PAGE, intensive care unit, Hopital Ambroise Pare, 92104 BOULOGNE, FRANCE.

If human death is defined by brain death, its diagnosis needs medicolegal criteria based on clinical examination and EEG. However this evaluation could be difficult because technical or physiological limitations might impair the interpretation, especially after barbiturate and/or hypothermia. Since brain death is characterized by an intracranial circulatory arrest, methods assessing this phenomenon are warranted. Among these methods, conventional or isotopic cerebral angiography, doppler technique, appears the most promizing but it cannot easily performed everywhere.

The technique of jugular oximetry affords continuous measurement of 02 saturation in the jugular bulb (Sj 02). For this technique, a catheter is introduced percutaneously into the internal jugular vein by retrograde cannulation and a fiberoptic catheter is inserted until its tip is in the jugular bulb. SjO2 measurements yield information on global cerebral oxygenation reflecting the net balance between oxygen supply and demand. The cerebral extraction of oxygen (CE02) is defined as SaO2 - SjO2.

We studied comatose adult patients (Glasgow score < 6) with sedation, paralysis and mechanical ventilation.

Early detection of brain death is recognized by very low values of SjO2 indicating cerebral perfusion arrest.

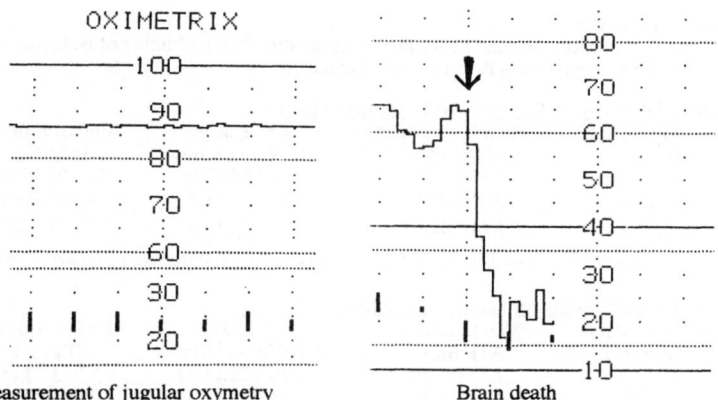

Stable measurement of jugular oxymetry   Brain death

In conclusion jugular oxymetry is promising in detecting cerebral ischemia and brain death during intensive care of head injured patients.

MODIFICATIONS OF UW SOLUTION CAN IMPROVE METABOLIC AND CELLULAR
PROTECTION OF HEARTS DURING LONG TERM HYPOTHERMC STORAGE:
EVALUATION BY P-31 MAGNETIC RESONANCE SPECTROSCOPY AND
BIOCHEMICAL ANALYSES.

M. BERNARD, T.CAUS, M. SCIAKY, J.R. MONTIES* and P.J. COZZONE
Centre de Résonance Magnétique Biologique et Médicale (CRMBM), Faculté de Médecine and *
Service de Chirurgie Cardiaque, CHU Timone, Marseille, France

Introduction:
University of Wisconsin (UW) solution has been reported to enhance cold storage preservation of
the heart. However, this solution is characterized by a high K^+ concentration and no Ca^{2+}, which
has been shown to be deleterious for the heart. In this study, we compared three different heart
preservation solutions: standard UW (I), Fabiani solution (II) (moderate K^+ concentration) and a
modified UW solution (III) containing Ca^{2+} and providing a Mg^{2+} mediated arrest.

Methods:
Isolated isovolumic rat hearts were arrested with one of the cardioplegic solutions (6 to 9 hearts in
each group) and then subjected to 5 or 12 hours of cold storage (4°C) in the same solution. An
additional period of 50 minutes of ischemia at 15°C was applied to the 5 hours groups, with
intermittent cardioplegic infusion. All hearts were reperfused for 60 minutes at 37°C. Function was
assessed during control and reflow. High energy phosphates and intracellular pH were followed
during all the experimental time course by P-31 Magnetic Resonance Spectroscopy (MRS) at 81 MHz
on a Bruker-Nicolet WP-200 spectrometer. Creatine kinase, Pi, lactate and purines were measured in
the effluents using biochemical assays and HPLC.

Results and conclusion:
The modified UW solution afforded better preservation after 5 and 12 hours of ischemia as shown
by the different indexes displayed in the two following tables:

Table I: Representative results for hearts with 5 hours ischemia.

	End of ischemia ATP (mM)	30 min reflow ATP (mM)	CK leakage (IU/60min reflow)	End of reflow RPP(%)
I	2.68±0.95	3.67±0.65	129.98±13.99	38.92±13.76
II	3.02±1.01	3.19±0.89	110.91±21.62	44.65±10.62
III	7.21±1.11*	5.68±0.50*	83.52±16.23	52.99± 5.05+

Means±SEM.*p<0.05 vs I and II, +p<0.05 vs II (ANOVA). RPP=rate pressure product

Table II: Representative results for hearts with 12 hours ischemia.

	End of ischemia ATP (mM)	30 min reflow ATP (mM)	CK leakage (IU/60min reflow)	End of reflow RPP(%)
I	0.98±0.24	1.75±0.56	270.25±57.31	5.91± 3.09
II	1.67±0.88	1.16±0.44	323.41±37.52	0.00± 0.00
III	2.29±0.71	3.36±0.60+	110.44±14.95♦✢	50.03±12.36*

Means±SEM.+p<0.05 vs II,♦p<0.05 vs I,✢p<0.01 vs II, *p<0.01 vs I and II (ANOVA).

This new solution, denominated "CRMBM solution", might prove particularly useful in extending
the duration of cold preservation of human transplants by providing augmented protection of
metabolic stores and mechanical performance.

This work is supported by MRT (grant 650994) and CNRS (URA 1186).

HYPOPHYSIS THYROID AXIS DISTURBANCES IN HUMAN BRAIN DEAD DONORS
JJ COLPART, S RAMELLA, M BRET, B CORONEL, D DOREZ, A MERCATELLO,
A HADJ AISSA, JF MOSKOVTCHENKO - Lyon University Hospital

Hypothalamus and hypophysis as brain are included inside the inextensible cranial box. When brain dead process is going on, hypothalamus and hypophysis are destroyed. Hypothermia and polyuria are very well known as brain death symptoms. Some authors thought, according to experimental model, that hormonal depletion should be responsible of sudden cardiac arrest.

Novitzky showed thyroidian and corticosurrenal hormons decrease on monkey experimental model. Lyon University Hospital brain death center group already published a study performed in 76 potential brain dead donors which improved significant TSH decrease with 0,84 m UI/l versus normal values 2,18 m UI/l and T3 active biological thyroidian hormon decrease with 0,98 nmol/l versus normal value 1,8 nmol/l.

T4 or T3 supply therapies give divergent hemodynamic results however T3 replacement seems to increase Adenosine Triphosphate (ATP) levels.

This seria in 75 potential donors shows a significant increase of reverse T3 which could explain a peripheral break T4-T3 conversion and consequently the plasmatic low dosages of T3 which has the main biological activity in energetic metabolism and catecholamines role.

Hormons	Number	Results	Normal means	
TSH (mUI/l)	76	0,84+ 0,82	2,18	P<0,001
T3 (nmol/l)	76	0,98+ 0,54	1,8	p<0,001
T4 (pmol)	76	16,1+ 4,7	18	p=0,01

Significant low T3 hormon level prevalent in brain dead
multi organ potencial donors population=80%

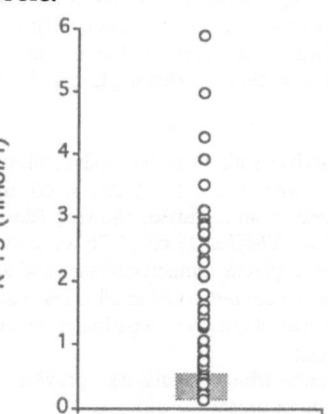

Significant increase of reverse T3 hormon level prevalent in brain dead multi-organ potential donors population

NORMOTHERMIC PRESERVATION OF "MULTIPLE ORGAN BLOCKS" WITH A NEW PERFLUOROOCTYL BROMIDE EMULSION.

E.J. Voiglio[1] , L. Zarif[2] , F. Gorry[1] , M.P. Krafft[2] , J. Margonari[1] , S. Balter[3] , X. Martin[1] , J.G. Riess [2], J.M. Dubernard [1].

1. Laboratoire de Recherches Chirurgicales, INSERM U281, Hôpital Edouard Herriot Pavillon P, 3   Place d'Arsonval, 69437 Lyon Cedex 03, FRANCE.
2. Laboratoire de Chimie Moléculaire, CNRS URA 426, Université de Nice-Sophia Antipolis, Parc Valrose,   06108 Nice Cedex 02, FRANCE.
3. Département d'Innovation et de Coordination Pédagogique, Université Claude Bernard - Lyon I, 8 avenue Rockefeller, 69373 Lyon Cedex 08, FRANCE.

Purpose:

To evaluate the efficiency of fluorocarbon emulsions as an oxygenating medium for the normothermic preservation of organs (Multiple Organ Blocks, MOB) a new perfluorooctyl bromide (perflubron) emulsion was compared to a mixture of modified Krebs' solution and blood.

Protocol:

The fluorocarbon emulsion used contained a low amount of egg yolk phospholipid (EYP) and was stabilized by a mixed fluorocarbon-hydrocarbon amphiphile $C_6F_{13}C_{10}H_{21}$ (F6H10) (perflubron/EYP/F6H10 90/2/1.4 % w/v). The MOB was composed of 'en bloc' removed heart-lungs, liver, pancreas, kidneys and bowels connected by the vascular system. Blood of 4 rat MOBs was replaced with 36% w/v of the new emulsion (EMOBs). 5 MOBs were perfused with a mixture of blood and albumin-containing Krebs' solution (KBMOBs). The following parameters were studied: electrolytes, acid-base balance, lactate and enzyme levels in arterious liquid, bile production and diuresis. Histologic examination of the organs was performed. Student's t test was used.

Results:

Survival with stable haemodynamics was in all cases longer than 210 min. The following parameters were lower ($p < 0.05$) at 60 and 120 min in EMOBs than in KBMOBs: lactate, amylase and creatine kinase, showing lesser suffering of the organs. Diuresis was also higher ($p < 0.05$) in EMOBs (5.65 ± 1.76 vs 0.94 ± 1.21 mg/min). There was no difference in bile production, aspartate aminotransferase and alanine aminotransferase levels. Electrolytes and acid-base balance were preserved in all cases, PaO2 was higher ($p < 0.05$) for the EMOBs than for the KBMOBs. Histological examination of the organs showed no necrotic lesions in EMOBs.

Conclusion:

Fluorocarbon emulsions provide significant improvement in the normothermic preservation of organs.

Financial support:
- Prix Antonin Poncet, Université Claude Bernard - Lyon I
- Hospices Civils de Lyon
- C.N.R.S. and I.N.S.E.R.M.
- Applications et Transferts de Technologies Avancées

EVALUATION OF A HIGH SODIUM - LOW POTASSIUM COLD-STORAGE SOLUTION USING THE ISOLATED PERFUSED RAT KIDNEY

S.G. Ramella, A. Hadj-Aïssa, A. Barbieux, J.P. Steghens, J. J. Colpart, P. Zech, N. Pozet
Hôpital E. Herriot et Université Claude Bernard, Lyon, France.

The isolated perfused rat kidney (IPK) model was used to assess initial renal function after 24h preservation in 3 different cold storage solutions : EuroCollins (EC), a solution prepared according to the formulation of Belzer's solution (High-K^+ UW) and a high Na^+ - low K^+ Belzer UW solution (High-Na^+ UW).

Glomerular Filtration Rate (GFR), Fractional Na reabsorption (FR_{Na}) and renal vascular resistances (RVR) were measured after 24h cold storage in each of the solutions during 60 min, and were compared to values obtained in a control group in which renal function was measured immediately after the kidneys have been harvested. ATP and Creatine Phosphate (CP) were measured in fresh renal tissu, in kidneys preserved for 24h in each solution, in control IPK, and in reperfused IPK after they have been preserved for 24h. Results concerning renal function are shown in the following table .

	Control	EC	High-K^+ UW	High-Na^+ UW
GFR µl/min/g	512.4 ± 41.5	25.0 ± 9.3*	49.4 ± 11.0*	52.2 ± 10.1*
TRNa %	92.2 ± 1.3	3.3 ± 1.7*	26.7 ± 4.9*§	58.2 ± 7.4*#
RVR mmHg/ml.min/g	4.2 ± 0.4	7.1 ± 1.7	5.3 ± 0.5	5.8 ± 0.5

* $p < 0.05$ vs Control, § $p < 0.05$ vs EC, # $p < 0.05$ vs High-K^+ UW

ATP and CP contents were decreased to ≈ 10% of basal values in all experimental groups after cold-storage (control ATP = 0.63± 0.01 µmol/g and control CP = 0.50 ± 0.07 µmol/g). Normothermic reperfusion of IPK after cold-storage induced a restoration of ATP levels, but CP content further decreased. There was no significant difference in ATP and CP content between cold-storage solutions, nor any correlation between metabolic and functional parameters.

In conclusion, this study showed that high-Na^+ version of Belzer's cold-storage solution seemed to be less deleterious to initial renal function than the original high-K^+ solution, at least after 24h cold-storage.

Organ preservation by vitrification

J.L. Descotes, E. Payen, E. Chapelier, JJ Rambeaud.
Service d'Urologie C.H.U. de Grenoble[1]

with collaboration of: J. Mazuer, J. Odin, A. Baudot, J.F. Peyridieu Centre de Recherches sur les très basses températures CNRS[2], P. Boutron, Labo L. Néel CNRS[3], A. Rossi, A. Ray, J. Verdetti, Labo de physiologie cellulaire cardiaque U.J.F[4], M. Decorps, C. Delon, R. Dupeyre, Equipe du GARN unité 318 INSERM.[5]

Introduction : In merging our various specialties, we try to solve the main problems in organ transplantation. These problems are linked to the weight of the urgency and to the limited time avilable to perform immunological tests necessary toimprove compatibility and to ensure a maximal transplant success.

Method : The only issue to increase the preservation time of organs is to significantly cool them (down to ~-150°C) to slow the metabolic reactions. It is the cryopreservation. Unfortunately any ice in the organ is deleterious. Therefore our goal is to vitrify the water contained in the organs. The vitrification is the "coagulation" of the liquid in an amorphous solid state, on the one hand by using cryoprotective agents that constrict the growth of crystals and, on the other hand by performing high cooling velocities.

Résults and discussions : We present the various domains that we have begun to study :

1) *Cryoprotectives solutions :* We have used 2,3-butanediol as cryoprotective agent, with respect to its weak toxicity and its strong tendency to favor the vitrification. Tests are undertaken on endothelial cells and on red blood cells (teams 3 and 4). Other tests of toxicity are made on the isolated rat heart cooled down to 4°C (team4). The vitrification conditions of cryoprotective solutions of Euro-Collins and 2,3-butanediol have been measured. Addition of different sugars to protect the cells has been studied. These conditions have been also determined on small pieces of perfused rabbit kidneys and rat hearts. We observed a noticeable improvement that we attributed to the presence of the strongly divided circulatory system (team 1,2 and 3). Finally the good diffusion of the cryoprotective agent during the perfusion of the rabbit kidney has been verified by RMI imaging (team 1,2 and 5)

2) *Thermal studies :* Optimization of the cooling conditions has been approached on model systems made of inorganic material that we rapidly cool down. The first results allowed us to define cooling techniques which are compatible with the vitrification constraints. Measurements are associated to numerical simulation and the results let us think that the vitrification of the rabbit kidney would not be so difficult (team1 and 2).

3) *Autotransplantation of the rabbit kidney :* In order to verify in a further step the viability of vitrified then reheated organs, a rabbit kidney transplantation has been developed. This surgical technique is now on the rails. It is performed in three steps : i)Harvesting of the right kidney ii) Perfusion of the kidney with the cryoprotective solution and cooling down to 4°C. iii)Discarding of the left kidney and transplantation of the right treated kidney. This graft is improved by using small prosthese that we have realized (team1 and 2). We have shown the importance of regulating the perfusion pressure on the variations with time of the resistance of the kidney (ratio pressure/flow). The aims of this work is to compare from the three point of view of the clinical, biological and histological aspects, two groups of rabbits submitted to the same protocol with or without cryoprotective agent.

Conclusion : The first results on the toxicity of the cryoprotective agent, their diffusion in the organ and the vitrification conditions let us think that we will be able to realize the vitrification of a small organ in a close future.

IMMUNOLOGICAL FACTORS TOGETHER WITH ISCHAEMIA RESULT IN PRIMARY NON-FUNCTION OF CADAVERIC KIDNEY GRAFTS

B.Łągiewska, M.Pacholczyk, W.Rowiński, K.Ostrowski, S.Cajzner, J.Wałaszewski
Department of General and Transplantation Surgery, Warsaw Medical School

It is generally believed that major ischemic damage results in primary non function of cadaveric renal graft after transplantation. A retrospective analysis of incidence and of the factors which might have been responsible for such complication among 461 patients (pts) who received cadaveric kidney transplant during last 9 years was carried out. In 191 pts (41.4%) the graft functioned immediately after transplantation (IF) and in 270 (58.6%) delay in renal function (DF) was observed. In most instances (229 pts) kidney regained function after 4-72 days after surgery. In 41 cases the graft never functioned. In all cases the best available recipient was chosen according to HLA (A,B and DR) typing, in the presence of negative cross-match. Several factors which might have contributed to the final outcome were assessed in all three groups and are shown in the table below.

renal function	IF	DF	NF
Age of donor (y) x±SD	33.8±12	33.8±14	35.1±18
Hypotension in donor before procurement (%)	26	54	68
Oliguria in donor at the time of retrieval (%)	7.5	41	38
Warm ischaemia time (min) x±SD	6.7±10	7.5±5	8.8±7
Anastomosis time (min)x±SD	29±8	32.1±11	31.9±10
Cold storage time (h) x±SD	24.6±8	26.6±9	25.6±8
No of common HLA in the donor and recipient (% of pts) HLA A,B 2 or more 1 HLA DR 2	 67.8 50.1 10	 65 44 9.4	 54 43 8.6
PRA % maximal last before Tpx	15.8 3	22.6 4.5	24.4 4.5

In all NF patients biopsy of the transplanted kidney was taken. Microscopical examination of the NF kidneys showed acute accelerated or acute vascular rejection in 23 cases (55%), necrosis due to ischaemia and infection in 10 patients (25%). In remaining 8 pts lack of function was due to technical errors.
Conclusion: In over 50% of cases primary non function of transplanted cadaveric kidney was due to immunological factors and not to ischaemia per se.

The new technique of rapid en bloc removal of both kidneys
in non-heart beating donors

Min Zhi-Lian   Wang Li-Ming
Department of transplantation, Chang Zheng Hospital
Shanghai 200003, China

Abstract

Kidney removal in cadaver of non-heart beating is different from that in cadaver of only brain death. The removal procedure must be simple, rapid and safe. This new tachnique confirmed a'fore'mentioned characteristics. The main procedure is: long cross incision of abdomen. Retroperitoneum mobilization of the left and right kidney and ureters (outside of Gerota's capsule). Making a hole at the root of mesentery.Shifting the left kidney and ureter to the rightside. Entirely removing of bilateral kidneys with its surrounding tissue after cutting the abdominal aorta and vena cava. Using 4℃ 250-300ml HCA solution to perfuse kidney through the renal artery until reanl cortex become pale. Tailoring the kidney, renal vessel and ureter, unnecessary tiseue and vessel should be removed and ligated. After this, kidney must be preserved in 4℃ HCA solution till being using (the longest storage time is fifty hours). From the begining of 1989 to the end of 1993, we carried out the new technique in non-heart beating donors for 516 times. The mean time of kidney removal and perfusion is about five minuts (3-7minutes) and three minutes (2-5minutes) respectively. The incidence of renal vessel, kidney and ureter injury is 2.4%. The utilization of kindeys is 99.3%. ATN post transplantation is about 2.2%. Renal function recovering time is about three days post transplantation. The new technique steps are fairly simple and easy to be operated rapidly. It is no need to mobilize renal vessel directly and unnecessary to isolate colon broadly and to divide pancreas. Therefore it is also safe. The new technique is quite suitable to be used for kidney removal in non-heart beating donors.

THE ANATOMIC FEASIBILITY STUDIES ON THE TECHNIQUE OF SPLITTING-LIVER TRANSPLANTATION (SLT)

WEN Zhi-Xiang, XIA Sui-Sheng, LIU Deng-Gui
(Institute of Organ Transplantation,Tongji Medical University,
430030 Wuhan Hubei,China)

Abstracts,
This article states the possibility of SLT through 30 liver divisions and X-ray imaging.
1. The divisions of hepatic pedicle
Three main vessels(portal veins,bile ducts and hepatic arteries)are located in pedicle. According to their structures,they were classified into different types (three types for both portal veins and bile ducts,two types for hepatic artery).
The majority of the livers(n=25) was in Type I portal vein structure. In this Type,left branches of portal veins were longer than the right,the former was 2.6±0.3cm (mean value), the latter 1.7±0.4cm. The rests were Type II(n=3) and Type III (n=2). For all 30 livers, we divided the portal veins by cutting off the Left branches. After division,the shortest left branch was 0.9 cm long.
In bile ducts classification,Type I was common (n=26),Type II (n=3) and Type III (n=1) were few. Cutting off the left bile duct was chosen in Type I, II, III. After separation, there were 2 livers to be found with 0.5cm long left bile duct. If transplanted, Roux-Y technique could be selected for the bile duct reconstruction.
24 livers had Type A hepatic artery structure in which the right branches were longer than the left (mean value 3.1±0.6cm VS 2.4±1.0cm). Other 6 livers with Type B structure. Right branches were cut off for 30 liver's arterial divisions. The remnant of right branches in Type B was 2.1cm (mean value), no influence on arterial anastomosis.
2. The divisions of hepatic veins
Middle hepatic vein is very important in the divisions of hepatic veins. In 29 livers, left and middle hepatic veins or their common trunks with Inferior Vena Cava (IVC) cuff were cut from IVC. Only one liver was the left hepatic vein with IVC cuff. Right hemi-livers contained IVC,but the left didn't. If the left was transplanted, the recipient's IVC would be preserved.
3. The status of intra-hepatic portal veins,bile ducts and hepatic veins.
Parenchymal divisions were referred to the main fissure. No injuries were found on the segmental portal viens and bile ducts by 40 hemi-livers X-ray imaging. Only 6 livers had injuries on the distant parts of the middle hepatic veins.
4. The size of hemi-livers
The size of the right hemi-livers was larger than the left (mean value 780±130g VS 400 ±60g). No doubt, the right hemi-livers were enough for the recipient's need. How about the left hemi-livers? The answer is definite. Left hemi-livers could resolve more serious dismatch between adult donor and child recipient.
In a word,SLT is a widely practical technique from anatomic views.

COMBINED KIDNEY TRANSPLANTATION (Tx) WITH HEART, LIVER OR PANCREAS

A.C. Marrast, J.L. Touraine, J.M. Dubernard, G. Dureau, O. Boillot, J.L. Garnier, J. Finaz, C. Pouteil-Noble, P. Paillard, N. Lefrancois.
Pavillon P, Hôpital E. HERRIOT, Lyon, France.

Surgical technologies and immunosuppressive treatment refinment allow to practice simultaneous or differed multiple Tx for a same patient (pt).

Out of 15 combined kidney and heart Tx, 8 were successful. The small incidence of kidney or heart rejection should autorize to lower immunosuppression. Tx for pts with poor physic conditions must be discussed.

Out of 8 combined kidney and liver Tx, 7 were successful. Kidney or liver rejection incidence was low. Problems were viral recurrence on the hepatic graft and oxalate lithiasis recurrence on the kidney despite liver Tx. Vaccination and anti viral therapy should permit inhibition of viral replication.

219 combined kidney and pancreas Tx were performed from 1977 to 1994 in 204 pts, with a 73 % pt survival. Pancreas and kidney survivals were similar when a total duodenopancreatic Tx with bladder drainage was performed. Pancreas graft survival was improved using this duodenopancreatic Tx as compared to segmental pancreas Tx with chemical Wirsung duct obstruction. Kidney rejection incidence was higher in case of combined Tx as compared to isolated kidney Tx.

These results plead for developpement of combined Tx. Immunosuppressive regimens must be adjusted to each kind of Tx in order to reduce adverse effects.

COMBINED HEPATIC AND RENAL TRANSPLANTATION IN PRIMARY HYPEROXALURIA
TYPE I : REPORT OF FOUR CASES.

A. Déglise-Favre[1], G. Manganella[2], D. Samuel[1], H. Bismuth[1]

Centre Hépato-Biliaire[1] - Hôpital Paul Brousse - 94800 Villejuif

Laboratoire d'Anatomie Pathologique[2] - Hôpital de Bicêtre - 94275 Le Kremlin-Bicêtre

We report the outcome of combined hepatic and renal transplantation in four patients affected by primary hyperoxaluria type I (PHI), an autosomal recessive inborn error of glyoxylate metabolism. All patients had typical history of PHI : recurrent urolithiasis, irreversible nephrocalcinosis leading to end-stage renal failure, extra-renal oxalate deposition, and had been on dialysis for more than one year. In all patients, the diagnosis was established by enzymologic analysis of native liver biopsies (Department of Chemical pathology, Middlesex Hospital, London).

, After transplantation, all patients received conventional immunosuppressive regimen consisting of prednisone, azathioprine, antilymphocyte globulins replaced by cyclosporine A after fourteen days. Hyperdiuresis, large fluid intake and dialysis were used to prevent calcium oxalate deposition in the renal graft. A renal biopsy was performed in all patients between 3 and 8 weeks post-transplant : oxalate deposition in tubular lumina and cells was found in all of them ; three patients had histologic features of cyclosporine nephrotoxicity : two had tubular damage (isometric tubular vacuolization) and a third one had small vessel damage (myocyte vacuolization, sub-endothelial hyaline deposits). Those three patients had been treated with nephrotoxic antibiotics for systemic infection. The last patient had no signs of cyclosporine nephrotoxicity on two early renal biopsies but showed slight vascular and interstitial cyclosporine chronic damage on a third renal biopsy one year after transplantation. No sign of acute rejection was found in any of the 7 renal biopsies performed in our four patients. Liver function remained stable except for an episode of acute liver rejection reversible after antirejection therapy. Two of our patients died from septic complications at 5 and 10 weeks post-transplant, two have a normal hepatic and renal function at 2,5 and 18 months follow up. In this patient a decrease of renal oxalate deposits was demonstrated histologically 12 months after transplantation.

In conclusion : the outcome of our small group of patients shows an increased risk of cyclosporine nephrotoxicity whose toxic effects are probably enhanced by oxalate crystals deposition in renal tubules. Treatment with nephrotoxic antibiotics should be avoided because of increased vulnerability of renal tubules in hyperoxaluric patients. The low rate of acute rejection episodes and the high mortality in our patients confirm the results of larger series. Combined hepatic and renal transplantation in hyperoxaluric patients ought to be performed before the constitution of extensive systemic oxalosis because prolonged oxalate precipitation can jeopardize the kidney graft.

*RISKS, COMPLICATIONS AND TREATMENTS
IN GRAFT RECIPIENTS*

HCV RNA IN PATIENTS UNDERGOING KIDNEY TRANSPLANTATION

G.Lunghi, A.Archenti, R.Cardone, A.Aroldi*, A.Pagano
Laboratorio di Virologia, Ospedale Maggiore di Milano
*Divisione di Nefrologia, Ospedale Maggiore di Milano

Chronic liver disease is common in patients undergoing kidney transplantation. Infection caused by hepatitis B virus, often associated with unfavorable clinical outcome, decreased after introduction of efficient measures of profilaxis and hepatitis B vaccine, in contrast it became apparent that many transplant recipients had chronic liver disease related with hepatitis C. In these patients prevalence of anti HCV antibodies reported from several studies ranged from 6.2 to 65.8 %, depending on the use of I or II generation immunoassays, but no many dates are available about prevalence of HCV RNA , which detect viremia and can identify patients with active infection. The aim of this study was to determine prevalence of HCV RNA and clinical correlations in patients undergoing kidney trasplantation at the Ospedale Maggiore of Milano between 1976 and 1991. 216 patients positive for anti HCV by ELISA and RIBA II (ORTHO Diagnostic Systems, Raritan N.J.) were studied. Serum liver biochemical parameters were assayed every 3 months. Nested PCR for the detection of HCV RNA in serum was performed using primers of the 5`UTR. All samples were also tested for IgM anti c22 (Abbott Labs. IL/USA) to verify the presence of this marker in chronic disease. 197 patients (91.2%) were HCV RNA positive (the rate of HBsAg positivity in the same population was 13.6%).IgM anti c22 were positive in 49 patients(22.6%) , all patients except 1 were HCV RNA positive too. No important correlation between increased ALT levels and presence of IgM anti c22 or HCV RNA was found. These data suggest that: a) prevalence of active HCV replication is high in kidney transplant recipients; b) these patients may have significant liver disease despite normal ALT levels; c) although IgM anti c22 were always found in HCV RNA positive patients , the use of this marker as indicator of disease activity needs more studies.

INDICATION FOR TRANSPLANT AND EFFICACY OF ITRACONAZOLE IN ASPERGILLUS FUMIGATUS INFECTION RECONSIDERED.

L. Van Elslande, E. Cassuto-Viguier, J. R. Mondain, J. C. Bendini, J. Bracco, M. Gari-Toussaint, M. Franco, H. Gaid, D. Barrillon.

Department of Nephrology, Hôpital Pasteur, 06000 Nice, France.

A patient born in 1945, B chronic hepatitis since 1982 and HCV hepatitis, hemodialysed for polycystic kidney disease, received primary renal transplantation in 1984. Non observance for immunosupressive treatment led to rejection and the patient returned to hemodialysis in1988 december.

Despite these facts and surimposed malnutrition, a second renal transplant was performed in 1992 june with early acute rejection treated by methylprednisolone pulse. On maintenance immunosuppressive treatement (azathioprine, prednisolone and cyclosporine) transient leucocytopenia and CMV infection treated by gancyclovir happened two month later.

In 1992 december, he presented a shoulder osteo-arthritis and a dermo-hypodermal lesion of the thigh. Clinically, there was no antecedent trauma to the region of the affected joint and skin.There was neither fever nor chills. Physical exam revealed diffuse tenderness and limitation of motion. The shoulder radiograph and MRI showed important osteo-arthritis, destructive lesions with synovial thickening and massive joint effusion. Aspergillus was isolated directly from the synovial fluid described as turbid. Skin lesion of the thigh was nodular and histology showed filaments whose culture grew Aspergillus fumigatus. Laboratory evaluation showed increased sediment rate, moderate leukocytosis, Serologic tests for aspergillus fumigatus were negative. Lungs and sinus X rays, bronchoscopy were normal. Technetium bone scan only showed increase uptake at the right shoulder. MIC antifungal agents study showed a large superiority of itraconazole which was prescribed to the patient (400 mg/d). Progressive decrease of stiffness and swelling then appeared. Concommitant monitoring and reduced dosage of ciclosporin were necessary because of strong interactions mediated by cytochrome P-450. Chronic hepatitis, recent rejection treatment with methylprednisolone pulse and previous leukocytopenia secondary to ganciclovir treatment for cytomegalovirus disease were supposed to be host risk factors of this unusual fungal infection presentation.

Despite of treatment by Itraconazole the patient died in 93 november because of dissemination of aspergillus infection with cutaneous and neurological localisations (prebulbar extradural empyema).

Setting the host risk factors (chronic B and C hepatitis, malnutition, non observance for immunosupressive treatment leading to rejection) and organ shortage, should we reconsider indications for transplant in this kind of patient?

OUT-CENTER DIALYSIS AND RENAL TRANSPLANTATION.

E. DELAWARI, M. LAVILLE, W. ARKOUCHE, E. ABDULLAH, R. SIBAI, J. TRAEGER.

A.U.R.A.L. & PAV P HÔPITAL EDOUARD HERRIOT. LYON - FRANCE.

Between 1974 and July 1992, we received in AURAL 430 new patients, aged 43,5 ± 15,9 years, for the treatment by Dialysis in out-Center structures. The sex ratio was 130 females and 300 males.

The causes of renal failure were : chronic glomerulonephritis 44,8%, nephrosclerosis 15,47%, chronic interstitial nephritis 15,01%, polycystic kidney disease 7,39%, diabetes 7,16%, systemic diseases 3,7%, nephronophtisis 2,31%, renal dysplasia 2,31%, indeterminated 1,85%.

369 patients (85,81%), aged 41,5 ± 14,2 years, were treated by Hemodialysis (HD); and 61 patients (14,19%), aged 57 ± 17,5 years, were treated by Peritoneal Dialysis. The treatment was applied at home in 258 cases (60%), and in self-dialysis units in 172 cases (40%).

On July 1992, 122 patients (28,37%) remained treated in AURAL. Sixty patients (13,95%), aged 57,6 ± 13,6 years, were dead during the period of treatment in AURAL. Sixty-six patients (15,35%) were transfered towards other stuctures of dialysis' treatment. One hundred and eighty patients (41,86%), aged 39,2 ± 12,2 years, were transplanted for a first time. Until this period, the candidates of transplantation treated in AURAL were treated only by HD.

The followed table, shows the distribution of 355 HD-patients and 61 PD-patients, as their age at the beginning of dialysis :

Age/Years	nb/HD	Failing/HD	nb/PD	Failing/PD
10 - 20	22	0	4	0
20 - 30	63	4	3	2
30 - 40	75	7	3	1
40 - 50	79	15	5	4
50 - 60	75	17	14	11
60 - 70	35	7	18	11
70 - 80	6	1	12	5
80 - 90	0	0	2	1

In the group of 355 HD-patients, the survival was at : 95% after 3 years, 91% after 5 years, 85% after 8,5 years, 81% after 10 years, 80% after 11 years, 75% after 13 years.
In the group of 61 PD-patients, the survival was at : 56% after 3 years, 40% after 5 years, 25% after 8 years, 19% after 11 years.

The out-center dialysis is of importance in the treatment of the chronic renal failure. The successful collaboration with the transplantation team, assures a good preparation of the candidates of transplantation.

SPONTANEOUS REGRESSION OF A METASTATIC ADENOCARCINOMA TRANSMITTED BY A CADAVER KIDNEY GRAFT : SUPPORT FOR "IMMUNOTHERAPY" ?

VINCENT F.[1], LEVY V.[1], GLOTZ D.[2], DUBOUST A.[2], BARIETY J.[2]

1: Intensive-Care-Unit, Institut Gustave Roussy, rue Camille Desmoulins, 94805 Villejuif Cedex, France; 2: Nephrology Unit, hôpital Broussais, 96 rue Didot 75014, Paris, France.

Actual approach in the treatment of melanoma or renal cell carcinoma consists in use of Interleukine 2 or Interferon α.We report the first histologically proved regression of a renal adenocarcinoma, involving a kidney allograft, after incomplete surgery and withdrawal of immunosuppression, without adjuvant therapy.

M[r]. A., a 50-years-old white man, underwent cadaveric renal transplantation on January 1988, for treatment of chronic renal failure secondary to autosomal-dominant polycystic kidney disease. The donor was a previously healthy 40-years-old man died of cerebral trauma. Macroscopic examination of both kidneys was normal. Immunosuppression regimen consisted in cyclosporine A and prednisolone. History was uneventful, except for pyelonephritis. In January 1992, after a new episode, echography and computed tomography revealed a hypoechogenic, hypodense lesion in the graft Simple echographic follow-up was instituted. The size of this lesion increased, with apparition of lymph nodes along the right iliac primary artery, confirmed by magnetic resonance imaging, leading to a surgical exploration on May 12, 1993. Renal tumor was confirmed, associated to adenopathies along the renal and right iliac vessels. Removal of the kidney with perinephretic fat was achieved. Histological diagnosis was a clear cell carcinoma with invasion of the perinephric fat, renal vein and regional nodes. Lymph node preleved at the primary iliac artery bifurcation was also involved. Persistence of abnormal adenopathies was radiologically confirmed. Immunosuppression was withdrawled. The patient returned to regular haemodialysis. No adjuvant therapy was performed. He remained febrile. Infectious disease was ruled out. Hypothesis of rejection of remnant neoplastic cells was sustained and non-steroidal anti-inflammatory drugs (NSAIDs) were introduced. Apyrexy was achieved. Three months after tumorectomy, sigmoidectomy was performed for infectious sigmoiditis. During surgical procedure right iliac region was explored. Multiples biopsies were done including remaining graft's artery and vein. There was no macroscopic or histological evidence of carcinoma. Eleven months after graft removal the patient remains well. There is no evidence of metastatic disease. NSAIDs are tapered and he remains apyretic. The recipient of the controlateral kidney remains alive without evidence of malignancy.

We expected that neoplasia was present in the graft before transplantation Its cells exprimed donor's antigens. After discontinuation of immunosuppression, rejection of the remnant allograft's cells (most neoplastics) occurred. Our patient was therefore submitted to "spontaneous immunotherapy" following T cells activation related to the discontinuation of immunosuppression. Recent report (1) suggests the possibility to induce remission of metastatic melanoma, after creation of only one mismatch between normal and neoplastic cells by direct gene transfer with DNA-liposome complexes encoding a foreign major histocompatibility complex protein. HLA mismatches between donor and recipient were 1 A, 2 B, 1 Dr., supporting this new therapeutic. Our observation suggests that successful treatment of melanoma or renal cancers may be best achieved obtaining "exogenous" (Interleukine 2 for instance) and "endogenous" immunomostimulation.

(1) Nabel GJ, Nabel EG, Yang ZY, Fox BA, Plautz GE, Gao X, Shu S, Gordon D, Chang AE. Direct gene transfer with DNA-liposome complexes in melanoma : expression, biologic activity, and lack of toxicity in humans. *Proc Natl Acad Sci USA* 1993 ; 90 : 11307-11311.

POSTTRANSPLANT MALIGNANT LYMPHOMAS (PTL) TREATED WITH DOXORUBICIN-BASED CHEMOTHERAPY

Altieri M, Maloisel F*, Herbrecht R*, Sosa Cl*, Chenard MP**, Lioure B*,
Woehl-Jaegle ML, Ellero B, Boudjema K, Jaeck D, Oberling F*, Wolf Ph.
Service de Chirurgie viscérale et de Transplantation, * Service d'Onco-Hématologie,
** Service d'Anatomopathologie
CHU Hautepierre, 67098 Strasbourg cédex, FRANCE.

PTL after solid organ transplantation are a serious complication occuring in 1-18% of patients. Between 1978 and february 1994, 1000 transplantations were performed and eleven secondary lymphoproliferative disorders were observed (1.1%). Seven of them were high-grade lymphoma and required chemotherapy.

Material and methods : 4 males and 3 females of mean age of 38 years (range 17 to 54) underwent 3 liver, 3 kidney, and 1 pancreas+kidney transplantation. Median number of organ rejection was 2 (range 0 to 3). Diagnosis of lymphoma was performed 28 months after transplantation (range 5 to 84, med 26). In all cases, it was immunoblastic lymphoma and one was immunophenotype T. Transplanted organ was involved in 4 cases and lymphoma staging was 6 stage IV and 1 stage I.
After diagnosis and staging, initial management was reduction of immunosuppression by discontinuing azathioprine and reducing corticosteroid and ciclosporine.
ACVBP regimen as described in LNH93 french protocol was used with reduction of dose. Patients received intravenously on day 1 : doxorubicin 50 mg/m^2 ; cyclophosphamide 1g/m^2 ; vindesine 2mg/m^2 ; bleomycin 10mg ; methotrexate 15mg IT ; and prednisone 60mg/m^2/d for 5 days. Three patients received G-CSF 5μg/kg from day 7 to day 17. Treatment cycles were repeated every 21 days.
Patient's disease stage was redetermined after 3 and 6 cycles. In case of progression or relapse, a MIV regimen was used. Patients received daily for 2 days ifosfamide 1500mg/m^2 ; vepeside 120 mg/m^2 ; and on day 1 mitoxantrone 12 mg/m^2.

Results : 34 cycles were performed and all patients received at least 3 cycles (range 3 to 6). Disease went into a complete (2)(CR) or partial (4) remission (PR) after 3 cycles in 6 cases. Patients in PR received 3 additional cycles and underwent in CR. 5 patients remained in CR 1 to 56 months (mean 20 months) after the end of therapy. One patient relapsed at 25 months and underwent as the patient in progression, the MIV regimen.
The non responding patient was in CR after 6 cycles of MIV and received 3 additional cycles. However, the relapsing patient was in progression after 6 cycles of MIV and died of progressive lymphoma.

Toxicity : Haematological grade 4 toxicity was noted in 8 cases (23.5%) and complicated in 5 cases of grade 3 infection (14%). In one case, patient developped a vascularitis related to CMV infection and was treated by gancyclovir. One case of neurological grade 3 and one case of renal grade 3 toxicities were also noted. No treatment-related death was noted.

Conclusion : PTL is a serious complication of organ transplantation. Few reports describe the effectiveness of chemotherapy in PTL. This small series demonstrates that cytotoxic chemotherapy induces an acceptable toxicity in this type of patient. However, it demonstrates that ACBVP with dose adjustements and G-CSF induces a high rate of complete remission (85%). ACVBP regimen gives comparable response rate to CHOP and Promace.

MALIGNANCIES IN CHILDREN WITH RENAL REPLACEMENT THERAPY (RRT)

S. Carl, M. Wiesel, A.-M. Wingen, O. Mehls, G. Staehler

Depts. of Urology and Paediatrics, Transplant Centre, University of Heidelberg, Germany

Introduction: Statistical evaluations of the outcome of children after start of RRT do not demonstrate the high incidence of malignancies found in adults. But, as the end of childhood usually is defined to be 15 years of age, all children older than 15 years and still in pediatric care escape from these statistics. Therefore, the true incidence of malignancies in patients starting RRT in childhood is not known.

Patients and Methods: We analysed the clinical course of 155 patients who started RRT in our pediatric unit between January 1980 and December 1993. Complete data of 152 patients were available.

Results: Median age at start of RRT was 11,5 (0,02 - 20,3) years. 39 % suffered from glomerular diseases (61 % focal segmental glomerulosclerosis), 39 % from hypo- dysplasias or uropathies and 22 % from other diseases (35 % nephrophthisis). First choice of treatment was peritoneal dialysis (PD) in 55 %, hemodialysis (HD) in 43 % and transplantation (TPL) in 2 %. in December 1993 after an observation period of 5,2 years (0,01 - 12.7) per patient 58 % of the patients were living with a functioning graft, 16 % were on PD, 11 % on HD and 15 % had died. 3/23 deaths were due to lymphomas. In 4 children malignancies were diagnosed and cured before RRT (renal carcinoma, retinoblastoma, Wilm's tumor, ureteral sarcoma) without recurrence during 16,3 - 25 years after diagnosis of malignancy. In 6 patients malignancies were diagnosed 6,1 (2,0 - 14,9) years after start of RRT (4 lymphomas, 1 dysgerminoma, 1 carcinoma in acquired renal cystic disease) at the age of 20,4 (7,7 - 26,5) years. One boy after 2 years of dialysis developed B-cell lymphoma, which was resistant to chemotherapy. In two patiens B-cell lymphoma was diagnosed 0,2 and 0,5 years after TPL with multiple rejection crises and high dosage of immunosuppressive therapy. Another patient developed T-cell lymphoma 8 years after successful grafting. In the last three patients lymphomas were not treated and diagnosed at autopsy. Dysgerminoma and renal carcinoma were cured by surgery at the age of 22,8 and 26,5 years, after more than 10 years of RRT.

Conclusions: Cured malignancies in children are no contraindication for RRT. Malignancies on RTT seem to be rare before the age of 15 years, but, are more frequent thereafter. Patients starting RRT in childhood probably have the same high incidence of malignancies as adults.

ENDOTHELIAL ACTIVATION IN XENOGRAFTS' REJECTION: EVALUATION OF THE ROLE OF HEPARAN-SULPHATE.

Di Stefano R., Bonanomi G., Scavuzzo M., Pinna A.*, Donati D., Mosca F.
Institute of General and Experimental Surgery, University of Pisa, Pisa - Italy -
* Institute of Pharmacology, University of Pisa, Pisa - Italy -

Endothelial activation plays an important role in discordant xenogenic rejection. The process is thought to be initiated by antigen-antibody recognition and complement cascade that lead to activation and damage of endothelium as the main target of rejection. One aspect of endothelial activation is the loss and release of a proteoglycan like heparan-sulphate (HS) from cellular surface. The anticoagulant and fibrinolytic activity of heparan-sulphate is well documented but other properties of HS need further investigation.

In the present study we have tested the effects of heparan-sulphate administration on survival and histology of heterotopic cardiac xenografts from Guinea-pig to Lewis rat. In vitro, we have obtained cell cultures from rat aortic rings and tested the action of different concentrations of HS on endothelial migration and proliferation.

Subcutaneous injections of not fractionated HS have been admnistered to donors and hosts at 100mg/kg/die starting three days before surgery. Another way of administration has been the perfusion of explanted hearts before transplantation with Krebs-Henseleit added with heparan-sulphate at 3gr/l of concentration by a Langendorff apparatus.

Results have been a significant prolongation of graft mean survival time in treated group versus control group ($24,2 \pm 4,4$*min vs $13,6 \pm 2,2$ min; * $p < 0,01$ vs control) and a better conservation of cardiac tissue. Perfusion of isolated heart with HS before transplantation has lightly prolonged survivals but not significantly as to parenteral way alone ($27,5 \pm 2,1$ min).

Thoracic aorta has been drawn after median thoracotomy to Lewis rats and then have been delicately removed fat, connective tissue and intercostal branches. The vessel has been cuted in little rings of about 1 mm. of thickness that have been subsided on the bottom of wells covered with fibrin. Culture medium was: DMEM, HamF12, bovine serum 10%, antibiotics and ε-aminocaproic acid to inhibit fibrinolysis. Heparan-sulphate has been added at 10, 75, 150, 300, 450 μg/ml. Cultures were incubated at 37°C, 95% O_2, 5%CO_2 and observed daily with an inverted microscope.

Observation on 12th day showed that endothelial sprouts were similar in controls and in wells incubated with 10 and 75 μg/ml. On the contrary, higher concentrations (150, 300, 450 μg/ml) inhibited in a dose-dependant way endothelial migration and proliferation.

The effects of HS on migration and proliferation of endothelial cells suggest that this molecule has a role in the control of cell activity that is dependant on its concentration and probably its binding to cell surface. It is likely that suitable doses of HS can control endothelial activation by binding to cell surface and hampering access of ligands like growth factors, antibodies and inflammatory mediators.

In conclusion, heparan-sulphate might be an adjuvant therapy to immunosuppressive drugs in the prevention of discordant xenograft rejection and further investigations are needed to understand its mechanism of action.

SYSTEMIC IL-10 RELEASE, AFTER A SINGLE PRE OR PER OPERATIVE LARGE DOSE OF ATG-FRESENIUS IN HUMAN KIDNEY TRANSPLANTATION.

Y SAINT HILLIER, B HORY, E RACADOT*, C BRESSON, D DAVID, F AL FREIJAT, P VAUTRIN, V FOURNIER, E BERGER, M JAMALI.
Service de Néphrologie - Transplantation rénale - C.H.R. Saint Jacques et Centre Régional de Transfusion Sanguine* - 25000 Besançon - France.

IL-10 is a key cytokine with pleiotropic effect secreted by B cells, cells of the macrophage lineage and also TH0, TH1, TH2 subset. Initialy described as "cytokines synthesis inhibitor factor", producted by TH2 cells, IL-10 inhibits IL-2 and INF gamma production by TH1 cells. IL-10 has the ability to suppress MHC II expression and thereby the antigen presentation capacity of monocytes/macrophages. IL-10 also down regulated IL-12 and the production of free oxygene radicals produced by actived macrophage. IL-10 is a chemotactic attractant for CD8⁺ T cells. These multiple suppressive effects on various effector phase of the immune response of IL-10 corrobore the finding that IL-10 is a "natural" immunosuppressor. Systemic effect on all T cells and monocytes occure concomittantly and if IL-10 is present several hours before and on time of transplantation, this realise a veritable "preincubation", a "bath" of IL-10, leading perhaps to tolerance induction and anergy.

Patients and methods : In thirty one consecutive cadaverics kidneys transplantations performed between 1er june 1993 and 31 mars 1994, we measured at many time serum IL-10 level. In all patient (18 M - 13 F, 48 ± 13 years old, extreme 22 to 70, 25 first, 4 second and 2 third graft), the analysis were performed before, during and after the infusion of ATG-FRESENIUS (a rabbit polyclonal anti Human T Lymphoblast gammaglobulin derived from JURKAT Cells line) and then every day during hospitalisation. An ATG-FRESENIUS infusion, is given in 3 hours pre or intra operative before the reimplantation, on a peripheric or central catheter, in all patients, at 9 mg/kg. In the 25 cases of first graft, ATG infusion is unique, while in 6 hyperimmunised or retransplanted patients, ATG is continued at lower doses 3 mg/kg/j four days only.

The corticotherapy is given at 500 mg just before the ATG, 40 mg three days, 30 mg to day 20 and then 20 mg to day 30, Ciclosporine at 6 mg/kg/d at day 5 or more precocely if creatinine have falled of more than 30 %, Azathioprine at 3 mg/kg/d at day 0 and then adapted with leucopenia

Results

All patients had no detectable level of IL-10, after pulse of methylprednisolone and before ATG FRESENIUS. The production of IL-10 begin very rapidly within 15 minutes. The mean level of IL-10, for the 31 patients is respectivly of 764, 730, 386, 85, 7 pg/ml just before, 30 minutes, 6, 12, 24 hours after declampage.

There is no IL-10 release after the other infusions of ATG FRESENIUS during the four days of treatment.

Only one patient with Wegener disease does not produced IL-10 (Max at 90 pg/ml) and have irreversible reject, even after OKT3 treatment, who required transplantectomy at day 33.

The tolerance of ATG F was excellent without any cytokines syndrome release. All patients are alive with creatinine level at 158 µmol/l and only 7/31 (22 %) have rejected, controled by corticosteroïd or OKT3 and their last creatinine is at 151 µmol/l.

Conclusion

IL-10 is release in the circulation, rapidly, for several hours, after a single large doses well tolerated of ATG FRESENIUS. This protocol's interest is to produce maximal natural immunosuppression when the recipient is most likely to respond to the new organ, with systemic IL-10 production during hours, before or just after the graft, associated with lymphocytes depletion (results to published) with only a single infusion of ATG FRESENIUS.

PROLONGATION OF SKIN ALLOGRAFT SURVIVAL IN MICE FOLLOWING ADMINISTRATION OF NEW 20-EPI VITAMIN D3 ANALOGUES.

Raymond Pamphile[1], Paule Veyron[2], Lise Binderup[3] and Jean-Louis Touraine[2] :
1: Laboratories LEO S.A.78180 Montigny. 2 : Transplantation and Clinical Immunology, Pavillon P, Hopital Ed. Herriot, 69437 Lyon, cedex 03, France. 3 : LEO Pharmaceutical Products: DK-2750 Ballerup, Denmark.

A new class of vitamin D analogues characterized by an altered stereochemistry on carbon 20 of the side chain of the molecule has been synthetized in order to have a better profile on hypercalcemia than Calcitriol, the biologically active form of vitamin D3 (1,25 dihydroxyvitamin D3 : (1,25 (OH)2 D3)) . Discovery of high affinity receptors for vitamin D in monocytes and activated T and B lymphocytes has led to the finding that this hormone plays an important role in the regulation of the immune system. Use of 1,25 (OH)2 D3 in the immunological field is limited because of its low therapeutic index. We have tested 3 of them (MC1288, MC1301, MC1357) for their capacity to delay the rejection of skin allograft in CBA recipient mice transplanted with C57 BL/6 donor mice. The mean survival times and serum calcium obtained with these 3 analogues were compared with vehicle and with cyclosporin A (CsA). Results are presented in the table below :

	DOSES	ADMINISTRATION	POPULATION	SURVIVAL	SERUM CALCIUM
VEHICLE		PO	9	11,7 ±1,7	80,0 ±2,8
CSA	20 mg/kg/day	PO	11	15,3 ±1,9	89,7 ±9,8
MC1288	0,02 µg/kg/day	IP	11	14,2 ±1,1	85,7 ±10,9
	0,1 µg/kg/day	IP	10	18,6 ±1,3	95,2 ±8,7
	0,2 µg/kg/day	IP	10	22,2 ±1,0	100,4 ±15,3
MC1301	0,02 µg/kg/day	IP	11	13,6 ±2,0	76,1 ±8,9
	0,1 µg/kg/day	IP	9	16,3 ±2,4	82,3 ±8,7
	0,2 µ g/kg/day	IP	11	19,6 ±1,4	100,4 ±7,4
MC1357	0,02 µg/kg/day	IP	10	13,3 ±1,5	82,7 ±6,5
	0,1 µg/kg/day	IP	11	16,3 ±1,7	88,1 ±5,7
	0,2 µg/kg/day	IP	10	20,0 ±3,2	80,2 ±11,2

In this transplantation model, the profile of these three analogues led us to look to active new compounds, without hypercalcemia effect, to prevent graft rejection.

A model for self tolerance induction based on intrathymic anergy, reversible in the absence of the tolerogen.

A. Aitouche and J-L Touraine

INSERM U80, Hôpital Edouard Herriot, Place d'Arsonval, 69437 Lyon, France.

It is believed that the primary role of the thymic epithelium is to serve as an environment in which T cell precursors differentiate into mature T cells as well as to selectively promote maturation of those T cells deemed to be "useful" by virtue of their affinity for self. However the evidence that thymic epithelium can also induce tolerance has come from several recent studies which addressed this question. The mechanism is clonal anergy rather than deletion.

Here we propose a model where we postulate that thymic epithelium tolerizes all positively selected T cells. This means that all early thymic migrants are inactivated. How this postulate could be accorded with the subsequent acquisition of immunocompetence in the extrathymic compartment against foreign antigens and pathogens ?.

The answer has come from recent studies from many groups among which ours. In vivo isolation of anergized T cells in an environment free from the tolerogen (antigen to which they are anergic) provokes a lost of anergy. While the persistence of the tolerogens contributes to keep T cells in their inactive state. Self antigens, including those that are not expressed in the thymus and organ specific antigens, are present in the periphery. Therefore, anergic T cells bearing autoreactive TCRs are prevented from exerting their harmful effect by a continuous or episodic contact with persisting autoantigens. However, T cells bearing TCRs with a specificity to foreign antigens and pathogens that are absent from the body loose their tolerance and return to a normal functional status. A subsequent contact with a specific antigen would result into an immune response. APC non-degradable and sequestred autoantigens by their structural and anatomical barriers are not allowed to interact with their specific T cells and thus behave like foreign antigens. Their specific T cells recover from their anergy to a normal functional status. A subsequent contact with relevant antigens may result in autoimmunity.

In conclusion, this model does not conflict with the notion that tolerance is maintained by a serial of fail-safe mechanisms. It introduces the well known notions of intrathymic epithelium-induced T cell unresponsiveness and the reversibility of anergy in the absence of the tolerogen.

SUPPLEMENTAL POSTERS

BREAKING THE DONOR AGE BARRIER TO FACE THE ORGAN SHORTAGE IN LIVER TRANSPLANTATION

Luca Aldrighetti, M.D.[1], Ignazio R. Marino, M.D.[1], Howard R. Doyle, M.D.[1,2], Cataldo Doria, M.D.[1], Carlo Scotti-Foglieni, M.D.[1], Judith A. Kovalak R.N., M.S.N.[1], Andreas G. Tzakis, M.D.[1], John J. Fung, M.D., PhD.[1] and Thomas E. Starzl M.D., PhD.[1]

[1]Division of Transplantation and [2]Section of Computational Medicine, Pittsburgh Transplantation Institute, University of Pittsburgh and the Veterans Administration Medical Center, Pittsburgh, PA 15213, USA

Introduction

As of March 31, 1994, there were 34,493 patients in the United Network for Organ Sharing (UNOS) waiting list (1), up from 13,115 in December 31, 1987, an increase of 263%. Of these, 3,264 awaited liver transplantation (OLTx), up from 449 in 1987 (727% increase). The supply of organ donors, on the other hand, underwent a marginal increase between 1988 and 1990 (from 4,085 to 4,514), and has remained relatively stable (4,531 in 1991, 4,521 in 1992 and 4,849 in 1993). Consequently, while the need has increased dramatically, we observe with mounting concern the persistent wastage of available organs, and the death of potential recipients. Many routes have been explored in an attempt to remedy this situation, including the development of artificial organs (2), utilization of living donors, even for extra-renal organs (3), xenotransplantation (4,5), and non-heartbeating donors (6,7). However, a more immediate impact on organ shortage could be effected by changing the current donor selection criteria to include the so-called *marginal donors* (i.e. cardiac arrest, prolonged CPR, older age).

Materials and methods

The case material consists of 467 adult OLTx: 54 from donors aged between 60 and 79 years old (Group I), and 413 from donors less than 60 years of age (Group II). All grafts were flushed with UW solution. Group I and Group II were compared in terms of fraction of donors that were on pressors (defined as dopamine infusion > 10µg/kg/min or need for a continuous infusion of epinephrine or norepinephrine), pitressin, and that required CPR prior to procurement. They were also analyzed in terms of ICU length of stay, AST, ALT, cold ischemic time, mean recipient age and recipient UNOS status (UNOS status is a measure of severity of disease, according to UNOS candidate classification. Status 1: patient may wait at home; Status 2: patient may wait at home but needs medical support; Status 3: patient needs to be in the hospital; Status 4: patient requires life support). Continuous data are presented as the mean ± SEM, and categorical data as frequencies. Means were compared using a two-tailed t-test, and frequencies were compared using Pearson's chi-square. Survival analysis was performed using the method of Kaplan-Meir. The significance level was set at a $p < 0.05$.

Results

Mean donor age for Group I was 65.3 ± 0.6 (range: 60 -79), vs. 35.8 ± 0.7 (range 7-59) for Group II. In Group I there were 29 donors between 60 and 64, 17 between 65 and 69, and 8 between 70 and 79. There was no difference in the fraction of donors that were on pressors, pitressin, or that required CPR prior to procurement. The two groups were also comparable when evaluated for ICU length of stay, AST, ALT, cold ischemic time, mean recipient age, and recipient UNOS status (Table 1).

Table 1. Comparison of the two groups (donor age ≥ 60 yrs and < 60 yrs) for various donor selection criteria

Donor data	Group I (n=54) Donor age ≥ 60	Group II (n=413) Donor age < 60	Significance
Pressors (%) [see text]	35.1%	41.0%	n.s.
Pitressin (%)	22.2%	32.0%	n.s.
CPR (%)	13.0%	17.7%	n.s.
ICU length of stay (days)	3.05±2.86	3.62±5.07	n.s.
ALT (U/l)	35.96±3.52	51.96±3.29	p=.001
AST (U/l)	52.64±5.49	77.18±4.22	p=.001
Cold ischemia time (hrs)	13.20±0.51	13.36±0.19	n.s.
Mean recipient age (yrs)	53.9±1.3	50.5±0.6	n.s.
Recipient UNOS status:			
status 2	16.7%	15%	n.s.
status 3	40.7%	42.9%	n.s.
status 4	42.6%	42.1%	n.s.

Twelve patients (22.2%) underwent retransplantation in Group I, while 35 (8.5%) underwent retransplantation in Group II (p=.0016). The indications for retransplantation in Group I were: primary non function in 6 cases, severe ischemic injury in 3 cases, suprahepatic vena cava stenosis in 1 case, bile cast syndrome in 1 case, and rejection in 1 case. The indications for retransplantation in Group II were: primary non function in 12 cases, severe ischemic injury in 5 cases, hepatic artery thrombosis in 9 cases, portal vein thrombosis in 1 case, rejection in 6 cases, hepatitis in 1 case, and bile cast syndrome in 1 case. The 1-year actuarial graft survival was 55.6% in Group I and 74.8% in group II (p=.0001). The 1-year actuarial patient survival was 72.2% in Group I and 81.7% in Group II (p=.014). There were no differences between successful and failed grafts, in either the young or older donor groups.

Discussion

The evaluation of every single potential donor based on physiological and biochemical data, instead of pre-set rigid criteria, allows an expansion of the organ donor pool. Patients with cardiac arrest and prolonged CPR have been found acceptable by post-CPR physiological and biochemical criteria, and their organs have been successfully transplanted (8).

The donor age deserves special mention since, when assessing for specific organ donation, chronological age is less important than the physiological age. The liver seems, in a certain way, to be protected from aging. Its great functional reserve, regenerative capacity, and large blood supply are the key factors in delaying aging of the liver, as compared to other organs (9). Based on a positive preliminary clinical experience (10), we have been routinely using grafts from older donors. However, our results show that, although older donor livers can be used to face the present organ shortage, they do not function as well as livers from younger donors, and their use should probably be limited to selected recipients (i.e., those in urgent need of OLTx). Retransplantation should be considered early when an older donor liver fails to function promptly, considering the high number of primary-non-functions and severe ischemic injuries in Group I patients.

In conclusion, we believe that, given the current organ shortage crisis, it is mandatory to continue to use older donors. Unfortunately, we still cannot accurately identify preoperatively those grafts that are more likely to fail, and further studies will be required to answer this question.

References

1. UNOS Update 10(4)29-30, 1994
2. Galletti PM: Bioartificial organs. Journal of Artificial Organs 16(1):55-60, 1992.
3. Caplan A: Must be my brother's keeper? Ethical issues in the use of living donors as sources of livers and other solid organs. Transplant Proc 25(2):1997-2000, 1993.
4. Starzl TE, Fung JJ, Tzakis AG, Todo S, Demetris AJ, Marino IR, Doyle H, Zeevi A, Warty V, Michaels M, Kusne S, Rudert WA, Trucco M: Baboon to human liver transplantation. Lancet 341:65-71, 1993.
5. Marino IR, Tzakis AG, Fung JJ, Todo S, Doyle HR, Manez R, Starzl TE: Liver xenotransplantation. In Braverman MH, Tawes RL (ed.): Surgical Technology International, A Medical Corporation Publishing, San Francisco, CA, 1993, pp 139-144.
6. Anaise D, Rapaport FF: Use of non-heart-beating cadaver donors in clinical organ transplantation. Logistics, ethics and legal consideration. Transplant Proc 25(2):2153-2155, 1993.
7. Casavilla A, Ramirez C, Shapiro R, Nghiem D, Miracle K: Experience with liver and kidney allografts from non-heartbeating donors. Transplantation, in press.
8. Yanaga K, Tzakis AG, Starzl TE: Personal experience with procurement of 131 liver allografts. Transplant Int 2:137-142, 1989
9. Popper H: Aging and the liver. In Popper H, Levy GL (eds): Progress in liver disease, vol VIII. Grune & Stratton, New York, 1985, pp 659-683.
10. Teperman L, Podesta L, Mieles L, Starzl TE: The successful use of older donors for liver transplantation. JAMA 262:2837, 1989.

SUCCESSFUL TRANSPLANTATION OF PEDIATRIC DONOR KIDNEYS IN ADULT RECIPIENTS

Kirste G., Blümke M., Pisarski P.
University Hospital Freiburg, Surgical Department, Transplantation Center,
Hugstetter Straße 55, 79106 Freiburg i.Br., Germany

Pediatric kidneys of donors below the age of three have been very restrictly used in adult recipients and in pediadtric recipients as well. It has been argued that renal mass might be insufficient for adult recipient. Moreover the rate of technical difficulties and problems is high.

A new technique of paratopic positioning of pedriatic kidneys en bloc has been developed. Both donor aorta and donor vena cava can be prolonged by an interpositional graft of the distal part of both donor vessels. This prolongation of the aorta and vena cava allows a paratopic positioning side to side to recipient aorta and vena cava without any king-king of torsion at the renal vessels. Using this technique 12 patients have had transplants at the Freiburg University Hospital Transplant Center without any major problems. Renal mass has been sufficient, when choosing normal weighted adult recipients.

Pediatric donors should be used in the same way as adult donors. It is not yet clear whether this technique can be used in pediatric recipients in the same way.

PUBLIC CAMPAIGN TO INCREASE DONOR AVAILABILITY IN A REGIONAL TRASPLANT CENTER

Kirste G., Blümke M., Schaub F., Dreier R.
University Hospital Freiburg, Surgical Department, Transplantation Center,
Hugstetter Straße 55, 79106 Freiburg i.Br., Germany

At the beginning of 1994 the availability of donors decreased in the Federal Republic of Germany by nearly 30 %. The reason for the decrease seems to be the negative influence of publications in the yellow press, public discussion about brain death criteria and some extremly critical case reports as well as reports on commercialism in organ donation.

It seems to be necessary to increase positive information about transplantation and to increase the awareness in the public about transplantation as a treatment of choice in several endstage organ diseases.

At the University Hospital Freiburg a public campaign in the region of the University Hospital and local donor hospitals was started with medical information in all local newspapers of the area, TV-reports and radio interviews. All broadcasting stations were supplied with information about transplantion and organ procurement. Moreover commercial advertising on the radio with short radio spots presented by VIP's or by patients suffering endstage renal disease were sent out. Posters were presented in a number of public places.

The succes of the whole campaign can not be calculated in numbers of donors so far. The number of positive responses was extremely high with frequent phone calls every day during the time of the campaign. Since then three organ procurement procedures have been undertaken after relatives approached the doctors with the question whether organ donation would be possible. Based upon our past experience, this is an extremely rare event.

Conclusion
Public advertising of organ procurement as the basis for transplant medicine seems to be necessary in the future to increase the awareness in the public and to counteract influence of negative presentations in the media.

MORPHOLOGIC FINDINGS IN BASELINE RENAL TRANSPLANT BIOPSIES

R. Cahen[1], F. Dijoud[2], C.Couchoud[1], M. Devonec[3], P. Trolliet[1], P. Adeleine[4], J.P. Fendler[3], P. Joubert[3], P. Perrin[3], B. François[1]
[1]Service de Néphrologie, Centre Hospitalier Lyon-Sud, 69310 Pierre-Bénite
[2]Laboratoire d'Anatomie Pathologique, Hopital Debrousse, Lyon
[3]Service d'Urologie, Hopital de l'Antiquaille, Lyon
[4]Laboratoire d'Informatique Médicale des Hôpitaux de Lyon

A prospective study was undertaken to determine the incidence of preexisting lesions in renal grafts and their possible influence on renal function after transplantation.

Since January 1992, 53 kidney transplant biopsies have been performed at the time of transplantation, before revascularization. Fifty two donors were cadaveric and 1 was living related. They had a mean age of 38 years (range 10-62); 38 were male. All recipients were treated with the same quadruple sequential immunosuppressive protocol. Morphological investigations included light microscopy and immunofluorescence study on a frozen specimen (n=15), using standard techniques.We looked for possible correlations between histological findings, donor age and serum creatinine level at 3, 6 and 12 months post transplant.

An adequate specimen was available for light microscopy in 50 cases (at least 5 glomeruli and 5 vascular sections). Only 14 (28%) biopsies were considered completely normal. Thirty six (72%) revealed non specific lesions, scored as slight in 23 and marked in 13 cases. These non specific lesions consisted of either vascular changes (intimal fibrosis, arteriolar hyalinosis) in 8 cases, tubulointerstitial changes (fibrosis, inflammation, tubular atrophy) in 5 cases, or the association of both changes in 23 cases. No significant glomerular lesion was seen. Immunofluorescence was negative once and showed vascular deposits of complement C3 in 14 cases, associated with non significant glomerular IgA deposits in 3 cases. No specific histopathological lesion was detected.

Donor age was significantly higher in the group with renal lesions as compared to the group with normal biopsies (42 vs 26 years; p<0.001). Before the age of 40 years, 48% of biopsies were normal, while after 40 years, 92% of biopsies revealed pathological changes. The mean serum creatinine levels at 3 months (136 vs 142 µmol/l), 6 months (134 vs 139 µmol/l) and 12 months (136 vs 135 µmol/l) were comparable in the patients transplanted with normal or abnormal grafts, whether the lesions were slight or marked. Furthermore, there was no difference between the 2 groups with normal and abnormal biopsies for the following parameters: donor sex, recipient age and sex, HLA matching, cold ischemia and anastomotic times, requirement of dialysis after transplantation (7 vs 19%), incidence of acute rejection (36 vs 29%).

In conclusion: (1) Nearby 3 out of 4 renal grafts showed preexisting non specific lesions on pretransplant biopsies. (2) These changes were strongly related to donor age. (3) However, neither these lesions, nor donor age could be shown to influence renal function in the first 12 months after transplantation.

SYSTEMIC IL-10 RELEASE, AFTER A SINGLE PRE OR PER OPERATIVE LARGE DOSE OF ATG-FRESENIUS IN HUMAN KIDNEY TRANSPLANTATION.

Y SAINT HILLIER, B HORY, E RACADOT*, C BRESSON, D DAVID, F AL FREIJAT, P VAUTRIN, V FOURNIER, E BERGER, M JAMALI, H BITTARD**.
Service de Néphrologie - Transplantation rénale - Service Urologie** - C.H.R. Saint Jacques et Centre Régional de Transfusion Sanguine* - 25000 Besançon - France.

IL-10 is a key cytokine with pleiotropic effect secreted by B cells, cells of the macrophage lineage and also TH0, TH1, TH2 subset. Initialy described as "cytokines synthesis inhibitor factor", producted by TH2 cells, IL-10 inhibits IL-2 and INF gamma production by TH1 cells. IL-10 has the ability to suppress MHC II expression and thereby the antigen presentation capacity of monocytes/macrophages. IL-10 also down regulated IL-12 and the production of free oxygene radicals produced by actived macrophage. IL-10 is a chemotactic attractant for $CD8^+$ T cells. These multiple suppressive effects on various effector phase of the immune response of IL-10 corrobore the finding that IL-10 is a "natural" immunosuppressor. Systemic effect on all T cells and monocytes occure concomittantly and if IL-10 is present several hours before and on time of transplantation, this realise a veritable "preincubation", a "bath" of IL-10, leading perhaps to tolerance induction and anergy.

Patients and methods : In thirty one consecutive cadaverics kidneys transplantations performed between 1st june 1993 and 31 march 1994, we measured at many time serum IL-10 level (Elisa Innotherapie). In all patient (18 M - 13 F, 48 ± 13 years old, extreme 22 to 70, 25 first, 4 second and 2 third graft), the analysis were performed before, during and after the infusion of ATG-FRESENIUS (a rabbit polyclonal anti Human T Lymphoblast gammaglobulin derived from JURKAT Cells line) and then every day during hospitalisation. An ATG-FRESENIUS infusion, is given in 3 hours pre or intra operative before the reimplantation, on a peripheric or central catheter, in all patients, at 9 mg/kg. In the 25 cases of first graft, ATG infusion is unique, while in 6 hyperimmunised or retransplanted patients, ATG is continued at lower doses 3 mg/kg four days only.
The corticotherapy is given at 500 mg just before the ATG, 40 mg three days, 30 mg to day 20 and then 20 mg to day 30, Ciclosporine at 6 mg/kg/d at day 5 or more precocely if creatinine have falled of more than 30 %, Azathioprine at 3 mg/kg/d at day 0 and then adapted with leucopenia

Results
All patients had no detectable level of IL-10, after pulse of methylprednisolone and before ATG FRESENIUS. The production of IL-10 begins very rapidly within 15 minutes. The mean level of IL-10, for the 31 patients is respectivly of 764, 730, 386, 85, 7 pg/ml just before, 30 minutes, 6, 12, 24 hours after declampage.
There is no IL-10 release after the other infusions of ATG FRESENIUS during the four days of treatment.
Only one patient with Wegener disease does not produced IL-10 (Max at 90 pg/ml) and have irreversible reject, even after OKT3 treatment, who required transplantectomy at day 33.
The tolerance of ATG F was excellent without any cytokines syndrome release. All patients are alive with creatinine level at 158 µmol/l and only 7/31 (22 %) have rejected, controled by corticosteroïd or OKT3 and their last creatinine is at 151 µmol/l.

Conclusion
IL-10 is release in the circulation, rapidly, for several hours, after a single large dose, well tolerated of ATG FRESENIUS. The protocol interest oftis is to produce maximal natural immunosuppression when the recipient is most likely to respond to the new organ, with systemic IL-10 production during hours, before or just after the graft. associated with lymphocytes depletion (results to published) with only a single infusion of ATG FRESENIUS.

CITIC 1994

The feasibility of organ preservation at warmer temperatures
Lauren Brasile, Jolene Clarke, Ernie Green and Carl Haisch
VEC TEC, Inc., Schenectady, NY, Alliance Pharmaceutical Corp., San Diego CA and East Carolina University, Greenville, NC

Hypothermia has represented the foundation of organ preservation, since it was demonstrated that hypothermia reduces the metabolic needs of an organ. At approximately 4°C, the utilization of oxygen is only 5% of that at normothermia. The inability to supply oxygen lead to our current reliance on hypothermia. A new perfusate has been developed which can be used without traditional hypothermia. An increased PO_2 is provided by a perfluorochemical emulsion (PFOB, Alliance Pharmaceutical Corp.). The available oxygen can be more effectively utilized because preservation at warmer temperatures (25°C & 32°C) means the cell membranes are in a more normal fluid state. We have demonstrated that kidneys can be preserved at warmer temperatures with stable flow dynamics, O_2-consumption and diuresis for time periods of at least 18 hours. METHODS-Fifty canine and 40 bovine kidneys have been studied, at two temperatures (25°C & 32°C) for time periods ranging from 3 to 18 hours. The kidneys were pumped on a modified Max-100 at mean pressures ranging from 60-90 mmHg, resulting in vascular flow rates of 80-150cc/min. The renal perfusions were conducted at PO_2 of 170-185 Torr to deliver oxygen at 7.7ml/min. RESULTS-The kidneys pumped at 25°C and 32°C demonstrated stable flow dynamics and diuresis for time periods of at least 18 hours. The renal metabolism occurring at the two temperatures was monitored as described below.

METABOLIC FUNCTION AFTER SIX HOURS OF EX VIVO PRESERVATION*

	Group 1 - 25°C	Group 2 - 32°C
O_2-consumption+	4.8ml/min	5.7ml/min
diuresis	143.1cc/hr	123.3cc/hr
histology	normal	normal
perfusate glucose conc.**	72mg/dl	0

---

* - specimens collected after 6 hours of perfusion and represents the mean from experimental data in each group
** - starting glucose concentration: 165mg/dl
\+ - calculated using the method of Fick

Autotransplantation studies have demonstrated the immediate function of warm preserved canine renal autografts. After 6 hours of ex vivo preservation at warm temperatures, canine renal autografts were transplanted via an end-to-side anastomosis of the renal artery to the aorta and the renal vein to the vena cava. The untreated, contralateral kidney was nephrectomized at the time the transplantation. In no case did the peak posttransplant serum creatinine exceed 2.5mg/dl; and in some cases the serum creatinine did not rise above 1.4mg/dl.

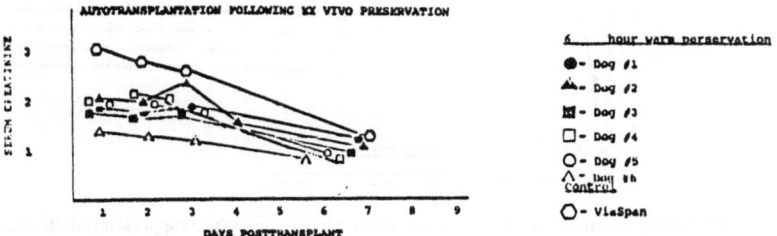

CONCLUSIONS-These studies demonstrate that kidney preservation at warm temperatures is feasible. A benefit of preserving renal allografts at warmer temperatures will be the opportunity to evaluate the functional potential of an allograft, prospectively. The further development of warm preservation technology may also present the opportunity to perform immunomodulation protocols and ultimately to initiate a repair process in warm ischemically damaged organs.

In Situ Preservation Without Traditional Hypothermia
Lauren Brasile, Jolene Clarke, Ernie Green and Carl Haisch
VEC TEC, Inc., Schenectady, NY, Alliance Pharmaceutical Corp., San Diego, CA and East Carolina University, Greenville, NC

The shortage of organs for transplantation has lead to an expansion of the donor pool into the nonheartbeating cadaver (NHBCAD) population. The ability to in situ preserve organs from NHBCAD at warm temperatures could present the opportunity to perform in situ flushing without the current use of extreme hypothermia with solutions containing high K^+ concentrations. We have developed a preservation solution which can be used to preserve kidneys without traditional hypothermia. The perfusate consists of a modified tissue culture medium and is supplemented with a perfluorochemical emulsion (PFOB, Alliance Pharmaceutical Corp.). We evaluated if the perfusate could be used to in situ preserve renal auto- and allografts at near physiologic temperatures. METHODS-Model 1: An in situ model was developed which provided for kidney preservation while allowing for animal survival. The limitation to the model was that the aorta and vena cava below the renal vessels would be ischemic. Therefore, this in situ model could be used for only three hours of in situ preservation. Using an abdominal approach, two dogs were anesthetized and cannulas were placed in the aorta and vena cava. The vasculature above and below the kidneys was occluded. The vasculature was flushed with the new perfusate until the hematocrit was <1%. The perfusate was then recirculated during the period of in situ preservation at 37°C using a pulsatile pump. The cannulas were then removed and the blood vessels were repaired. Model 2: To extend the period of in situ preservation past three hours, an allotransplant model was used. The allotransplant model involved in situ preservation of the kidneys in two euthanized dogs. Following a period of six hours, one kidney from each was allotransplanted into a canine recipient. This involved an additional 30 minutes of warm ischemia without perfusion during reanastomosis. The native kidneys were nephrectomized at the time of allotransplantation. The control experiment entailed two hours of warm ischemia at normothermia without in situ perfusion. RESULTS-Diuresis continued throughout the in situ preservation in all four test dogs. The results with both models demonstrated excellent renal function following three and six hours of in situ preservation. A control kidney experiencing two hours of warm ischemia, without perfusion, was irreversibly damaged.

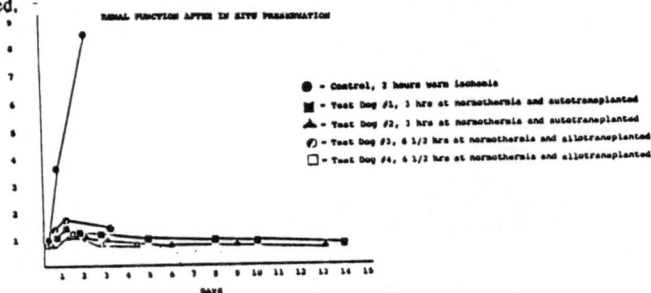

CONCLUSIONS-These preliminary results suggest that in situ preservation which supports metabolic function may be feasible with warm temperature preservation technology. The ability to in situ preserve organs at warm temperatures with a solution compatible with life, may help in expanding the organ donor pool by more effectively utilizing NHBCADs.

NAME INDEX

Abdullah, E. 359
Adeleine, P. 373
Aguyao, M.T. 331
Aitouche, A. 366
Al Freijat, F. 364
Al Freijat, F. 374
Albrechtsen, D. 73
Aldrighetti, L. 369
Altieri, M. 361
Antoniadis, A. 338
Archenti, A. 357
Arkouche, W. 359
Aroldi, A. 357

Backman, U. 73
Bagou, G. 127
Balter, S. 346
Bandini, S. 329
Barbieux, A. 347
Barcikowska, B. 340
Bariety, J. 360
Barrillon, D. 358
Barrou, B. 336
Baude, C. 127
Bauldoff, G.S. 267
Benalia, H. 336
Bendini, J.C. 358
Benoit, G. 328
Benoit, S. 103
Bensadoun, H. 328
Berger, E. 364
Berger, E. 374
Bernard, M. 344
Bertocchi, M. 277
Bertoni, E. 329
Binderup, L. 365
Bismuth, H. 353
Bitker, M.O. 336
Bittard, H. 374
Blümke, M. 371
Blümke, M. 372
Blanchet, P. 328
Blancho, G. 121
Blangero, M. 333

Boillot, G. 352
Boillot, O. 127
Boisriveaud, C. 332
Boissonat, P. 261
Boissonat, P. 281
Bonanomi, G. 363
Bonnefoy, E. 281
Borsarelli, J. 333
Botti, G. 333
Boudjema, K. 361
Bouttin, B. 143
Bouttin, B. 330
Bracco, J. 358
Brasile, L. 375
Brasile, L. 376
Bresson, C. 364
Bresson, C. 374
Bret, M. 143
Bret, M. 345
Buelow, R. 213
Busson, M. 327

Cabrer, C. 67
Cabrer, C.A. 191
Cahen, R. 373
Cajzner, S. 349
Calmus, Y. 317
Cantarovich, D. 121
Cardone, R. 357
Cardoso, J. 317
Carl, S. 362
Carmellini, M. 329
Carrington, C.A. 309
Cassuto-Viguier, E. 358
Caus, T. 344
Chéreau, Ch. 317
Chabrol, B. 127
Champsaur, G. 261
Champsaur, G. 281
Chapellier, E. 348
Charpentier, B. 328
Chassignolle, J.F. 111
Cheliakine, Ch. 103
Chenard, M.P. 361

Chossegros, P. 261
Chuzel, M. 111
Clarke, J. 375
Clarke, J. 376
Cloix, P. 197
Cochat, P. 337
Cochat, P. 99
Cohen, B. 3
Colpart, J.J. 143
Colpart, J.J. 330
Colpart, J.J. 345
Colpart, J.J. 347
Colpart, J.J. 41
Coronel, B. 345
Coronol, B. 143
Couchoud, C. 373
Cozzi, E.C. 309
Cozzone, P.J. 344
Cuzin, B. 287

Déglise-Favre, A. 353
Daemen, J.-W. 55
Daguin, P. 121
Dantal, J. 121
David, D. 364
David, D. 374
David, L. 337
David, L. 99
Davies, E.A. 85
Dawahra, M. 197
Dawahra, M. 99
De Meester, J. 3
Decaris, J. 328
Decaux, A. 328
Delafosse, B. 127
Delawari, E. 359
Depret, J. 328
Deschênes, G. 103
Descotes, J.L. 348
Deteix, P. 253
Devictor, D. 328
Devonec, M. 373
Di Stefano, R. 363
Dijoud, F. 373
Donati, D. 363
Donnolly, P. 334
Donnolly, P. 335
Dorez, D. 143
Dorez, D. 345
Doria, C. 369
Doyle, H.R. 369
Dreier, R. 372

Drouet, J.C. 333
Dubernard, J.M. 197
Dubernard, J.M. 261
Dubernard, J.M. 287
Dubernard, J.M. 346
Dubernard, J.M. 352
Dubourg, L. 337
Dubourg, L. 99
Duboust, A. 360
Duncker, G. 49
Dureau, G. 111
Dureau, G. 261
Dureau, G. 352
Dureau, G. 61

Elkhammas, E.A. 85
Ellero, B. 361
Ellingson, L. 213

Fagalde, Alcides 27
Felipe, C. 167
Felipe, C. 179
Fendler, J.P. 373
Ferguson, R.M. 85
Fernandez, E. 331
Finaz, J. 352
Fournier, V. 364
Fournier, V. 374
Foust, D.E. 267
François, B. 373
Franco, M. 358
Fung, J.J. 369

Gaid, H. 358
Gakis, D. 338
Gambiez, L. 317
Garcia-Fages, L.C. 191
Garcia-Fages, L.C. 67
Gare, J.P. 111
Gare, J.P. 261
Gari-Toussaint, M. 358
Garnier, J.L. 261
Garnier, J.L. 352
Garwood-Gowers, A. 334
Garwood-Gowers, A. 335
Gilgenkrantz, H. 297
Gille, D. 127
Giral, M. 121
Glanville, L. 213
Glotz, D. 360
Gorry, F. 346
Graber, M.C. 127
Green, E. 375

Green, E. 376
Griffith, B.P. 267
Gruessner, A.C. 77
Gruessner, R. W.G. 77
Guillot, B. 330
Guttmann, R.D. 235
Guttmann, R.D. 243

Hadj-Aïssa, A. 337
Hadj-Aïssa, A. 345
Hadj-Aïssa, A. 347
Hadj-Aïssa, A. 99
Haisch, C. 375
Haisch, C. 376
Henry, M.L. 85
Herbrecht, R. 361
Hors, J. 327
Hory, B. 364
Hory, B. 374
Hourmant, M. 121
Houssin, D. 317

Igoudin, L. 213
IJzermans, J.N. 339
Imvrios, G. 338

Jaeck, D. 361
Jaime Caro, J. 243
Jamali, M. 364
Jamali, M. 374
Jegaden, O. 111
Joubert, P. 373

Karam, G. 121
Kirste, G. 371
Kirste, G. 372
Kootstra, G. 55
Kopp, C. 127
Kovalak, J.A. 369
Krafft, M.P. 346

Łagiewska, B. 349
Langford, G.A. 309
Lao, M. 340
Laville, M. 359
Le Sant, J.N. 121
Lea, A. 334
Lea, A. 335
Lebranchu, Y. 103
Lefrancois, N. 352
Levy, V. 360
Lioure, B. 361
Liu Deng-Gui 351

Løkkegaard, H. 73
Long, D. 127
Luciani, J. 336
Lunghi, G. 357

Maillefaud, B. 330
Maloisel, F. 361
Manganella, G. 353
Manyalich, M. 191
Manyalich, M. 67
Manzetti, J.D. 267
Margonari, J. 346
Marino, I.R. 369
Marion, A. 330
Marrast, A.C. 261
Marrast, A.C. 352
Martin, X. 197
Martin, X. 261
Martin, X. 337
Martin, X. 346
Matesanz, R. 167
Matesanz, R. 179
Mattiuz, P. 329
Mehls, O. 362
Mercatello, A. 143
Mercatello, A. 345
Mercier, I. 213
Micaud, C. 330
Michalak, G. 340
Michielsen, P. 33
Mikaeloff, P. 111
Min Zhi-Lian 350
Minarro, D. 330
Ming Yin 55
Miranda, B. 167
Miranda, B. 179
Mondain, J.R. 358
Monties, J.R. 344
Mornex, J.F. 277
Mosca, F. 329
Mosca, F. 363
Moskovtchenko, J.F. 143
Moskovtchenko, J.F. 330
Moskovtchenko, J.F. 345
Moulin, A.M. 223
Mouquet, C. 336
Mulder, P.P. 339

Najarian, J. S. 77
Navarro, A. 135
Naya, M.T. 167
Naya, M.T. 179
Neidecker, J. 281

Nicita, G. 329
Ninet, J. 261
Ninet, J. 281
Nivet, H. 103

Obadia, J.F. 111
Oberling, F. 361
Opelz, G. 161
Ostrowski, K. 349

Pacholczyk, M. 349
Pagano, A. 357
Page, B. 343
Paillard, P. 352
Pamphile, R. 365
Papagiannis, A. 338
Papanikolaou, V. 338
Paradis, I.L. 267
Parchoux, B. 337
Payen, E. 348
Perrin, P. 373
Persijn, G.G. 3
Pinna, A. 363
Pisarski, P. 371
Pouletty, P. 213
Pouteil-Noble, C. 261
Pouteil-Noble, C. 352
Pozet, N. 347
Pradella, F. 329
Price, D. 334
Price, D. 335

Racadot, E. 364
Racadot, E. 374
Raffaele, P. M. 19
Rambeaud, J.J. 348
Ramella, S. 345
Ramella, S.G. 347
Richard, C. 328
Richards, A.C. 309
Riess, J.G. 346
Rindi, P. 329
Rizzo, G. 329
Robin, J. 281
Romano, P. 327
Romano, P. 332
Romano, P.J.-P. 11
Rosati, A. 329
Rosengard, A. 309
Rowiński, W. 349
Rowinski, W. 340

Saïd M.H. 99

Saalmela, K. 73
Sagnard, P. 127
Saint Hillier, Y. 364
Saint Hillier, Y. 374
Salvador, L. 191
Salvador, L. 67
Salvadori, M. 329
Samuel, D. 353
Sanchez, J. 191
Saury, G. 143
Saury, G. 330
Scavuzzo, M. 363
Schütt, G. 49
Schaub, F. 372
Sciaky, M. 344
Scotti-Foglieni, C. 369
Segers, A. 213
Sibai, R. 359
Sosa, C.L. 361
Soulillou, J.P. 121
Staehler, G. 362
Starzl, T.E. 369
Steghens, J.P. 347
Sutherland, David E.R. 77
Sykes, M. 301

Taddei, G. 329
Tajra, L. 197
Takoudas, D. 338
Terasaki, P.L. 93
Tesi, Raymond J. 85
Thévenet, F. 277
The Teams of Hôpital G. de Clocheville 103
Tosi, P.L. 329
Touraine, J.-L. 365
Touraine, J.-L. 366
Touraine, J.L. 261
Touraine, J.L. 352
Traeger, J. 359
Traeger, J. 41
Trolliet, P. 373
Tzakis, A.G. 369

Valero, R. 191
Valero, R. 67
Van Elslande, L. 358
Van Minh, T. 207
Van Steenberge, P. 339
Vanpouille, N. 213
Vautrin, P. 364
Vautrin, P. 374
Veyron, P. 365
Via, J.M. 331

Viars, P. 336
Viedma, M.A. 331
Vincent, F. 360
Voiglio, E.J. 346

Wałaszewski, J. 349
Wait, S. 243
Walaszewski, J. 340
Wang Li-Ming 350
Weill, B. 317
Weimar, W. 339
Wen Zhi-Xiang 351
White, D.G. 309
Wiesandanger, T. 277

Wiesel, M. 362
Wingen, A.-M. 362
Woehl-Jaegle, M.L. 361
Wolf, Ph. 361
Wujciak, T. 161

Xia Sui-Sheng 351

Yannoutsos, N. 309
Yuge, J. 93

Zarif, L. 346
Zech, P. 347